SMALL ANIMAL SURGICAL NURSING

Skills and Concepts

SMALL ANIMAL SURGICAL NURSING
Skills and Concepts

Second Edition

Marianne Tear, MS, LVT
Program Director
Veterinary Technology Program
Baker College
Clinton Township, Michigan

With *570* illustrations

3251 Riverport Lane
St. Louis, Missouri 63043

SMALL ANIMAL SURGICAL NURSING, SKILLS AND CONCEPTS,
SECOND EDITION

ISBN: 978-0-323-07735-4

Notices

Knowledge and best practice in this field are constantly changing. As new research and experience broaden
our understanding, changes in research methods, professional practices, or medical treatment may become
necessary.

Practitioners and researchers must always rely on their own experience and knowledge in evaluating and
using any information, methods, compounds, or experiments described herein. In using such information
or methods they should be mindful of their own safety and the safety of others, including parties for
whom they have a professional responsibility.

With respect to any drug or pharmaceutical products identified, readers are advised to check the most
current information provided (i) on procedures featured or (ii) by the manufacturer of each product to be
administered, to verify the recommended dose or formula, the method and duration of administration,
and contraindications. It is the responsibility of practitioners, relying on their own experience and
knowledge of their patients, to make diagnoses, to determine dosages and the best treatment for each
individual patient, and to take all appropriate safety precautions.

To the fullest extent of the law, neither the Publisher nor the authors, contributors, or editors, assume
any liability for any injury and/or damage to persons or property as a matter of products liability,
negligence or otherwise, or from any use or operation of any methods, products, instructions, or ideas
contained in the material herein.

ISBN: 978-0-323-07735-4

Library of Congress Cataloging-in-Publication Data

Small animal surgical nursing : skills and concepts / [edited by] Marianne Tear. — 2nd ed.
       p. ; cm.
    Rev. ed. of: Small animal surgical nursing / Sara J. Busch. c2006.
    Includes bibliographical references and index.
    ISBN 978-0-323-07735-4 (pbk. : alk. paper)
    1. Dogs—Surgery—Nursing. 2. Cats—Surgery—Nursing. 3. Veterinary surgical nursing. I. Tear,
Marianne. II. Busch, Sara J. Small animal surgical nursing.
    [DNLM: 1. Dogs—surgery. 2. Cat Diseases—nursing. 3. Cats—surgery. 4. Dog Diseases—
nursing. 5. Perioperative Nursing—methods. SF 991]
    SF991.B92 2012
    636.089′70231—dc23

                                                                    2011016157

Vice President and Publisher: Linda Duncan
Publisher: Penny Rudolph
Acquisitions Editor: Teri Merchant
Publishing Services Manager: Catherine Jackson
Senior Project Manager: Mary Pohlman
Designer: Ashley Eberts

Printed in China

Last digit is the print number: 9 8 7 6 5 4 3

CONTRIBUTORS

Paige A. Allen, MS, RVT

Instructional Technologist
College of Veterinary Medicine
Purdue University
West Lafayette, Indiana

Teri Raffel, CVT

Instructional Assistant
Madison Area Technical College
Veterinary Technician Program
Madison, Wisconsin

Ann Wortinger, BIS, LVT, VTS (ECC, SAIM)

Program Chair
Veterinary Technology
Sanford-Brown College
Dearborn, Michigan

To CMT—my rock and my safe haven

PREFACE

Surgery is one of the most complex and interesting tasks a veterinary technician can orchestrate. While we are not allowed to perform surgery, we can help to ensure that our animal patients and our veterinarians come through the experience healthy and happy. In a busy clinic it is easy to get overwhelmed and feel task saturated; add the daunting task of taking care of animals under anesthesia and even a seasoned technician can crack under the stress. With a little careful planning and fore-thought many of the variables can be removed.

The intricate dance that exists when a veterinarian and a technician work together to help animals is truly an amazing thing to watch. There is a lot of nonverbal communication and trust that takes place. Unfortunately, it takes a while to learn the steps and it can seem impossible sometimes. My hope with this book is to help those new to the profession by giving them a firm foundation in small animal surgical nursing, and help those who have been in the field by giving them a quick reference.

The book begins with setting up the facility, including the surgical suite and instruments, and then moves through patient and personnel prepping. Each chapter has been expanded, including additional illustrations. Text boxes have been included to give a quick reference to key ideas. Key terms in the chapter are defined in the glossary at the end of the book. The technician's role in pain management has also been expanded in this edition, reinforcing the important role technicians play in patient advocacy.

With all that said, there is not a better profession in the whole world. Go forth, have fun, and never quit learning because you have the distinct responsibility for making a difference every single day!

Marianne Tear

ACKNOWLEDGMENTS

This edition would not be possible without the hard work of contributors. I was energized by your dedication and zeal for the subject matter.

As with everything in this profession it builds on the knowledge and work of those who came before. Without the first endeavor, the second attempt is never possible; to all of those who contributed to the first edition a heartfelt thank you.

Margi, this is your fault, but thank you for the push and for always being the voice of reason and logic – especially all those times I didn't want to listen. Teri, you are a saint and an angel. There are not words for the thanks I owe you.

Without the constant encouragement and unconditional love of my parents, Kathy and Tom Robson, I would not be the person I am today. "Do whatever you want, but make sure you do it to the best of your ability" is a mantra I try to live by every day. (Some days I'm more successful than others.)

Christopher, thank you for taking care of everything, allowing me time to devote to this project. Your love and support make all things possible. I would be lost without you.

Finally to my kids, the four-legged and the two-legged variety. Molly, Gehrig, Brosius, Zach, Morticia, and Dewy (and the parakeets and chickens), you inspire me to learn more and be a better person so I deserve your adoration. And my two-legged children, my students, you come into my life in 2-year increments and help me learn and grow.

Marianne Tear

CONTENTS

Preoperative Room Considerations

Teri Raffel

LEARNING OBJECTIVES

After studying this chapter, the reader will be able to:
- Explain the ideal layout of a surgery suite and adjacent areas.
- Differentiate between nonmovable (permanent) and movable equipment in a surgery room.
- Explain the cleaning of the equipment located in the surgery room.
- Describe the steps used to manufacture surgical instruments.
- Describe the function of an anesthesia machine.
- List the individual components of an anesthesia machine.
- Describe the method for performing a leak check of an anesthesia machine.
- Describe the difference between rebreathing and non-rebreathing circuits and the indications for their use.
- Describe how to calculate the size of rebreathing bag to be used.
- Describe the use of different oxygen flow rates and the indications for their use.
- List the common surgical instruments used in general, orthopedic, and ophthalmic surgery in veterinary medicine.
- Describe the different styles of suture needles.
- Describe the characteristics of suture material.
- List examples of suture material and their main properties.
- List examples of equipment used perioperatively in veterinary surgery.

One of the most challenging and rewarding activities that a technician can participate in is surgery. In order to ensure positive, successful outcomes, careful preparation is imperative. It is the technician's responsibility to ensure that everything is in order before the surgeon can begin his or her portion.

For elective (non–life-threatening) procedures the facilities should be properly prepared. Preparations include the room, the equipment, and the instruments. Once all this has been accomplished the animal can be prepared for the procedure.

Layout of the Surgery Suite

The American Animal Hospital Association (AAHA) recommends three distinct and separate areas for a surgical facility: the preparation area, the scrub area, and the surgery room. Although AAHA certification is not a legal requirement for veterinary facilities, a surgical facility should create the best environment for the patient. In addition, some state licensing boards have specific requirements regarding surgical facilities that a veterinary hospital must meet to pass inspection and to receive authorization to offer surgery.

Preparation Area

Ideally, the preparation area should be adjacent to the surgery room. The "prep" room can be used for patient preparation and the storage of surgical supplies. AAHA also recommends placement of storage and cabinets in the prep area, not the surgery room. The surgeon can use the preparation area to scrub and gown for surgery if a separate scrub area is not available. It is ideal to have a separate anesthesia machine for the prep room so that cross-contamination does not occur when the machine is moved from one room to another. The prep area is used for clipping the patient. Procedures classified as "dirty" should be done in the prep area. Procedures such as abscessed wound care, débridement of old wounds, and treatment of impacted anal sacs are often defined as "dirty."

Scrub Area

The scrub area may be a small area with the scrub sink, autoclave, and room to gown and glove (Figure 1-1). This is a transitional area where the veterinarian and technician can prepare to move into the surgery room. Adding the autoclave to the space makes it a dual-purpose area that works well for personnel, because the counter area would not be in use for pack preparation while the surgeon and assistant are gowning and gloving for surgery.

Surgery Room

Ideally, the surgery room is a separate room that should be used only for surgery. The AAHA recommends that the surgery room be easily cleanable and be closed off as needed. Closing the door minimizes traffic, maximizes

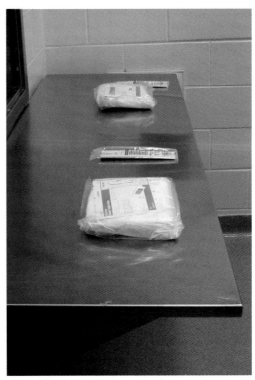

FIGURE 1-1 Gowning table. Note the absence of clutter on the table and the sufficient space to allow two people to gown and glove simultaneously.

cleanliness, and helps ensure that the surgery room is used only for aseptic procedures. The room should be a "dedicated" room reserved for clean surgical procedures. It should be used only for surgery, not for other types of procedures that may introduce bacteria into the room. The surgery room should be large enough that personnel can easily move around the surgery table without contaminating the surgical field or the surgeon. If present, cabinets should be off the floor and constructed of nonporous material. Keeping cabinets off the floor allows for adequate cleaning underneath and prevents dust and debris from collecting around the base of the cabinets. The cabinets that hold sterile supplies should have doors that can be closed to protect the packs and other supplies from dust, debris, and other contaminants (Figure 1-2).

The surgery room should also be free of clutter and items that may collect dust or harbor bacteria. It should have a door that can be closed, and this door should be opened only when necessary to limit the amount of traffic and air flow in and out of the room. "Tacky mats," which have a strong adhesive coating for dirt removal, historically have been used to decrease the amount of debris entering the surgery room. However, the U.S. Centers for Disease Control and Prevention (CDC) found that tacky mats in operating rooms do little to minimize the overall degree of floor contamination. If possible, the air pressure should be greater in the surgery room to reduce the influx of bacteria from the rest of the veterinary facility.

FIGURE 1-2 "Pass-through" storage cabinet.

FIGURE 1-3 Surgery light. Note that the shiny surface of the lamp is dust free.

FIGURE 1-4 Surgery table.

Equipment Cleaning

Different types of equipment are located in a surgery room. Some equipment is nonmovable (i.e., permanently affixed), and some is movable. Cleaning of these pieces of equipment varies according to their use and design.

Nonmovable (Permanent) Equipment

Permanent items are pieces of equipment that are attached to the floor, wall, or ceiling in the surgery room. These pieces are usually not moved from the room because of their weight or the physical difficulty of moving them. These items should be wiped down daily before surgery with a cloth dampened with isopropyl alcohol or some other disinfectant to remove any dust that may have accumulated. The surgery room should never be dry dusted. Nonmovable pieces of equipment include the following:
- Surgery lights (Figure 1-3)
- Surgery table (Figure 1-4)
- Radiographic view box

Movable Equipment

Movable pieces of equipment can be transported to other areas of the hospital. Movable items should not leave the surgery room, but in many veterinary facilities, they serve dual purposes and are moved to other areas of the hospital. If these items must be moved, they must be cleaned and disinfected thoroughly before being returned to the surgery room. Movable equipment items include the following:
- Anesthesia machine (Figure 1-5)
- Monitoring equipment:
  - Electrocardiogram (ECG) machine (Figure 1-6)
  - Blood pressure (BP) cuffs and monitors
  - Airway tubes and monitors
- Heating pads
- Intravenous (IV) drip stand (or IV pole)
- Instrument table, mayo stand (Figure 1-7)
- Suction unit
- Cautery unit
- Kick bucket (Figure 1-8)

General Cleaning Instructions

All equipment should be wiped daily before surgery with the appropriate cleaning or disinfecting solution. It is important to follow the manufacturer's instructions because improper cleaning or use of inappropriate solutions may damage the equipment. The CDC states that the manufacturers of medical equipment should provide care and maintenance instructions that are specific to the equipment. This information should include the equipment's compatibility with chemical germicides, whether it can be immersed for cleaning, and how it should be

FIGURE 1-5 Anesthesia machine.

FIGURE 1-6 ECG (electrocardiography) monitor.

FIGURE 1-7 Mayo stand, or instrument table.

FIGURE 1-8 Kick bucket. Kick buckets are cleaned after every surgery and prepared with a new plastic liner before every surgery.

decontaminated. The CDC also states that in the absence of any instructions from the manufacturer, items that are considered noncritical (stethoscopes, BP cuffs, knobs of equipment) can be cleaned and then disinfected with alcohol.

Anesthesia Machine

One purpose of an anesthesia machine is to deliver inhalation anesthesia to the patient and then remove the unneeded gases from the patient and the surgery suite. Generally this is accomplished with the use of a corrugated tubing system. The inhalation anesthetic gas is delivered to the patient through oxygen molecules (i.e., oxygen is the carrier gas for the anesthetic gas). Another purpose of an anesthesia machine is to deliver oxygen (O_2) as the sole gas, as in cardiopulmonary resuscitation (CPR). For the anesthesia machine to perform as intended, it must do the following:

1. Deliver O_2 at a controlled rate.
2. Vaporize (turn a liquid into a gas) a designated concentration of liquid anesthetic, mix the anesthetic with oxygen, and deliver the mixture to the patient.
3. Remove exhaled gases from the patient, then dispose of the gases through a scavenging system or recirculate them (after removing the carbon dioxide) to the patient.

FIGURE 1-9 Basic anesthesia machine.

FIGURE 1-10 Basic double-vaporizer anesthesia machine.

The ability of the anesthesia machine to function properly depends on the equipment being in good repair and properly maintained.

Anesthesia machines are configured in many forms, depending on the manufacturer. Well-known producers of anesthesia machines include North American Matrix (Figure 1-9), Drager (Figures 1-10 and 1-11), and Ohmeda Medical. Some machines are designed with the simplest intent of delivering inhalation anesthesia (see Figures 1-9 and 1-10). Others have accessories and the ability to provide automatic ventilation, multiple inhalation gas choices (e.g., nitrous oxide, isoflurane, sevoflurane), and space for placement and storage of monitoring devices (see Figure 1-11). Regardless of the machine's appearance, the basic function remains the same.

Components

The anesthesia machine has many components working together to perform its intended function properly. To best understand how the machine works, it is necessary to identify and understand each component. This basic information not only provides a working knowledge of the machine, but also assists the technician with troubleshooting problems in the event of a malfunction. Tracing the oxygen flow through the machine allows a view of all the components of the machine.

FIGURE 1-11 Complex anesthesia machine with multiple vaporizers, storage for monitoring devices, and a ventilator.

Oxygen Source

The oxygen source can be a localized cylinder or a large, centrally located source (Figure 1-12). Cylinders are available in different sizes; the two most common sizes are the "E" and "H" tanks. The "E" tanks are smaller and generally

FIGURE 1-12 Large "H" tanks as an oxygen source.

FIGURE 1-13 Oxygen flowmeter. Note the gradations for measuring oxygen flow. The float is shown at the bottom of the flowmeter. The fast flush valve is to right of the regulating knob.

attached to the machine, whereas the "H" tanks are larger and generally stand alone away from the anesthesia machine, often chained against a wall. Tanks are color-coded for easy recognition (green in the United States, white in Canada) and have a pressure reading of 2200 pounds per square inch (psi) when full. When opening a tank, personnel should remember the rule of "righty tighty, lefty loosey." When turning the valve clockwise (to the right), the tank is being closed; turning the valve counterclockwise (to the left) opens the tank. Using 100% O_2 from an oxygen source is justified because (1) the O_2 acts as a carrier for the vaporized anesthetic gas and delivers it to the patient, and (2) anesthetized patients have a decreased tidal volume, so an increased O_2 concentration will compensate for the decrease in tidal volume.

Pressure-Reducing Valve
The first pressure-reducing valve in the system should be found near the oxygen source tank. This valve reduces the pressure leaving the tank and entering the machine to 40 to 45 psi. The lower-pressure gas is carried through the source lines to the anesthesia machine.

Flowmeter
Next in the flow of O_2 is the oxygen flowmeter (Figure 1-13). The flowmeter further reduces the pressure of the gas to 15 psi. This is very close to atmospheric pressure and is well tolerated by patients. The flowmeter regulates how much O_2 is entering the system and being delivered to the patient. O_2 flow is measured in liters per minute (L/min) or milliliters per minute (mL/min). The O_2 flow is regulated by a knob at the bottom of the flowmeter. Personnel must take care to avoid excessive tightening of the

knob when turning off the flow. When reading the flow-meter, the "float" needs to be properly read. Ball floats are read on the scale where the middle of the ball sits on the graduations. Floats with a point are read at the top of the float. Graduations on the flowmeter may be in 100-mL increments until the 1-L level, then in 500-mL increments thereafter.

Fast Flush Valve
Next in the order of O_2 flow through the machine is the fast flush valve. On many anesthesia machines the oxygen flush valve is found near the oxygen flowmeter. The fast flush valve allows quick infusion of only O_2 into the breathing circuit. This infusion can occur because, with a vaporizer "out of the circle," the vaporizer is bypassed with the tubing arrangement of the machine. The fast flush valve should never be used with a non-rebreathing system for two reasons. First, the pressure of O_2 coming out of the system is too high and may harm the patient. Second, the non-rebreathing systems use such a high O_2 flow that the valve's purpose becomes moot; the high flows result in O_2 levels similar to those achieved with the fast flush valve. The fast flush valve should never be used if the pressure relief, pop-off, valve is closed. This could lead to a dangerous increase in pressure in the patient's lungs and atelectasis.

During the recovery phase, the fast flush valve is frequently employed to dilute residual anesthetic gases that remain in the system. Flushing the system of residual gases will hasten the patient's recovery because less anesthetic gas is present.

TABLE 1-1	Comparison of Precision and Nonprecision Vaporizers	
	Precision Vaporizer	Nonprecision Vaporizer
Temperature compensation	Output not affected by ambient temperature in most models	Output affected by ambient temperature
Flow compensation	Output not affected over a wide range of oxygen flow rates	Output affected by oxygen flow rate
Back-pressure compensation	Changes in back pressure do not affect output	Changes in back pressure affect output
Maintenance requirements	Requires periodic factory recalibration and cleaning	Minimal; can be done by hospital staff
Cost	High	Minimal
Anesthetics commonly used	Isoflurane, sevoflurane, halothane (i.e., those with high vapor pressure)	Methoxyflurane (i.e., those with low vapor pressure); isoflurane and halothane with low-flow techniques
Control over anesthetic concentration	Precise; given as a percentage	Not precise; given as a control lever setting (1-10)
Position relative to anesthetic circuit	Out of circle (VOC)	In circle (VIC)

From McKelvey D, Hollingshead KW: Veterinary anesthesia and analgesia, ed 3, St Louis, 2003, Mosby.

Vaporizer

The vaporizer is usually found next when tracing O_2 flow. The vaporizer inlet is the point where the O_2 enters the vaporizer to carry anesthetic gas molecules to the patient. The vaporizer outlet is the point at which the O_2 and anesthetic gas leave the vaporizer to enter the circuit. (Up to this point, the O_2 flow has been "out of the circle," assuming the anesthesia machine being used has the vaporizer out of the circle. The "circle," or circuit, is the loop that the gases travel to cycle in and out of the patient when a rebreathing ["recycling"] system is used.) The primary function of the vaporizer is to house or hold liquid anesthetic and to vaporize that liquid into a gas form that can be delivered to the patient in a controlled manner. The vaporizer is likely the most expensive component of the anesthesia machine and therefore must be used appropriately.

Vaporizers are calibrated internally for a specific type of inhalation anesthetic. Only the type of anesthetic for which the machine has been calibrated should be used in the vaporizer. All designs of vaporizers have some style of indicator window at the base of the unit. This window allows determination of the amount of liquid anesthetic remaining in the machine. Once the level reaches a half to one quarter remaining, liquid anesthetic should be added to avoid running out during a procedure. If the vaporizer does need to be filled while the machine is in use, personnel must be sure to turn off the vaporizer before filling it. This action prevents the anesthetic from bubbling out and contaminating the environment with anesthetic fumes. Some vaporizers have two indicator windows, one to show anesthetic level and one to show when to refill. Vaporizers have some type of device to determine the amount of anesthetic being delivered to the system. Depending on the type of

vaporizer, this amount is determined as a percentage or just a setting on the dial.

Vaporizers should be serviced annually to ensure a properly functioning mechanism. In the event that a vaporizer needs to be shipped for servicing, it should be drained of any liquid anesthetic to avoid any accidental spill or leaks during shipping.

Both precision and nonprecision vaporizers are available (Table 1-1). However, nonprecision vaporizers are infrequently used now.

Precision vaporizer. The precision vaporizer has many advantages over the nonprecision style (Figure 1-14). Precision vaporizers are used with high-vapor-pressure anesthetics and are always found out of the circle. The liquid phase of a high-pressure anesthetic vaporizes easily and quickly and must be delivered in a controlled state. If uncontrolled delivery occurs, the concentration of the drug in the carrier gas could easily become excessive and dangerous. Three factors affect vaporizer function and are compensated for in the precision vaporizer: (1) temperature, (2) gas flow rate, and (3) back pressure. First, if the room temperature is cold, the amount of volatile anesthetic vaporized may be less than the amount indicated on the dial. In a warm room, however, the amount of anesthetic vaporized may be much higher, and therefore a higher level will be delivered to the patient than indicated on the dial setting. The precision vaporizer is constructed with insulation to the liquid anesthetic chamber, so the problems with temperature are eliminated.

The second factor that the precision vaporizer compensates for is the carrier gas flow rate. The O_2 flow rate can affect the amount of vaporized anesthetic delivered to the patient. Extremely high flows (>10 L/min) or extremely low flows (<500 mL/min) are difficult to compensate for, and therefore they should not be used

FIGURE 1-14 Isoflurane precision vaporizer.

FIGURE 1-15 Nonprecision vaporizer. (From Thomas JA, Lerche P: Anesthesia and analgesia for veterinary technicians, ed 4, St Louis, 2011, Mosby.)

FIGURE 1-16 Anesthesia machine components (a), unidirectional inspiratory valve; (b), negative-pressure relief valve; (c), unidirectional expiratory valve; (d), pop-off valve; (e), manometer.

routinely. In a vaporizer that is compensated, the amount of vaporized gas will match the amount indicated on the dial. As the O_2 flow rate is reduced from 300 to 200 to 100 mL/min, the reliability of the dial setting becomes more questionable. Because the flow is reduced, less fresh gas is being delivered. Even though the amount of vaporized gas being sent to the circuit is constant, the amount of gas delivered to the patient is reduced. Vaporizer settings for lower O_2 flow rates need to be adjusted to deliver the amount of anesthetic gas that is actually desired.

The third factor affecting vaporizer function and compensation is back pressure. Vaporizers exposed to pressurized gas may release additional anesthetic agent, increasing the concentration in the circuit. This occurs when an animal is "bagged." Modern precision vaporizers are designed to adjust for any increase in pressure so that the amount of anesthetic released is not affected.

Precision vaporizers are designed to eliminate or reduce the effect of these three factors on the liquid anesthetic and its vaporization. Precision vaporizers have a dial that shows, in a percent unit, the amount of anesthetic that is being delivered to the circuit.

Nonprecision vaporizer. Nonprecision vaporizers are seen less and less in veterinary medicine with the development of safer inhalant anesthetics that require precision vaporizers. Inhalants usually used in nonprecision vaporizers are not even available anymore. A nonprecision vaporizer is basically a glass canister that allows liquid anesthetic to vaporize at an uncontrolled rate (Figure 1-15). This uncontrolled vaporization is the main reason that only anesthetics with low vapor pressure should be used in this type of vaporizer. Low-vapor-pressure liquid anesthetics are those that vaporize slowly. This slow

vaporization means that a level of approximately 4% concentration is the maximum that will be reached in the carrier gas. This level of anesthetic is relatively safe for most patients because of the high blood gas solubility and the drug's slow onset of action. The construction of the nonprecision vaporizer does not permit compensation for the three factors that affect anesthetic vaporization. The lack of compensation results in less accurate delivery of the anesthetic occurs, increasing the risk to the patient.

Unidirectional Inspiratory Valve

The unidirectional inspiratory valve, also called the inspiration valve or flutter valve, is a component of anesthesia machines designed to allow movement of gases in only one direction (Figure 1-16A). It consists of a thin, plastic circular piece (wafer) that moves (flutters) each time the patient inspires. As the patient inspires, the gases are moved through this valve, then through corrugated tubing, and are delivered via the endotracheal tube to the patient.

Negative-Pressure Relief Valve

The next part in many anesthesia machines is the negative-pressure relief valve (Figure 1-16B). This valve is primarily intended as a safety device. If negative pressure is detected in the system, this valve will allow room air to enter the system. Negative pressure may occur, for example, if the oxygen source is empty. Without this safety device, the patient would be without oxygen. The negative-pressure relief valve allows room air into the system, thereby providing 21% O_2 rather than no O_2. Negative pressure may also result if an active scavenging system is being used with the vacuum set too high or if the O_2 flow rate is too low.

Corrugated Breathing Tubing and Y-Piece

Gases pass through the tubing as the patient inspires and expires. This corrugated tubing is available in a variety of materials, lengths, and diameters. Although there is no formula to determine the size of tubing to use, shorter tubing with a smaller diameter generally is used for smaller patients, weighing 7 to 20 kg. Larger tubing is used with patients weighing more than 20 kg. It is important to remember that this tubing is not unidirectional; tube ends can be placed on either the inspiratory valve or the expiratory valve. The unidirectional valves determine gas flow direction. The tubes come together at a Y-piece that connects to the patient either via the endotracheal tube or mask.

Unidirectional Expiratory Valve

The unidirectional expiratory valve functions on the same premise as the inspiratory ("inhalation") valve, except it works with expired gases (Figure 1-16C). As the patient exhales, the gases travel though the corrugated tubing to the unidirectional expiratory valve. As with the inspiratory valve, a wafer of plastic moves or "flutters" as the expired gases pass through the valve. The movement of these two valves is also a good indicator of the patient's respiration for the anesthetist.

Adjustable Pressure Relief Valve ("Pop-off" Valve)

The adjustable pressure relief valve is generally located close to the unidirectional expiratory valve (Figure 1-16D). The pop-off valve has several functions in the anesthesia machine. First, it can act as a vent. When in the completely open position, the pop-off valve prevents buildup of pressure in the system. This is important because if pressure builds up in the system, the alveoli of the lungs expand and may rupture, leading to atelectasis. Second, the pop-off valve can be used to determine flow rate techniques (e.g., low flow). When varying degrees of

"open" are used (i.e., pop-off valve is partially opened), different O_2 flow rates can be used. Higher flow rates need to be used with a wide-open pop-off valve, and lower flow rates can be used with the valve partially closed or "closed," meaning mostly closed. (The only time the pop-off valve should be completely closed is when "bagging" the patient, and even then it is only temporarily closed because the patient cannot breathe against a closed pop-off valve.) Any level of closure is dangerous because the pressure may build in the system and cause alveolar damage.

Manometer

The manometer is the pressure gauge of the anesthesia machine (Figure 1-16E). This component only measures the pressure in the system; the manometer does not regulate the pressure. The pressure reading of the system, as indicated by the manometer, is useful information because it gives the anesthetist a good indication of the pressure in the patient's lungs. The unit of measure for the manometer is in centimeters of water (cm H_2O). Some manometers may have a double scale, one in cm H_2O and the other in millimeters of mercury (mm Hg). Personnel must be careful to read the correct scale because the graduations between the units are not the same and therefore display different information. For example, 20 mm Hg of pressure is approximately at the same graduation as 33 cm H_2O, but a reading of 33 cm H_2O is a dangerous pressure for a patient. It is a rare situation that would require the pressure reading on the manometer to exceed 20 cm H_2O, even when "bagging" the patient. Normal resting pressure, with the pop-off valve open, should read 0 cm H_2O. The manometer and the pop-off valve have a direct relationship; the more closed the pop-off valve, the higher the pressure reading on the manometer.

Rebreathing Bag (Reservoir Bag)

The rebreathing bag is a rubber bag that may serve different purposes depending on the circuit with which it is being used. One purpose, when the bag is being used with a rebreathing system, is to allow the patient to rebreathe some of the exhaled gases stored in the rebreathing bag. The level of fullness of the bag adjusts as the gases enter and leave the circuit. The reservoir bag deflates as the patient inspires and inflates as the patient expires. This movement is a good indication of respiratory rate that the anesthetist can monitor. An indirect level of respiratory quality can also be assessed on the basis of how much of the bag is deflated with each breath (i.e., shallow breaths are evident as barely moving the bag).

Another purpose of the rebreathing bag, regardless of the circuit, is to allow manual ventilation of the patient ("bagging"). Whether as an alveolar expanding "sigh" or as a resuscitative measure, being able to provide manual ventilation to the animal is essential. When providing artificial ventilation, the first step is to close the pop-off valve. Then, the rebreathing bag is squeezed to a pressure no greater than 20 cm H_2O on the manometer, and the

BOX 1-1	Calculation for Size of Rebreathing Bag

5 × Tidal volume = Bag size in milliliters (mL)
Tidal volume calculated as 10 mL/kg of body weight.
or
Body weight in pounds × 30 = Bag size in milliliters (mL)

FIGURE 1-17　Various rebreathing bags.

pop-off valve is immediately opened. It is important to ventilate the patient with as normal a respiratory character as possible. For example, a pattern of longer inspiration and then quick expiration best simulates a "normal" breath.

With the rebreathing bag storing excess gases and providing backup quantities of gases to be inspired, the proper size bag must be used. One formula to calculate bag sizes is simple and relies on the tidal volume of the patient (Box 1-1). Tidal volume is calculated as 10 mL/kg of body weight and is the volume of air inhaled during a normal breath at rest. That volume is then multiplied by a factor of 5 to ensure that enough gas will be available for the patient in the event of a full, deep breath. Another formula takes the animal's body weight in pounds and multiplies it by a factor of 30 to determine the correct bag size.

Rebreathing bags are available in several sizes, ranging from 0.25 to 5.0 L for small animals (Figure 1-17). After calculating the volume needed, the bag is selected. If the calculation does not correspond to a bag size, round up to the next size to ensure the minimum volume required is provided (see Box 1-2 for examples).

Carbon Dioxide Absorber

As the patient exhales, the waste gases pass either to the carbon dioxide (CO_2) absorber or to the scavenger. The CO_2 absorber is a canister that contains a material made of either barium hydroxide lime (Baralyme, A-M Systems, Everett, WA) or sodium hydroxide lime (Sodasorb, WR Grace, Columbia, MD). The crystals absorb the exhaled CO_2, and the resulting chemical reaction produces heat,

BOX 1-2	Examples of Rebreathing Bag Calculations

Example 1: 40-kg Patient
5 × (40 kg × 10 mL/kg) = Volume (mL)
5 × 400 mL = Volume (mL)
2000 mL, or 2 L
Use a 3.0-L rebreathing bag because volume needed is equal to bag size.
or
40 kg = 88 lb
88 lb × 30 = 2640 mL, or a 3-L bag

Example 2: 16-kg Patient
5 × (16 kg × 10 mL/kg) = Volume (mL)
5 × 160 mL = Volume (mL)
800 mL
Use a 1-L rebreathing bag because 800 mL is less than 1000 mL (1 L).
or
16 kg = 35.2 lb
35.2 lb × 30 = 1056 mL or a 1-L bag

FIGURE 1-18　Carbon dioxide (CO_2) canister. The machine is in use with a patient attached. Partially depleted crystals are evident by the color change at the top of the canister.

water, and a color change. The crystals have a pH indicator added to allow for the color change. Once the crystals have undergone the chemical reaction, they are depleted. Fresh crystals are easily crushed, but depleted crystals are very hard and may exhibit a color change from white to violet (Figure 1-18). When isoflurane is used, the color change may be evident only while the crystals are exposed to the anesthetic gas. Once the vaporizer is turned off, the color will disappear. Generally, crystals are disposed of and replenished when 50% of the crystals in the canister display a color change. Crystal density should also be evaluated to determine when to change the canister. The hours of use should be tracked, rather than a set time frame of every week or every 2 weeks, to determine when to replenish the crystals.

When the crystals are replaced, the old material can usually be disposed of in the regular trash, but the local health department may have other guidelines or ordinances; these can be consulted if disposal options are unclear. New crystals should be added to the canister in increments, and the canister should be shaken to settle the crystals. About ½ inch of air space is left at the top of the canister to allow proper gas flow over the crystals.

Scavenging System

It is important to use some type of system to evacuate waste gases from the anesthesia machine and out of the surgery suite. Two types of scavenging systems are available: active and passive. Active scavenging systems are mechanical devices attached to the anesthesia machine and then connected to a general building source that produces a vacuum to remove the gases. These systems are generally incorporated into the building plans for a new facility. The centrally located vacuum in this system removes the gases from the anesthesia machine and then evacuates the waste out of the building. Anesthesia machines require a local vacuum control on the machine as well as hosing to connect to the central source, similar to the oxygen hose used to connect with the general oxygen source.

Passive scavenging systems rely on gravity to remove the gases from the system. Anesthetic gases are the heaviest of the expired gases and naturally gravitate to the lowest point. Tubing attached to the pop-off valve can carry the anesthetic waste gas either to an activated-charcoal canister attached to the base or stand of the machine or to an outside wall vent (Figure 1-19). Wherever the canisters are attached, it is important that they be suspended so that air can circulate through the vents found on the bottom of the canisters. If the canisters are placed on the floor, these vents are effectively plugged. To ensure that the canister is effectively scavenging the waste gases, its use needs to be monitored and documented. The canister should be weighed with a gram scale before its first use and before being suspended on the machine. After each use the canister should be reweighed and the weight recorded on the canister. Once the unit has gained 50 grams (g) from the initial weight, it should be disposed of because it will no longer adequately absorb the waste gas. Canisters can be disposed of in the regular trash. Hoses from the pop-off valve that attach to an outside wall vent should be no longer than 20 feet; longer hoses would compromise the system's function. Scavenging to a vent limits the mobility of the anesthesia machine, but this arrangement is appropriate if the machine remains

FIGURE 1-19 Activated-charcoal scavenger canister for waste anesthetic gas.

in the same area all the time. Scavenging of waste gas to the floor without any type of collection or evacuation is inappropriate and should not be done.

Leak Testing

Properly functioning equipment is extremely important in anesthesia. Technicians are responsible for maintaining equipment and should take this responsibility seriously. In addition to the use of a scavenging system, leak checking the machine aids in reducing and eliminating any gas that may be inappropriately leaving the system. Before every use, the anesthesia machine should be checked for a system leak. If the machine was cleaned or replenished or if hoses or bags were changed, the potential exists for a leak in the system. Box 1-3 outlines the steps for performing a machine leak check. Machine leak checks should be performed only with a rebreathing circuit. If a non-rebreathing system is required for the patient, once the machine leak check is completed, the machine can be converted to the appropriate system.

Any area on the machine has the potential for leaking, but some sites are more likely than others to develop leaks. One of the first places to check is the pop-off valve. This valve must be completely closed when doing the leak check. If the pop-off valve is left open, there is no way for pressure to build up in the system. Even if the pop-off valve is only partially closed, a leak will result, so complete closure of this valve is critical. Another common place for leaks is the rebreathing bag or the corrugated hosing. Many of these products are intended as single-use items, but the economics of veterinary medicine often

BOX 1-3 Steps for Performing an Anesthesia Machine Leak Check

1. Connect oxygen hose to oxygen source or turn on local oxygen source.
2. Attach circuit to be used.
3. Check vaporizer for adequate level of liquid anesthetic.
4. Securely occlude patient end of circuit with thumb, palm of hand, or cork.
5. Completely close pop-off valve.
6. Depress fast flush valve until a pressure reading of 40 cm H_2O registers on the manometer.
7. Observe needle of manometer for declining movement, which would indicate a leak.
8. If there is no leak, proceed to step 12.
9. If there is a leak, turn on oxygen flow to 200 mL/min.
10. If leak is corrected—indicated by a stable needle on the manometer—no further action is needed. Proceed to step 12.
11. If leak is not corrected, perform machine maintenance to determine location of leak (see text for possible locations of leak). Correct leak.
12. Without removing the occlusion from the patient end of the circuit, open the pop-off valve. The rebreathing bag should deflate.
13. Remove hand, thumb, or cork from circuit end.
14. Check scavenging system to ensure that connections are intact.
15. Completely open pop-off valve.

FIGURE 1-20 A, Large-diameter rebreathing circuit. B, Small-diameter rebreathing circuit.

FIGURE 1-21 Universal F rebreathing circuit (a) connects to the endotracheal tube; (b) connects to the inspiratory valve; (c) connects to the expiratory valve.

dictate their reuse. Anesthetic gas can degrade the integrity of the rubber in these items, and areas of thinning or microscopic holes can develop. If the leak is isolated to the bag or hoses, these items should be discarded and replaced with new equipment. Another place for a leak is the occluding of the Y-piece. If the Y-piece is not fully occluded with a finger or the palm of the hand, a leak may persist.

Other, more subtle areas of the anesthesia machine that may leak include the metal rings on the inspiratory and expiratory valves. If removed or loosened for cleaning purposes, the rings may not have been securely replaced and fully tightened. Another "hidden" place for a leak is the CO_2 absorber. When the canister is removed to replenish the crystals, the tightening mechanism may easily be left a little loose. Finally, all the tubing on the machine is continually exposed to the detrimental effects of anesthetic gas, which may lead to small, barely detectable holes in the tubing.

Regardless of the location of the leak, it needs to be corrected before the machine is used.

Breathing Circuits

The size of the patient determines the breathing circuit that should be used to deliver anesthetic gases. There are two types of circuits: rebreathing and non-rebreathing.

Rebreathing Circuit

The rebreathing circuit is useful because it allows the recirculation of some expired anesthetic gases and permits a lower flow of oxygen because some of the gases are rebreathed. This circuit is used with patients that have a body weight greater than 7 kg. The traditional circuit is two corrugated hoses connected at one end by a Y-piece (Figure 1-20A-B). The hosing can be plastic or rubber, and the Y-piece can be plastic or metal. The open end of the tubing is placed on the inspiratory and expiratory valve openings on the anesthesia machine.

An alternative to the traditional rebreathing circuit is the Universal F circuit (Surgivet, Waukesha, WI) (Figure 1-21). This circuit is used with patients weighing more than 7 kg and offers some distinct advantages over the traditional circuit. The design of the inspiratory tube inside the expiratory tube allows the inspired gases to be warmed by the expired gases surrounding the tube. The single-tube design is also beneficial in offering less con-

FIGURE 1-22 **A,** Modified Jackson Reese non-rebreathing circuit. **B,** Modified Mapleson D non-rebreathing circuit.

BOX 1-4	Oxygen Flow Rate Values

Rebreathing System: Patients >7 kg*
Induction: 3 L
Maintenance: 25-50 mL/kg/min, but not less than 500 mL/min
Recovery: 3 L

Non-rebreathing Systems: Patients <7 kg†
Induction: 200 mL/kg/min
Maintenance: 200 mL/kg/min
Recovery: 200 mL/kg/min

*Large-breed patients (<60 kg) may require higher induction and recovery flows (3-5 L/min).
†Formulas range with recommendations from 130 to 300 mL/kg/min; however, 200 mL/kg/min is typically used.

gestion at the head and mouth. This advantage is especially appreciated during a dental prophylaxis.

Non-Rebreathing Circuit

The non-rebreathing circuit is used so that none of the gases are rebreathed. Patients weighing less than 7 kg benefit the most from the use of this circuit because of the low gas resistance. The use of this circuit requires high flows of oxygen to ensure adequate levels of anesthetic.

A major advantage of the non-rebreathing system is that it has low resistance for breathing for the patient. Fresh gases are constantly being provided to the patient with minimal effort required of the animal. The design and high flows of the non-rebreathing system allow the gases to be "delivered" at the endotracheal tube, and the patient merely breathes a normal respiration and takes in fresh, new gases.

The disadvantage of the non-rebreathing circuit is the expense incurred because of the amount of oxygen used. Figure 1-22 shows two examples of non-rebreathing circuits.

Oxygen Flow Rates

Depending on the type of breathing circuit used, different O_2 flow rates should be employed. Providing adequate oxygen to the patient is critical, but using an excessive amount of oxygen is wasteful.

Rebreathing circuits generally use a high O_2 flow rate for induction and recovery, with large-volume delivery of gas. This perpetuates a speedy induction and assists in a quick recovery. Maintenance flows for rebreathing circuits are significantly less than the induction and recovery flow rates. Only enough oxygen to match the patient's tidal volume is needed, because in addition to the fresh gas being supplied, the patient is rebreathing some of the gases already in the system. Usually a buffer is added in calculating the flow to allow for large breaths that may be given to or taken by the patient (Box 1-4).

Non-rebreathing systems also use high O_2 flow rates (see Box 1-4), but the flows remain at a constant high flow whether the patient is undergoing induction, maintaining the desired depth of anesthesia, or recovering. Continuous high flow rates are necessary to provide adequate gases to the patient. Smaller patients cannot rebreathe any of the gases because of the difficulty in moving that much air with each respiration. Fresh gases need to be provided to these patients at all times.

Summary

Anesthesia can be a stressful time for the veterinary technician. However, a thorough understanding of the components of the machine, the flow of gas through the machine, and the options available to deliver the anesthetic gases to the patient can reduce the stress level and can even make surgery a rewarding part of the technician's day.

Perioperative Equipment

Many pieces of equipment besides surgical instruments are critical to the success of a surgical procedure. Whether related to providing patient comfort, assisting the surgeon, or monitoring anesthesia, each item is an integral part of the process.

Patient Warming Devices

Circulating warm-water blankets are used frequently with surgical patients and critically ill patients. The circulating warm-water blanket is a good way to provide a heated

FIGURE 1-23 Circulating warm-water blanket.

FIGURE 1-24 Hard pad for circulating warm water.

FIGURE 1-25 Hot Dog Warming Controller and Blanket (Augustine Temperature Management, Eden Prairie, MN).

A relatively new device available for thermoregulation is a Hot Dog Warming Controller and Blanket (Augustine Temperature Management, Eden Prairie, MN; Figure 1-25). This system uses electricity to warm the pad but does not pose the same threat for thermal burns as a traditional heating pad poses. The Hot Dog Blanket has a sensor in the pad to regulate the heat generated. The pads are not puncture proof but are not harmed if punctured by a cat claw or other penetrating object. Pads are available in a variety of sizes, and cleanup is easily accomplished by spraying the pads with any commonly used disinfectant.

Another option for thermoregulation of the surgical patient is the use of forced warm air (Figure 1-26). One example is the Bair Hugger (Arizant Inc., Eden Prairie, MN). The pad is placed around the patient, then "inflated" with warm air. A variety of pads are available to best suit the size of the patient. The constant flow of warm air that envelops the patient is very effective at maintaining or increasing their body temperature. Although expensive, this pad is a viable alternative or addition to a circulating warm-water blanket. The pad is not puncture proof, but there is less risk of puncture because the pad is not placed near the animal until the patient is anesthetized.

Surgical Lights

The lights used in the surgery room can make a huge difference for the surgeon. Adequate lighting is imperative. Many brands and styles of lights are available. Single-beam lights that have a mechanism for a wide lateral as well as a vertical range of motion are desirable. Ceiling or wall-mounted lights are a much better choice than the standing floor models. If installed in the ceiling, the lights are out of the way and easily manipulated. Removable

surface on which the patient can lie during surgery (Figure 1-23). The heated surface helps prevent the loss of body heat to a cold metal surface, thereby diminishing the hypothermia that so often occurs during surgery. Water blankets are available in a variety of sizes, and some are considered disposable. Unless damaged by a patient, water blankets can be used repeatedly. A cat's claw, a misplaced towel clamp, or even a set of teeth can easily puncture holes in the water blanket, making it unusable. Single puncture holes or small tears can be repaired with use of a vinyl patch kit in some cases, but more often the best solution is disposing of the blanket.

One alternative to constantly replacing the water blanket is using a hard heated pad (Figure 1-24). This pad, made of acrylic plastic glass (Plexiglas), operates on the same principle as the disposable pad and connects to many currently available circulating water pumps. The hard heated pad also is available in a variety of sizes. The main advantage to this style of heating system is the pad itself, because the acrylic plastic glass is puncture proof.

FIGURE 1-28 The surgeon is able to manipulate and position the lights as needed if the handles have been sterilized.

FIGURE 1-26 A, Forced hot-air unit being used on a surgery patient. B, Forced hot-air unit being used on a recovering patient.

FIGURE 1-29 Solid-top, adjustable surgery table.

FIGURE 1-30 Split-top, heated surgery table.

FIGURE 1-27 Removable, sterilizable surgery light handles.

light handles that can be autoclaved are a helpful feature because once wrapped and sterilized, the handles can be aseptically opened and placed on the sterile field (Figure 1-27). The surgeon or surgical assistant can then place the handles on the lights, allowing either person to adjust the lights directly (Figure 1-28).

Surgery Table

It is also important to have a quality surgery table. Many different types are available depending on the size of the

surgery room and financial constraints. A tabletop can be a solid surface or can be designed in a split-surface style. The solid-top model is generally less expensive and can be more difficult to work with because fluids pool on the tabletop and can soil the patient (Figure 1-29). The split-top table has the double advantage of (1) a tray under the space in the table to collect any fluid that may run off the surgical field and (2) the ability to be adjusted to help maintain the patient (especially large, deep-chested dogs) in dorsal recumbency (Figure 1-30).

FIGURE 1-31 Basic cautery unit with ground plate (*left*) and foot pedal (*right*).

FIGURE 1-33 Electrocautery applied directly to the tissue to be cauterized.

FIGURE 1-32 Cautery unit with option of hand or foot control.

FIGURE 1-34 Electrocautery applied indirectly to the tissue to be cauterized through an instrument grasping the tissue.

Another available feature in surgery tables is the incorporation of a heated tabletop. This heated surface aids in thermoregulation and eliminates the need for a circulating water blanket under the patient. Surgery tables should also have the capability to be raised and lowered and to tilt in one direction. Hydraulics or electric power can be employed to accomplish variation in height, whereas manual effort is generally required to tilt the table.

Electrosurgery

The use of electricity, transmitted through a special hand piece to cut or coagulate vessels, is very advantageous in surgery. Hemostasis is vital during surgery, and cautery is an important tool available to accomplish it. Both single-use and reusable cautery hand pieces are available. A member of the sterile team activates a hand piece by pushing switches or buttons on the hand piece or by stepping on a foot pedal (Figures 1-31 and 1-32).

Electrosurgery can be either monopolar or bipolar. When monopolar electrosurgery is used, a ground plate must be placed under the patient. When the hand piece is activated, the electric current passes through the patient to the ground plate and then is diverted away from the patient. The ground plate must have sufficient contact with the patient to transmit the current properly to the ground plate. A water- or saline-saturated sponge should be placed on the ground plate between the patient and the plate. Alcohol is never used to saturate the sponge because it may lead to patient burns or even fire. Bipolar electrosurgery utilizes a hand piece that resembles a thumb tissue forceps. As the hand piece is activated, the current passes from one tip to another, and therefore no ground plate is needed.

Monopolar electrosurgery can be used in one of two ways. First, the hand piece can be activated, and the tip of the hand piece can directly touch the tissue or vessel that needs cauterizing (Figure 1-33). Second, a hemostat can be placed on the tissue or vessel that needs to be cauterized. The hemostat is then elevated off the surgical field so that the only metal touching the patient is the tip of the hemostat. The cautery hand piece tip can then be touched to the hemostat as the hand piece is activated. The metal of the instrument conducts the electric current, therefore cauterizing the tissue held in the clamp (Figure 1-34). Monopolar hand pieces can also be used with the appropriate tip, to make the surgical incision. Although wonderful at keeping bleeding to a minimum, an incision created with an electrosurgery unit takes longer to heal, because of the charring of the tissue. Bipolar electrosurgery hand pieces, by design, look like a thumb tissue forceps. Therefore they can pick up either tissue or a vessel that needs to be coagulated.

Charred material may build up on the tip of the hand piece, impeding the flow of current. It may be cleaned by scraping with a scalpel blade (away from the sterile field) or by using a commercially available "scratch pad."

Suction

Suction can be defined as the ability to remove fluid or air from an area by using either a manual or a mechanical device. Suction can be performed with a syringe, a bulb syringe, or a mechanical pump. For application in surgery, the mechanical pump is most frequently used. Suction is an extremely important tool in surgery and if unavailable can make the procedure increasingly more difficult and frustrating for the surgeon. Whether an abdominal, orthopedic, or neurologic procedure is performed, having suction available is essential. For abdominal procedures, suction can be used to remove abdominal fluid in the event of a hemoabdomen or uroabdomen. Abdominal lavage is a common practice after an exploratory procedure, and mechanical suction assists in the removal of the lavage fluid better than any other option. Lavaging a joint, flushing a septic site, and removing bone dust created while drilling screw holes for a fracture repair are examples of how suction is useful in orthopedic surgery.

There are also risks associated with suction, and veterinary personnel must understand these risks to prevent unnecessary trauma to the patient. The vacuum pressure of the suction is easy enough to control with a manual device, but care must be taken to use appropriate levels of vacuum with mechanical devices. In abdominal procedures, if the vacuum level is too high, omentum may become entrapped in the suction tip and may be damaged. A sufficiently strong vacuum that meets the needs of the surgical procedure without being excessive, is the goal. Inappropriately low vacuum settings will not adequately suction the fluid and debris on the field and will prove to be frustrating.

Suction Machines

Many different models of suction machines are available. Some models run on electric power; a motor is used to generate the vacuum (Figure 1-35). Other models require a central vacuum system to operate (Figure 1-36). Any type of machine requires some sort of bottle or receptacle for the collected fluid. Older models may still have glass jars, which can be dangerous and easily broken. Plastic bottles or canisters are more desirable. Usually the cover of the bottle has some type of "float" or safety device that will not allow fluid into the working mechanism of the suction machine if the bottles become too full.

In addition to the suction machine, a suction tip and tubing are needed. Suction tubing is available in 6- and 10-foot lengths (Figure 1-37). The tubing is usually prepackaged and sterilized for single-time use. After the

FIGURE 1-35 Electric, motorized suction machine.

FIGURE 1-36 Central vacuum, double-collection suction unit.

FIGURE 1-37 Disposable suction hose (*left*) and reusable foot-operated cautery pencil (*right*).

FIGURE 1-38 Suction tips. *Top to bottom*, Poole, Yankauer, Frazier. (From Fossum TW, Hedlund CS, Hulse DA, et al: Small animal surgery, ed 3, St Louis, 2007, Mosby.)

FIGURE 1-39 Plastic suction tip for orthopedic procedures.

package is opened onto the sterile field, one end of the tubing is attached to the suction tip (usually sterilized separately), and the other end is dropped off the field to be connected to the nonsterile suction unit. Because of the length of the tubing and the difficulty in cleaning appropriately, this is one piece of equipment that is truly disposable and should be discarded after surgery. If for some reason the tubing is not used after being opened, it can be resterilized. Ethylene oxide sterilization must be used because this vinyl tubing will not withstand steam sterilization.

Suction Tips
Different designs of suction tips are more appropriate for some procedures than others.

Poole. A Poole suction tip is a two-piece instrument best used to remove large volumes of liquid or fluid (Figure 1-38). The inner cannula can be used alone or in conjunction with the outer basket. The basket is designed with many holes to remove the liquid quickly without entrapping any tissue.

Frazier/Adson. The Frazier/Adson suction tip is a single tube with a fairly small opening (see Figure 1-38). Often there is a thumb hole to help control the amount of vacuum. This instrument is frequently used in orthopedic and neurologic procedures.

Yankauer. The Yankauer suction tip is also a single-tube design, but it is bulkier than the Frazier (see Figure 1-38). The Yankauer is a general-purpose suction tip.

Plastic Tubing Connector
Some surgeons have concerns that the abrasive metal tip of the Frazier suction tip may be traumatizing the bone or cartilage during orthopedic procedures. A good alternative is an Argyle Bubble connector (Figure 1-39). This plastic tubing connector fits securely into the suction hose and is small enough to be efficient and lightweight enough to be easy to use.

Surgical Instruments

Surgical instruments are a major investment for the veterinary hospital. It is important that instruments be used for their designed purpose. Improper use can damage or destroy instruments.

Manufacturing
Instruments are generally made of stainless steel, although some disposable models may be made of plastic. The stainless steel used is composed of iron, chromium, and carbon. Martensitic stainless steel has higher carbon content and is generally used for cutting instruments because the potential for hardness during the tempering stage is greater. Austenitic stainless steel has higher chromium content and lower carbon content. This metal is used for hemostats and needle holders. Austenitic steel is not as hard as martensitic steel, and as a result, tungsten carbide inserts are often added to the austenitic needle holders to increase their durability.

The following five steps are involved in the production of surgical instruments:
1. Forging: forming or shaping of an instrument by heating and hammering.
2. Milling: cutting a forged piece to produce a final product.
3. Tempering: hardening the instrument by slowly heating in a salt bath and then immersing in oil, or "quenching."
4. Passivation: using a chemical bath to remove the particles created from grinding and other foreign materials, strengthen the steel, and aid in rust protection.
5. Polishing: refining the surface to produce a shiny or matte finish.

Components
Veterinary surgery personnel must know the basic parts of surgical instruments to use, clean, and inspect them appropriately (Figure 1-40).

FIGURE 1-40 Basic components of a surgical instrument. (From Bassert JM, McCurnin DM, editors: McCurnin's clinical textbook for veterinary technicians, ed 7, St Louis, 2010, Saunders.)

FIGURE 1-41 Thumb-ring finger grip for ring-handled instruments. (From Fossum TW, Hedlund CS, Hulse DA, et al: Small animal surgery, ed 3, St Louis, 2007, Mosby.)

The first part of the instrument to identify is the jaw or tip. This area can be traumatic or atraumatic in design, depending on the intended use, and can be straight or curved. The jaw or tip can have serrations, teeth, or flat surfaces. Serrations can be horizontal, vertical, or a combination (e.g., Rochester Carmalt hemostatic forceps). The arrangement of the teeth can be 1 × 2, 2 × 3, and so on. Tips with a 1 × 2 configuration have one tooth on one side of the tip and two teeth on the opposite side. The teeth can also be arranged in rows (e.g., Adson Brown thumb tissue forceps). The tips or jaws can easily become damaged. Teeth and serrations of the tips or jaws should be thoroughly evaluated after each use to observe any defects that may have resulted from use. Blades are available on most types of scissors as curved or straight. Some types of scissors also have the option of blades with sharp or blunt tips. In a description or identification of instruments, the blades or tips can provide important information. For example, identifying an instrument as a "curved Metzenbaum dissecting scissors" defines the shape and type of scissors. Identifying an operating scissors as a "curved, sharp/blunt (s/b) operating scissors" reveals even more about the instrument.

The second important part of the instrument, the box lock, is present only on instruments with ring handles. The box lock is the joint or hinge of the instrument. This area absorbs great stress when the instrument is in use, and therefore the box lock must be inspected carefully to detect any cracks or evidence of degradation.

The third part of the instrument to identify is the shank (also referred to as the "shaft") or body of the instrument. This part is usually the longest area and determines the instrument's overall length. Instruments may range from 3 to 12 inches in total length depending on the length of the shank.

The ratchet is the next part of the instrument but it is found only on instruments with ring handles. The ratchet is a device with interlocking teeth that will lock an instrument jaw in a closed position. Degradation of this part of the instrument is usually seen as the inability of the ratchet to remain locked.

Some instruments also have ring handles, which serve as the means for using and controlling the instrument. Proper handling of an instrument with ring handles is achieved by placing the thumb and ring finger in the rings. The thumb ring should not advance beyond the first knuckle of the thumb, and the ring on the ring finger should not advance beyond the second knuckle. The index finger can rest on the shank to help stabilize the instrument (Figure 1-41).

General surgical instruments are available in a variety of sizes. Depending on the area of the body having surgery, shorter or longer instruments may make the task easier for the surgeon. For instance, needle holders may be found in sizes ranging from 4 to 12 inches. Thumb tissue forceps are also available in up to 12-inch lengths. Indications for use of the longer instruments include thoracic surgery on a deep-chested dog and an abdominal exploratory procedure on a large dog.

General Surgery Instruments

Scissors

Many types of scissors are available to the veterinary surgeon (Figure 1-42). As with all instruments, it is important that scissors be used only for their intended function.

Operating scissors. The intended use of operating scissors is to cut only inanimate objects (e.g., suture, paper drapes, and sponges). Its design can be straight or curved, and the blades can be sharp tipped or blunt tipped (Figure 1-43).

FIGURE 1-42 Surgical scissors. *(a)* Sharp/sharp straight operating scissors; *(b)* curved Metzenbaum dissecting scissors; *(c)* straight Mayo dissecting scissors.

FIGURE 1-44 Suture removal scissors.

FIGURE 1-43 Operating scissor tips. *Left to right,* Sharp/sharp, sharp/blunt, blunt/blunt.

FIGURE 1-45 Hemostatic forceps tips. *Left to right,* Halsted mosquito, Crile, Kelly.

Mayo dissecting scissors. The Mayo dissecting scissors is used when cutting large muscle masses, cartilage, or any other nondelicate tissue. The blades are thick and approximately one-third the instrument's length. The blades can be straight or curved.

Metzenbaum dissecting scissors. The Metzenbaum dissecting scissors is used for delicate surgical dissection. The blades are thin, delicate, and approximately one-fourth the instrument's overall length. The shaft is long and thin, and the blades can be straight or curved.

Suture removal scissors. Sometimes called a "suture scissors," the suture removal scissors usually is not found in the surgery pack but rather is stored in the treatment area or examination room. The suture scissors has one blade in the shape of a hook that cradles the suture to be cut (Figure 1-44). This instrument is designed to remove external sutures from the skin.

Hemostats

Although there are many types of hemostats, only five styles are typically used in veterinary surgery (Figure 1-45). As their name implies, hemostats are used to aid in controlling hemostasis in the surgical field. Hemostats can have jaws that are straight or curved and serrations that are horizontal, vertical, or a combination. Serrations also may be partial or may extend the full length of the jaw.

Halstead mosquito hemostatic forceps. The Halstead hemostat has small jaws with fine horizontal serrations that extend the entire length of the tip. The instrument is generally used to clamp small vessels (e.g., "skin bleeders").

Kelly hemostatic forceps. The Kelly hemostat is larger than the Halstead hemostat. The horizontal serrations are wider and only extend half the length of the jaw. The Kelly hemostat can be used for medium-sized vessels or small tissue masses.

Crile hemostatic forceps. The Crile hemostat is similar to the Kelly hemostat, with the difference being how far the serrations extend along the jaws. The Crile hemostatic forceps has serrations that extend the entire length of the jaw.

Ferguson angiotribe. Although not a true "hemostat," the Ferguson angiotribe is an extremely strong forceps

FIGURE 1-46 Hemostatic forceps tips. *Left to right*, Pean, Rochester-Carmalt, Ferguson Angiotribe.

FIGURE 1-47 Needle holders A, Derf; B, Olsen-Hegar; C, Mayo-Hegar. (Photo by John T. Miller.)

that is quite traumatic, with a crushing jaw design that has one raised jaw and one recessed jaw. This clamp can be used on vessels of almost any size and on any tissue that will not need to be viable in the body (e.g., uterine stump) (Figure 1-46).

Rochester-Carmalt hemostatic forceps. The Rochester-Carmalt hemostat is quite different from other hemostats. The instrument has both horizontal and vertical serrations on the jaw near the tip. The result is a checkerboard appearance at the tip of the jaw. This hemostatic forceps is usually about 8 inches long, making it a large instrument, and the jaw is approximately 3½ inches of the total length. It can be used to clamp large vessels or large tissue masses.

Rochester-Pean hemostatic forceps. The Rochester-Pean hemostatic forceps is a large hemostat (usually 8 inches in length) with horizontal serrations the entire length of the jaw. The jaw length is similar to that of the Rochester-Carmalt hemostatic forceps (≈3½ inches in length). The length is the factor distinguishing it from the Crile hemostatic forceps. This forceps can also be used to clamp large muscle/tissue masses or large vessels.

Needle Holders

Needle holders have very short jaws that have a roughened platform in the tips to allow for a secure grip of the suture needle (Figure 1-47). As previously mentioned, tungsten inserts may be used in the jaws of needle holders to increase instrument longevity. Needle holders are the only surgical instruments designed with the specific intent of holding metal. Therefore the needle holder is the only instrument that should be used to hold needles or to place scalpel blades onto scalpel handles.

Derf. The Derf needle holder is small in length and is used with small animals, with special species, and in extraocular ophthalmic procedures (considered too large for intraocular surgery).

FIGURE 1-48 Neelde holder tips. *Left*, Olsen Hegar; *right*, Mayo Hegar.

Olsen-Hegar. The Olsen-Hegar instrument is different from other needle holders in that it has scissors built into the jaws. This added feature is a time-saving device that allows the suture to be cut without having to reach for another instrument. The main disadvantage to having the scissors as part of this needle holder is that an inexperienced user may inadvertently cut suture material when trying to grasp the needle.

Mayo-Hegar. The Mayo-Hegar needle holder is a commonly used instrument available in a variety of lengths, depending on the surgical procedure and the surgeon's preference (Figure 1-48).

Crile-Wood. Although similar to the Mayo-Hegar needle holder, the Crile-Wood needle holder has a finer, more delicate jaw.

Scalpels

Scalpel blade handles. Scalpel blade handles are designed to hold scalpel blades for easier and safer use. Scalpel blades numbered 10 through 19 fit on the No. 3 scalpel handle (Figure 1-49). Blades numbered 20 through 29 fit on the No. 4 handle (Figure 1-50). Handles often

FIGURE 1-49 No. 3 scalpel blade handle.

FIGURE 1-50 No. 4 scalpel blade handle.

FIGURE 1-52 Scalpel blades. *Left to right*, 10, 11, 12, 15.

FIGURE 1-53 Thumb tissue forceps. *Left to right*, Russian, Debakey, 1 × 2.

FIGURE 1-51 The pencil grip used for holding a scalpel. (From Fossum TW, Hedlund CS, Hulse DA, et al: Small animal surgery, ed 3, St Louis, 2007, Mosby.)

FIGURE 1-54 The pencil grip used for holding thumb tissue forceps. (From Fossum TW, Hedlund CS, Hulse DA, et al: Small animal surgery, ed 3, St Louis, 2007, Mosby.)

have units of measurement on them to be used as needed. One such use may be as a reference marker for procedures requiring photographic documentation (e.g., mass removal, foreign body removal). Scalpel handles should be held in a pencil grip with the index finger on the noncutting edge of the blade to stabilize the scalpel (Figure 1-51).

Scalpel blades. The most common scalpel blade used in small animal surgery is the No. 10 (Figure 1-52). This blade is used primarily for skin incisions. A No. 11 blade is tapered to a pointed shape and is generally used to create a "stab" incision. The No. 12 blade resembles a hook, with the cutting edge on the inside curve, and is frequently used to declaw a cat. A No. 15 blade has the appearance of a No. 10 blade, but with only half the No. 10's length. The larger scalpel blades (Nos. 20 to 29) are generally reserved for use in large animal surgery.

Thumb Tissue Forceps

A thumb tissue forceps (casually referred to as a "pick-up") is an instrument used to grasp and retract tissue on a short-term basis (Figure 1-53). Instruments in this category resemble a tweezers, but thumb tissue forceps should never be referred to as "tweezers." A pencil grip is used to hold this instrument in the nondominant hand (Figure 1-54). The best control of pressure is achieved when the forceps is held as if it were a pencil. The shaft of a thumb tissue forceps is generally straight, but some designs have unique shapes to the shaft that help distinguish them from others (e.g., Adson, Bayonet). The tips can be toothed, smooth (atraumatic), or fairly traumatic in design.

DeBakey thoracic thumb tissue forceps. Originally designed as a cardiovascular instrument, the DeBakey thoracic thumb tissue forceps is an excellent example of an atraumatic forceps that should be used only on delicate tissue. The tips have no teeth but rather a ridge or groove design. These forceps are often used in thoracic, vascular, or neurologic procedures.

Tissue thumb forceps. The tissue thumb forceps has a straight shaft and can range in length from 5 to 12 inches. The tips can have 1 × 2 or 3 × 4 teeth.

Russian thumb tissue forceps. The Russian thumb tissue forceps has a very traumatic, bulky tip. This instrument is generally reserved for use on skin or tissue that is being removed from the animal.

Adson thumb tissue forceps. The Adson thumb tissue forceps has a very narrow tip that broadens to a ½-inch-wide shaft. The tips can be of various designs and are described as follows:

Adson dressing. The Adson dressing forceps tip has no teeth but does have flat, atraumatic serrations. This Adson style is generally used as an aid in placing or removing dressings on wounds.

Adson-Brown. The tip of the Adson-Brown instrument has two parallel rows of nine shallow teeth on both tips. A common general surgery tissue forceps, the Adson-Brown forceps can be found in most general instrument packs.

Adson 1 × 2. The tip of the Adson 1 × 2 Adson style has one tooth on one tip and two teeth on the other. The teeth interdigitate to grasp tissue firmly. It can be fairly traumatic if used on delicate tissue or too aggressively.

Allis tissue forceps. The Allis tissue forceps is neither a hemostat nor a thumb tissue forceps. Its intended use of grasping tissue in a fairly traumatic way makes it a unique instrument. This ring-handled instrument has tips that may have teeth configured in a 3 × 4 or 4 × 5 style (Figure 1-55). Because of its traumatic nature, the Allis tissue forceps is generally used to grasp tough tissue (e.g., linea alba) or tissue being removed from the animal (e.g., tumor, skin).

Retractors

Retractors are instruments used to deflect or retract tissue or other structures away from the surgical field where the surgeon is working. Retractors can be handheld (Figure 1-56), which require at least two sterile members of the surgical team, or self-retaining (Figure 1-57).

Handheld retractors. *U.S. Army.* This handheld retractor is a double-ended retractor with different lengths of blades on either end. It has no teeth on the blades and therefore causes little tissue trauma, other than pressure

FIGURE 1-55   Allis tissue forceps tips. (Photo by John T. Miller.)

FIGURE 1-56   Handheld retractors. *Top,* U.S. Army retractor; *bottom,* Senn double-ended retractor. (Photo by John T. Miller.)

FIGURE 1-57   Self-retaining retractors. *Left to right,* Gelpi, Jansen, Weitlaner. (Photo by John T. Miller.)

damage if applied too forcefully to the tissue (Figure 1-58).

Senn. The Senn retractor is also a double-ended handheld retractor. One end is a narrow, blunt blade, and the other end is a toothed, traumatic end. The teeth can be sharp or blunt, which may affect where it is used.

Self-Retaining Retractors

Gelpi. With its single, sharp-pointed tips, the Gelpi self-retaining retractor is a fairly traumatic instrument. It has limited use in soft tissue surgery but is extremely useful in orthopedic and neurologic surgery.

FIGURE 1-58 Handheld retractor ends. *Left to right,* Blunt Senn, Sharp Senn, U.S. Army.

FIGURE 1-60 Towel clamps. *Left to right,* Roeder, Backhaus, Lorna, Jones. (Photo by John T. Miller.)

FIGURE 1-59 Balfour abdominal retractor.

FIGURE 1-61 Dowling Spay Retractor. (U.S. Patent #7722639B2; Brian Dowling, DVM, Elma, WA.) (Photo by Dr. Dowling.)

Weitlaner. The Weitlaner self-retaining retractor has teeth in the jaw that can be blunt or sharp. Although it is used more often in orthopedic surgery, the blunt-toothed version can be used in some soft tissue surgical cases.

Balfour. The Balfour retractor is one of the few self-retaining retractors frequently used in soft tissue surgery (Figure 1-59). Available in adult and pediatric sizes, it is extremely useful for abdominal procedures. While keeping the abdominal walls in lateral retraction, it also has a third blade for cranial retraction as well. This widespread retraction provides excellent visualization of the abdominal cavity for the surgeon.

Towel Clamps

Towel clamps are instruments used to secure the sterile drapes to the patient during surgery or to secure the sterile drapes to one another (Figure 1-60). Towel clamps may have a penetrating design, which means the tips are sharp and pointed and are intended to pierce the patient's skin to hold the sterile drape in place. They also may have a nonpenetrating style, which is more likely to be used to secure one drape to another.

Backhaus. The most common style of towel clamp, the Backhaus has penetrating tips and is available in 3½- or 5½-inch sizes.

Roeder. The Roeder style is unique in that it has balls on the tips. The balls prevent the towel clamp from being placed too deeply into the tissue.

Jones. A penetrating towel clamp, the Jones is more delicate and lightweight than the other styles. Instead of the usual ratchet and ring handle, the Jones towel clamp has a squeeze-handle mechanism, which makes it convenient to use on smaller patients.

Lorna (Edna). Also known as the Edna nonpenetrating towel clamp, the Lorna, like the Backhaus, is available in 3½ and 5½ -inch sizes. The feature of nonpenetrating tips makes this an ideal clamp for securing second-layer drapes, whether cloth or paper, to the ground drapes.

Miscellaneous General Instruments

A few miscellaneous instruments are found in most veterinary surgical packs.

Snook spay hook. Some surgeons use the Snook spay hook to find and exteriorize the uterine horns when performing an ovariohysterectomy on dogs and cats.

Dowling spay retractor. The Dowling spay retractor was designed to assist the solo veterinary surgeon in performing an ovariohysterectomy on a canine or feline patient. By isolating the uterine horn with the retractor, the surgeon has better visualization and stabilization for ligation and excision (Figure 1-61).

Needle rack. The needle rack is a spring mounted on a metal base designed to store "eyed" free needles during the autoclaving process.

FIGURE 1-62 Groove director. (Photo by John T. Miller.)

FIGURE 1-63 Staple remover.

FIGURE 1-64 Stainless steel bowl for sharps or saline.

FIGURE 1-65 Doyen intestinal clamps.

Groove director. The groove director is designed to aid the surgeon in making incisions on the linea alba. This instrument provides a "channel" that the scalpel can follow, to avoid accidental incising of abdominal viscera (Figure 1-62).

Staple remover. When skin staples are used instead of suture, a special instrument is required to remove the staples (Figure 1-63). The staple remover has two "teeth" on one side and one tooth on the other. To use it properly, the two teeth are placed between the staple and the patient; the single tooth then presses into the top of the staple. This arrangement bends the staple, removing the edges from the skin.

Bowls. Every instrument pack should have at least one bowl. The bowls can be used for holding saline for lavage or for storing sharps during the procedure to help keep the instrument table safe and clean (Figure 1-64).

Soft Tissue Surgery Instruments

Many instruments are available for use in soft tissue surgery. The use of specialized intestinal clamps, thoracic vascular clamps, or thoracic retractors can significantly enhance the efficiency with which the surgeon performs.

Intestinal Clamps

Intestinal clamps are varied in construction, and the type utilized in a procedure depends on the intended outcome

of the tissue being clamped. Tissue that is not viable or that is being removed can be clamped with a more traumatic clamp, like a Rochester-Carmalt forceps. Tissue that merely needs to be manipulated but will remain in the patient needs to be handled with more care. Intestinal forceps such as Doyen intestinal forceps (Figure 1-65) and Babcock intestinal forceps allow handling of the delicate tissue without traumatization or compromise of blood flow. Due to similarities in appearance and construction, it is easy to confuse the Babcock intestinal forceps and the Allis tissue forceps (Figure 1-66). It is the responsibility of the veterinary technician to keep the two forceps separate and to understand the differences between the two very unique instruments.

Thoracic Instrumentation

Retractors. Thoracic surgery requires the use of appropriately designed instrumentation. A Finochietto retractor is designed to retract the thoracic wall. With the adjustable blades and sturdy construction, the

FIGURE **1-66** *Left,* Babcock intestinal forceps; *right,* Allis tissue forceps.

FIGURE **1-67** Punch biopsy instrument.

Finochietto is the retractor of choice for thoracic surgery. Two sizes are available; large, which is appropriate in animals larger than 10 kg, and small, which is appropriate for animals smaller than 10 kg. Malleable retractors, although hand held, may be of use in thoracic surgery as well. The wide variety of widths available and the ability to conform the retractor to whatever depth and shape is needed are a benefit. For instance, a wide malleable retractor would be an effective instrument to employ to retract the lungs within the surgical field.

Thoracic forceps. Depending on the procedure being performed, specific thoracic clamps can be very beneficial. Satinsky clamps, Cooley clamps, and 90-degree Mixter forceps are all examples of vascular instrumentation that can make a surgical procedure easier. With different angles of jaws and different tips, these clamps can be utilized to clamp off vessels in places that are difficult to reach with conventional clamps.

Biopsy Instrumentation
Special instruments have been created for the efficient collection of a tissue biopsy specimen. Depending on the type of tissue to be biopsied (i.e., liver, kidney, bone), different pieces of equipment should be utilized to encourage the best possible sample.

Punch biopsy. A punch biopsy instrument comes in a variety of sizes (Figure 1-67). Usually 2-mm, 4-mm, and 6-mm are available. The appropriate size to use is depends on the size of the tumor. The intent of the punch biopsy instrument is to collect a core sample from the suspicious tissue. A thumb tissue forceps and a Metzenbaum scissors are also needed when using a punch biopsy. The use of the punch biopsy is described in Chapter 7.

Needle punch biopsy. Needle punch biopsy instruments are currently manufactured by a variety of companies. Instruments are equipped with either a cutting or core biopsy needle and are available as manual and automatic devices. These instruments take a small piece of

tissue (approximately the size of a pencil lead) for microscopic evaluation. Ultrasound-guided biopsies of internal organs, including liver, spleen, kidney, and prostate, are often performed with these instruments. The technique for using these types of biopsy punches is somewhat complicated, and the surgeon and technician must have a thorough understanding of the mechanics of the instrument in order for it to work properly. Chapter 7 contains a detailed description of how to use this type of instrument.

Bone biopsy. Bone biopsy specimens are often collected using either a Michele Trephine or a Jamshidi biopsy needle. Both these instruments obtain a core sample from the tissue. The Jamshidi needle biopsy yields a smaller sample but is a less invasive procedure. The Michele trephine collects a larger sample of tissue, but higher risks are associated with its use because of the size of the sample. A description of the technique for using these biopsy instruments can be found in Chapter 7.

Orthopedic Surgery Instruments
Many types of orthopedic instruments are available. The instruments described here are the basics needed for orthopedic surgery and provide a starting point for building an orthopedic surgical instrument inventory.

Bone Holders
Bone-holding clamps are designed to hold bone fragments together until permanent fixation can be achieved. Bone holders can have pointed tips, toothed tips, or serrated tips (Figure 1-68). Bone holders are available in a variety of sizes and styles (Figure 1-69). Depending on the bone that is fractured and the type of fracture, certain styles of bone holders may be better suited than others.

Periosteal Elevators
The periosteal elevator is used to prepare the fractured bone for permanent fixation. As the name implies, the intended use is to elevate the periosteum from the bone so that the implants can be placed. Periosteal elevators are available in many shapes and sizes, with the most popular

FIGURE 1-68 Kerns bone-holding forceps. (Photo by John T. Miller.)

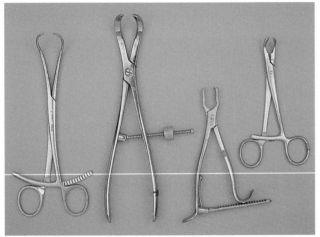

FIGURE 1-69 Bone-holding forceps. *Left to right,* AO reduction forceps, large speed-lock reduction forceps, Lane bone-holding forceps, small clamshell reduction forceps. (From Fossum TW, Hedlund CS, Hulse DA, et al: Small animal surgery, ed 3, St Louis, Mosby, 2007.)

FIGURE 1-70 Freer periosteal elevator. (Photo by John T. Miller.)

FIGURE 1-71 Periosteal elevators. *Left,* Synthes round edge; *right,* Synthes curved blade, straight edge. (From Fossum TW, Hedlund CS, Hulse DA, et al: Small animal surgery, ed 3, St Louis, 2007, Mosby.)

FIGURE 1-72 Single-action rongeur.

styles being the Freer elevator (Figure 1-70), the ASIF (Association for the Study of Internal Fixation) or Synthes elevator (Figure 1-71), and the Adson elevator.

Bone Rongeurs

Rongeurs have cupped tips with sharp edges and work with a squeezing action of the handles (Figure 1-72). Rongeurs are used to break up bits and pieces of bone for grafting purposes. Pieces of bone too small to reattach to the animal are broken down into small pieces and packed around the fracture lines to encourage new osteoblast formation and promote healing. Rongeurs can also be used to remove pieces of unnecessary bone.

Bone Cutters

Bone cutters have handles with squeezing and spring action, similar to those of rongeurs. Bone cutters have cutting-edged tips designed to cut through bone and to remove small pieces of bone.

Bone Curettes

Bone curettes are single-handled instruments that have a cupped tip surrounded by sharp edges. They are used to collect ("harvest") bone graft material or to shape and scrape bony surfaces.

Hand Chuck (Jacob's Chuck)

A hand chuck is designed to hold and drive intramedullary pins for repair of a fracture or for other orthopedic procedures requiring the use of pins (Figure 1-73). The

FIGURE 1-73 Hand chuck and key with extension piece.

FIGURE 1-74 Orthopedic drill. (Courtesy Synthes, West Chester, PA.)

hand chuck is a manual drill. It can hold wires with sizes from 0.035 inch and up to $\frac{3}{16}$ inch. The pins are held securely in the hand chuck when the key is used to tighten the chuck. An extension piece is available to protect the surgeon from the pin, which may extend beyond the end of the chuck.

Surgical "Power Tools"

Many types of surgical procedures require the use of "power tools." These tools can be powered by compressed nitrogen, batteries, or electricity. Fracture repair requires the use of a power drill to place implants. Neurosurgery requires the use of a specialized drill to remove the vertebral body bone. Even soft tissue surgery sometimes requires power tools. For example, a sternotomy for a thoracic surgery requires a power saw to open the sternum.

Some power devices are sold as individually functioning pieces, whereas others are available in sets that have interchangeable, multifunctional pieces. One available device has a pin driver, sagittal saw, and power drill in one set. This same set is also available in a larger/more powerful size to accommodate larger animals. Other styles of drills are available for use in neurosurgery. These drills have burrs, as opposed to drill bits, that attach to the hand piece to precisely shave or grind away the vertebral body bone. Some power tools are sold with their own sterilizing cases. The manufacturer's recommendations should be consulted for the best way to sterilize specific power tools, such as the Synthes orthopedic drill (Figure 1-74).

Internal Fixation Implants

Implants can be used for internal fixation of bone fractures, as curative measures for traumatic situations (e.g., tibial plateau leveling osteotomy, cranial cruciate ligament repair), and to correct congenital limb deformities. Many types of implants are available, from pins and orthopedic wire to standard dynamic compression plates (DCPs) and

FIGURE 1-75 Intramedullary pin set. (Photo by John T. Miller.)

specially designed bone plates. This section describes the basic types of implants and the equipment necessary to use them.

Intramedullary Pins

These implants are made of metal and range in size from $\frac{1}{16}$ to $\frac{1}{2}$ inch (Figure 1-75). Intramedullary (IM) pins are used to stabilize certain types of fractures or soft tissue in specific orthopedic situations. These pins can be smooth tipped or can have threaded ends. IM pins can be used alone or in conjunction with wire, plates, and screws. Pins can be placed with a hand chuck or a nitrogen air drill or electric drill.

Pin Cutter

A pin cutter is used to cut pins once they have been placed in the animal (Figure 1-76). Depending on the size of the pin, a squeeze-handle cutter or a bolt cutter may be needed.

FIGURE 1-76 Pin cutter. (From Sonsthagen TF: Veterinary instruments and equipment, ed 2, St Louis, 2011, Mosby.)

FIGURE 1-77 Orthopedic wire. (From Sonsthagen TF: Veterinary instruments and equipment, ed 2, St Louis, 2011, Mosby.)

Orthopedic Wire

Orthopedic wire is stainless steel wire designed for long-term implantation in a patient (Figure 1-77). This wire is sized from 16 to 30 gauge; the smaller the number, the larger (thicker) the wire. The most common sizes used in veterinary surgery are 18, 20, and 22 gauge, but the choice depends on the size of the patient, the procedure performed, and the expected stress level of the wound (and therefore its ability to heal). Wire can be used in conjunction with pins, plates, or screws. Wire twisters are used to secure the wire and are available in many styles (Figure 1-78). Previously used needle holders are often reserved for the purpose of securing wires as well.

Bone Plates and Screws

Bone plates are stainless steel (except for vertebral plates, made of plastic) and are designed to aid in the reduction of fractures and the repair of bone fragments. Plates are available in a wide variety of sizes (Figure 1-79). The size chosen by the surgeon primarily depends on the size of the patient, the particular bone being repaired and its size. Plates can have different shapes (e.g., straight, T-plates, L-plates), widths (e.g., 2.0, 2.7, 3.5 mm), and lengths (e.g., four, five, six holes). The width number indicates the size of screw that should also be used to secure the plate, and the length is defined by the number of holes available to be filled with screws. Accordingly, the larger the implant, the more expensive the piece. Bone screws are sized to

FIGURE 1-78 Wire twister. (From Sonsthagen TF: Veterinary instruments and equipment, ed 2, St Louis, 2011, Mosby.)

match the width of the plates. For example, a 3.5-mm plate would have 3.5-mm screws used with it. Bone screws also are sized by length. Screws can be anywhere from 6 mm to 45 mm long.

Bone plating specialty instrumentation. Many special instruments are needed to place bone plates and screws to hold the plates to the bone. Placement of the screws requires that a hole be drilled with the appropriate size drill bit. After the hole has been made, a depth gauge is used to determine the length of screw that will be needed. After that, a tap is used to prethread the bone so the screw "grabs" onto the bone more securely. A dedicated screwdriver is then used to place the screw. Other instruments, such as drill sleeves, tap sleeves, and countersinks, are also used to place a screw (Figure 1-80). Bone plates can be bent and conformed to the shape of the bone by a variety of methods. Either handheld bone plate benders or a tabletop plate bender can be utilized (Figure 1-81).

External Fixation Implants

External fixation implants are used, as their name implies, on the external surface of the skin to stabilize fractures. Often they are utilized for compound fracture repair.

FIGURE 1-79 External fixation kit. (From Sonsthagen TF: Veterinary instruments and equipment, ed 2, St Louis, 2011, Mosby.)

Bone plate   Bone screw

FIGURE 1-80 Bone plate and screws. (From Sonsthagen TF: Veterinary instruments and equipment, ed 2, St Louis, 2011, Mosby.)

FIGURE 1-81 Tabletop plate bender used to bend and form an implant (plate) to the bone surface. (Courtesy Synthes, West Chester, PA.)

Rods, clamps, and sometimes rings are used with this method of stabilization. This type of surgical intervention is quite complicated, and explanation of this technique is well beyond the scope of this text. Chapter 7 briefly describes the use of these devices.

Neurosurgery Instruments

Proper instrumentation is absolutely essential for neurosurgery. Whether it is a Hall air drill or delicate instruments, successful surgical outcomes can be enhanced when the appropriate tools are used. Rongeurs should be used to remove the articular facets of the vertebrae prior to bone removal with the drill. Double-action rongeurs are preferred over single-action rongeurs. A Hall air drill, or other pneumatic drill, is a drill that, with the use of burrs, removes the three layers of the lamina, thereby allowing exposure of the spinal cord. Once the inner cortical layer is removed, periosteum is visible. A dental spatula is useful in lifting the periosteum off the cord. Dural hooks are useful in retracting periosteum away from the cord. Depending on the procedure being done,

FIGURE 1-82 Ophthalmic surgery instruments. *(a)* Barraquer wire lid speculum; *(b)* curved 1 × 2 iris thumb tissue forceps; *(c)* straight iris scissors; *(d)* chalazion lid speculum; *(e)* Castroviejo locking needle holder; *(f)* Beaver blade handle; *(g)* Stevens tenotomy scissors; *(h)* curved baby Metzenbaum scissors. (Photo by John T. Miller.)

an ear curette, ophthalmic thumb tissue forceps, or iris spatulas may be needed.

Ophthalmic Surgery Instruments

Every veterinary surgical area should have a basic set of ophthalmic instruments available for use. These instruments are extremely delicate and expensive and should be handled with great care. Because of the nature of the tissue for which these instruments are routinely used, the tips are very fine, the shafts tend to be short, and the mechanism of use may be box lock or squeeze handle.

Beaver Blade Handle

The Beaver blade handle is used to hold Beaver scalpel blades (Figure 1-82F). Although some ophthalmic procedures can be performed using a No. 15 scalpel blade on a No. 3 handle, some intraocular procedures may require the use of a beaver blade.

Lid Speculum

An eyelid speculum may or may not be used, depending on the procedure performed. For intraocular procedures, a Barraquer wire speculum is often used to retract the eyelids away from the surgical site (Figure 1-82A). For lid procedures, a chalazion lid speculum may be used (Figure 1-82D). This instrument is most helpful in the removal of an eyelid tumor.

Lacrimal Cannulas

Both straight and curved lacrimal cannulas are available. These stainless steel cannulas can be used to flush lacrimal ducts. One end of the cannula is adapted to accept a syringe to allow for infusion of solution. The other end is blunt or bulb shaped to permit easy passage into the lacrimal duct (Figure 1-83).

FIGURE 1-83 Lacrimal cannulas. *Top to bottom:* Curved blunt, straight blunt, olive tip.

Thumb Tissue Forceps

Thumb tissue forceps are extremely delicate in design. Their function in ophthalmic surgery is the same as in general surgery. Gentle holding of tissue is imperative because the tips of these instruments are extremely delicate. It is crucial to handle the tissue of the eye and its associated structures in an atraumatic manner to avoid damaging the tissues. Examples of thumb tissue forceps are the iris 1 × 2 (Figure 1-82B), Bishop-Harmon, and Colibri.

Scissors

The scissors used in ophthalmic surgery may be miniature versions of general surgery instruments, such as the baby Metzenbaum dissecting scissors (Figure 1-82H). Others are specially designed and crafted for delicate eye surgery, such as the Castroviejo scissors. Many of the specialty scissors have a squeeze-action operation instead of the more traditional ring-handled mechanism. Two general-purpose utility scissors are typically used in ophthalmology: the Stevens tenotomy scissors (Figure 1-82G) and the iris scissors (Figure 1-82C). Compared with the Stevens tenotomy scissors, the iris scissors has a slightly longer blade, which tapers at a more constant rate from box lock to tip, as well as sharper points. Both of these scissors can be used to cut the extra-fine suture material used in ophthalmic surgery as well as tissue.

Needle Holders

The type of needle holder used depends on whether the surgical procedure is intraocular or extraocular. Extraocular procedures may be managed with a small (4-inch) Mayo-Hegar or Derf needle holder. Intraocular procedures may require a more delicate instrument, such as a Castroviejo needle holder (Figure 1-82E). As with the scissors, the specialty needle holders may have a squeeze-handle mechanism instead of the usual, bulkier ring-handle style.

Miscellaneous Ophthalmic Equipment

Hemostasis for ophthalmic surgery involves different concerns from those in general or orthopedic surgery. The delicate nature of the tissue surrounding the eye requires that materials other than sponges be used to perform hemostasis. For extraocular procedures (e.g., lid tumor, enucleation), regular, radiopaque surgical sponges are appropriate. For intraocular procedures (e.g., corneal laceration, lens luxation), a more delicate device is needed. Cotton-tipped applicators can be sterilized and used, or surgical spears (e.g., Weck-Cel cellulose sponge surgical spears, Medtronic, Inc., Jacksonville, FL) are available commercially (Figure 1-84). The spears have an arrow shape and permit pinpoint control of hemorrhages in a small working area.

Surgical Needles

Many sizes and shapes of surgical needles are available. The needle point, the needle body, and the needle eye are considered in the categorization of needles (Figure 1-85).

Needle Point

The needle point helps to determine the type of tissue in which the needle should be used. A taper-point needle has

FIGURE 1-84 Hemostatic tools for ophthalmic surgery. *Top*, Cotton-tipped applicators; *bottom*, Weck-Cel surgical spears (Medtronic, Inc., Jacksonville, FL).

a sharp point that pierces and penetrates tissues without leaving small cuts because the cross section is rounded. The round needle body associated with the taper point is best used in tissue when a sealed suture line is needed, such as for suturing intestine or other hollow organs. Any tissue that should not be traumatized or is not difficult to pass a needle through will tolerate a taper needle.

A taper-cut needle is a combination of a round, tapered body and a reverse cutting point. This type of needle is easily used with tough fibrous tissue and some cardiovascular procedures. A reverse cutting needle has three cutting edges on the point—the cross section is triangular, with one of the cutting edges being the outside of the curve—and it maintains that shape in the body and is stronger than the conventional cutting needle.

A cutting-edge needle also has three cutting edges on the point and body, but the third cutting edge is on the inside of the curve. This style of needle may be most traumatic because the cutting edge on the inside of the curve cuts toward the edges of the wound, compromising the strength of the tissue.

Needle Body

The shape of the needle body can also vary widely. Needles can be straight, circular, or curved. Straight needles, sometimes referred to as Keith needles, are available but have limited application in veterinary medicine. One procedure made easier by the use of a Keith needle is the placement of a purse-string suture in the anus. The straight shape of the needle makes it easier to avoid the anal glands by allowing superficial placement of the suture.

Curved needles can either be full curve, half curve, or double curve. Needles that are double curved have both ends curved in opposite directions. Double-curved needles are generally reserved for use in large animal surgery, especially bovine surgical closures.

Half-curved needles are classified as such because only half the body of the needle is curved. They are rarely used in veterinary surgery.

Full-curved needles have the entire body of the needle involved in the curve. Varying degrees of curvature can be found, based on the portion of a full circle that is involved. For example, a $\frac{3}{8}$-circle needle means that if a full circle were divided into eight equal parts, the continuous curve of three of those parts would be this shape. Likewise, a half-circle needle would mean that four continuous parts (or half the circle) would be the shape of the needle. Other common circular needle shapes are $\frac{1}{4}$-circle and $\frac{5}{8}$-circle.

Suture Attachment End

The final portion of the needle is the suture attachment end. Some needles have eyes, which can be single or French style. Single-eyed needles must have the suture material passed through the needle eye. Suture is threaded through the eye from the inside of the curve to the outside.

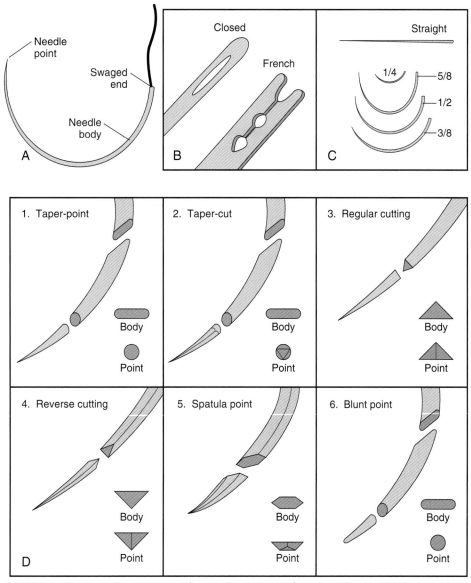

FIGURE 1-85 **A,** Basic components of a needle. **B,** Types of eyed needles. **C,** Needle body sizes. **D,** Needle body shapes. (From Fossum TW, Hedlund CS, Hulse DA, et al: Small animal surgery, ed 3, St Louis, 2007, Mosby.)

The threading of the needle results in a rather bulky portion of suture that must pass through the tissue, therefore creating excessive tissue drag and damage. The French-eyed needle has one complete eye and one split eye. The suture is passed through the complete eye and then pushed down through the split eye, which securely grips the suture.

The most atraumatic and therefore most common method of suture attachment is with the swaged needle, or eyeless needle. When the suture is manufactured, the needle and suture are attached to each other. With this type of attachment, the tissues undergo minimal damage because the point and diameter of the needle create the hole, and the suture simply follows along without causing further trauma. The ease of use and limited trauma of the eyeless needle make it the first choice of almost all veterinary surgeons.

Suture Material

The purpose of suture material is to hold together wound edges until the wound can withstand the stress of healing without additional support. Some examples of tissue instability that would require suture material are an intentional surgical incision, ligated vessels, and ligament, tendon, or muscle repair. Suture material is available in many forms, sizes, and colors. It is important to understand the terminology used when discussing suture to know the options available and to select the appropriate material for the procedure being performed. Although the technician will not be making the decision about which type of suture to use, he or she must have a working knowledge of the types of suture available (Table 1-2). The veterinary technician who can anticipate the type of suture that may be requested, on the basis of knowledge

TABLE 1-2	**Summary and Comparison of Common Suture Materials**					
Generic Name	Brand Name	Manufacturer	Absorbability	Multifilament or Monofilament	Color	Natural or Synthetic
Nylon	Ethilon	Ethicon, Somerville, NJ	Nonabsorbable	Monofilament	Black	Synthetic
	Dermalon	Davis & Geck, Danbury, CT	Nonabsorbable	Monofilament	Black	Synthetic
Polyester	Surgidac	USSC, Norwalk, CT	Nonabsorbable	Multifilament	Green	Synthetic
	Ethibond	Ethicon	Nonabsorbable	Multifilament	Green	Synthetic
Polyglactin 910	Vicryl	Ethicon	Absorbable	Multifilament	Purple/undyed	Synthetic
Polyglycolic	Dexon-Plus	Davis & Geck	Absorbable	Multifilament	Beige	Synthetic
Polypropylene	Surgilene	Davis & Geck	Nonabsorbable	Monofilament	Blue	Synthetic
	Prolene	Ethicon	Nonabsorbable	Monofilament	Blue	Synthetic
Polydioxanone	PDS	Ethicon	Absorbable	Monofilament	Violet/clear	Synthetic
Silk	Silk	Davis & Geck	Nonabsorbable	Multifilament	Black	Natural

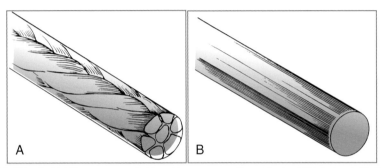

FIGURE 1-86   **A,** Multifilament suture. **B,** Monofilament suture. (From Meeker MH, Rothrock JC: Alexander's care of the patient in surgery, ed 12, St Louis, 2003, Mosby.)

and experience, will be an invaluable member of the surgical team.

Characteristics

Tensile Strength
Tensile strength is the amount of force in psi that the suture can withstand (as an untied fiber) before it breaks.

Memory
Memory is the ability or tendency of the suture to return to its original packaged form.

Flexibility
Flexibility is the ease with which the suture is manipulated, either by the surgeon or in the tissue. Flexibility is somewhat determined by the size (diameter) and the material used to make the suture. For example, silk has better flexibility than stainless steel.

Absorbability
Suture can be classified as either nonabsorbable or absorbable. Nonabsorbable suture is not broken down by the body and can remain intact in the body for at least 2 years. Absorbable suture can be broken down by the body

through different processes. During phagocytosis, leukocytes, usually neutrophils, are released and travel to the site of concern (incision) to ingest and destroy the microbes or, in the case of suture material, the foreign suture material. Suture is also absorbed through hydrolysis. The chemical compound in the suture is decomposed as it is exposed to water. Absorption of suture may begin as soon as 7 days after placement. Complete absorption may take 60 days to 2 years.

Capillarity
Capillarity describes the ability of the suture to allow microbes to "wick" (be carried) to the interior of the suture strand. This action can be curtailed if the manufacturer coats the suture at production to decrease the "wicking" action. Polytetrafluoroethylene (Teflon), wax, paraffin, silicone, and calcium stearate are substances used to coat suture. Generally, multifilament sutures are treated more often for capillarity than monofilament sutures.

Structure
There are two basic structure types of suture: multifilament and monofilament (Figure 1-86). Multifilament suture, also called braided suture, has two or more

strands braided together to form the single strand of suture. Monofilament suture is a single, solid strand of suture material. Monofilament suture material tends to have less "tissue drag," or friction, when it is being pulled through the tissues than multifilament suture material.

Knot Security

The ability of suture to hold the knots the surgeon has placed is imperative. Some types of suture materials hold knots better than other types. Usually, braided material has less knot slippage than monofilament suture. Once knots have been formed with the suture, they must stay secure. The slippage of a knot can result in the death of a patient if a knot that was around a major vessel slips, and the animal bleeds to death.

Color

Some sutures are dyed during the manufacturing process for easier identification after placement in the tissue. Suture material is available in dyed or undyed styles. Although not as great a concern with veterinary patients as with human patients, suture color should be considered in some cases. For example, if the patient is a black Labrador and both black nylon and blue polypropylene are available for the skin sutures, the blue sutures will be much easier to identify at suture removal in 10 days.

Origin of Material

Suture material is also classified by the origin of the material from which it is made. Natural suture material is a product made from fibers found in nature. Some examples are cotton, silk, and catgut (now made from sheep intestinal mucosa).

Synthetic material is other suture produced with the use of manufactured products. This group includes almost all the remaining suture not previously mentioned (e.g., nylon, polyglactin 910). Metallic suture is a small category of sutures and is limited to surgical stainless steel suture, which includes suture wire and staples.

The ideal suture material would have no knot slippage, would have high tensile strength, would be absorbable, would cause no tissue reactivity, would be easy to handle, and would be inexpensive. Unfortunately, no one "perfect" suture material exists, so the surgeon must consider all the characteristics of the material when deciding whether to use it for a particular procedure. In addition to the physical characteristics of the suture material, the surgeon must also consider the following criteria when selecting the suture type and size:

- Patient size.
- Area (tissue) of placement (skin vs. hollow organ).
- Strength required.
- Healing potential of the tissue.
- Importance of cosmetic appearance.
- Cost.

Sizing

Suture material is classified by size according to the United States Pharmacopeia (USP). The USP uses a numeric scale to denote size from fine to coarse. Hypodermic needles are classified by gauge, which indicates the diameter size of the needle. Intramedullary pins are classified by fractions of an inch to identify their size in diameter (e.g., $\frac{1}{8}$, $\frac{5}{32}$, $\frac{1}{4}$).

Suture is classified by the term *ought*. When sizing suture, the numeral "0" is used to represent "ought" or "zero." The more zeros in a size, the smaller is the suture. For example, "0000" (pronounced "four-ought") is the same as 4-0 (also pronounced "four-ought"). Similarly, "00" is the same as 2-0, which some refer to as "double-ought." Size 5-0 suture material is smaller in diameter (finer) than 3-0 suture. Whole numbers alone can also be used to identify the size of suture (e.g., No. 1, No. 2, No. 3). In the sizing of suture material, whole numbers used alone, that is, without any "oughts," increase in size with an increase in the number; the larger the number, the larger the suture. Suture is manufactured in a wide range of sizes, from 11-0 to No. 5. Smaller patients and more delicate tissue (ophthalmology or cardiovascular procedures) tend to use the small sizes, whereas the larger sizes are primarily used in large animal surgery.

Packaging

Most suture material is packaged as single-use items sterilized at the factory by the use of gamma radiation (Figures 1-87 and 1-88). Suture packaged and sterilized in this manner has a rather long shelf life, which is indicated by an expiration date on the box. Individual suture packs are

FIGURE 1-87 Single-use multifilament, absorbable, synthetic suture.

FIGURE 1-88 Single-use monofilament, nonabsorbable, synthetic suture.

opened on an as-needed basis, aseptically, onto the surgical field. Exposed but unused suture should not be resterilized but rather saved for use in nonsterile procedures (e.g., necropsy closure). If the inner suture pack was unopened and unused on the sterile field, resterilizing the package may be possible. Under no circumstances should suture be steam-sterilized. Any sterilization should be accomplished by the use of an ethylene oxide (EtO) sterilizer.

Another packaging option is to have long lengths (50-100 m) of suture placed on a reel or "cassette" by the manufacturer (Figure 1-89). Although economically a good idea, this method of storing suture material has a greater potential for contamination than individually packaged products. Also, a knot in the middle of the reel of suture is a common risk and can prove to be a difficult obstacle in removing suture from the cassette.

Staples

Internal and external staples are available for use in veterinary surgery and differ dramatically in cost, ease of use, and applicability.

External Staples

Skin (external) staples are stainless steel staples placed perpendicularly to an incision to close the wound (Figure 1-90A). If a patient has a history of postsurgical incisional licking or tissue reaction to other suture material, external staples may be a good option. Self-contained in a disposable stapling device, the staples can be placed quickly, significantly decreasing anesthesia time. Once placed in the skin, the staples take on a

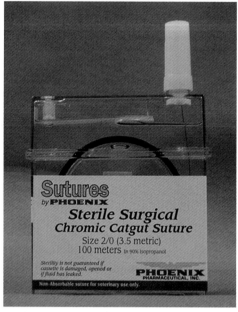

FIGURE 1-89 Cassette packaging of monofilament, absorbable, natural suture.

FIGURE 1-90 Surgical stapling equipment. **A,** Surgical skin stapler applies a single staple with each squeeze of the trigger (staple guns typically hold 25-35 staples). **B,** Gastrointestinal anastomosis (GIA) stapler. Staple cartridges are for one-time use and are purchased in presterilized packages. **C,** Thoracoabdominal (TA) stapler. Staple cartridges are purchased as for GIA stapler. Shown here with staple cartridge in place. (From Bassert JM, McCurnin DM, editors: McCurnin's clinical textbook for veterinary technicians, ed 7, St Louis, 2010, Saunders.)

unique shape to inhibit accidental removal. A special staple removal device is required to remove the staples safely and comfortably from the patient at the appropriate time.

Internal Staples

Specific soft tissue cases may benefit from the use of internal stainless steel staples. Internal staples may be most advantageous in certain thoracic cases (e.g., pulmonary resection, excision of tumors in certain locations). Thoracoabdominal (TA) staples are designed to place multiple rows of staples in tissue (Figure 1-90C). Special staples are also used with gastrointestinal procedures, such as gastrointestinal anastomosis (GIA; Figure 1-90B) and end-to-end anastomosis (EEA). A number may follow the initials of the staple type to indicate the length of the row of staples. For example, TA 90 is a row of staples 90 mm in length with the TA design. Special staplers are required for each of the different types of staples. Although expensive, these staples can save time in critical cases. The benefit must be weighed against the cost so that these staples are used judiciously.

Setting Up the Surgery Suite

After the surgery room has been appropriately cleaned for the start of the day, setup of the room may begin. It is most efficient to have a "case card" for each procedure performed by each surgeon. Each case card has listed on it all the supplies and equipment the surgeon will need for the procedure. It is important to minimize the traffic flow in and out of the surgery room, and having most if not all of the supplies in the room will accomplish this goal. Reducing the number of times the veterinary technician has to leave the room to retrieve something is also better time management. It is usually better to be over-prepared with supplies in the room than to constantly run out. In operating rooms at human hospitals, everything that enters the room, regardless whether it is used or not, gets thrown away at the end of the procedure. Fortunately this is not the case in veterinary surgery rooms. Unused items can be replaced on the storage shelf for use another day.

Types of Packs

A general soft tissue instrument pack will suffice for most surgical procedures, with the exception of ophthalmic surgery. Specialty instruments can be packaged separately or assembled together in a pack, whichever is better for the clinic. Retractors, periosteal elevators, rongeurs, and so on, can be packaged individually and opened on an as-needed basis. This arrangement gives flexibility to the surgical schedule, in that if only one instrument is needed, a whole pack does not need to be opened, thus avoiding the "down time" waiting for the pack to be reprocessed. Larger groups of instruments, such as multiple cardiovascular clamps or bone plating equipment, can be sterilized as a pack. It gives the surgeon the option of having many different instruments available to meet the needs of the case. Anything not stored in the room needs to be placed in the room prior to the beginning of surgery. It is important to remember those items not typically thought of as surgical supplies, for instance, urinary catheters, orogastric tubes, and medications. Forethought must be used, depending on the surgical procedure, to ensure that all necessary supplies are available.

Scheduling Surgical Procedures

When reviewing the surgical procedures planned for the day, it is important to remember to schedule them appropriately. A good rule to follow is to schedule cases from cleanest to dirtiest. It is also good to take into consideration the difficulty and anticipated length of each procedure. Surgeons and staff will be more fresh and alert in the morning than at 3 PM. More difficult cases should therefore be scheduled earlier in the day. In orthopedic cases, any joint replacement procedure should be scheduled first thing in the morning. In fact, the room should be set up the night before, and no traffic allowed into the room until the patient is wheeled in. Subsequent procedures for the day may be scheduled as follows: a metatarsal fracture, a cranial cruciate ligament (CCL) repair, and finally, a compound radial fracture repair. For soft tissue procedures, any noninfective intrathoracic procedures should go first, followed by clean abdominal, contaminated, and, finally, dirty procedures.

In addition to difficulty, length, and contamination, there are other things to consider when developing the daily schedule. Patient status is paramount in determining the schedule. Some patients may require an earlier time on the schedule even though it conflicts with some of the other parameters. Animals in critical condition that require surgery to survive obviously take precedence. Another consideration should be equipment needs and turnover. Scheduling three procedures back to back that will need the same equipment may not be the best idea. The potential for down time with the patient on the table while the equipment is cleaned and prepared must be considered. Given all things equal, procedures that need the same equipment should be spread out throughout the day to allow for reprocessing.

Conclusion

Time the veterinary technician spends readying the surgical suite and the necessary equipment prior to bringing the patient into the surgery room is important. Being ill prepared will compromise the patient, try the surgeon's patience, and overall prove to be a very inefficient use of time. Taking those few extra moments at the beginning of the day and of each case will ensure a smooth surgical event.

KEY POINTS

1. The surgery suite ideally should consist of a preparation area, a scrub area, and a surgery area.
2. The preparation area should be next to the surgery room and used for patient preparation and the storage of supplies.
3. Surgical procedures classified as "dirty" should be done in the preparation area, not in the surgery room.
4. The scrub area can also be used as the sterilization area and the place for gowning and gloving.
5. Ideally, the surgery room should be a separate room. (Some state licensing boards require the surgery room be a separate room.)
6. There should be minimal cabinets in the surgery room, and if possible, the cabinets should be mounted on the wall.
7. Permanent (nonmovable) equipment consists of surgery lights, surgery table, and radiographic view box.
8. Movable equipment consists of anesthesia machine, monitoring equipment (ECG, blood pressure, airway), heating pads, IV drip stand, instrument table or Mayo stands, suction unit, cautery unit, and kick bucket.
9. All equipment should be damp-wiped daily before surgery.
10. The manufacturer's instructions for cleaning of equipment should always be followed.
11. Proper use of surgical instruments is vital to maintain the health and usefulness of the instrument.
12. Every instrument needs to be evaluated frequently to assess its ability to function properly.
13. Each component of the anesthesia machine has a specific purpose and must be in good working order for the machine to function.
14. The flowmeter reduces the oxygen pressure to the atmospheric pressure of 15 psi, which is well tolerated by the patient.
15. The use of the fast flush valve should be avoided when a non-rebreathing system is used.
16. Only the liquid anesthetic for which a vaporizer has been calibrated should be used in the vaporizer.
17. The pressure reading on the manometer should not exceed 20 cm H_2O when a patient is being ventilated.
18. The CO_2 absorber removes carbon dioxide from the exhaled breath of the patient.
19. Appropriate scavenging of waste anesthetic gas is essential for the safety of the staff.
20. The use of a suture needle is determined by its shape.
21. All the characteristics of suture material should be considered before the decision is made as to type of material to use in any particular case.
22. External warming devices should be employed to help maintain patient body temperature during anesthesia.
23. Cautery can be activated by hand or foot control devices and can be monopolar or bipolar in function.
24. Suction tip styles vary widely and have recommended intended uses.
25. A No. 40 or 50 clipper blade should be used to remove hair from the surgical site.
26. Pulse oximeters measure the level of oxygen saturation of the blood.
27. Capnometry is the measurement of the level of exhaled CO_2; a normal reading is 35 to 45 mm Hg.
28. Blood pressure can be monitored by direct or indirect methods.

REVIEW QUESTIONS

1. Why is it important to use surgical instruments only for their designed purpose?
   a. To avoid damaging them.
   b. To protect their useful life.
   c. The high-quality instruments are expensive and should be handled with care.
   d. All of the above.

2. Why is it important for ratchets to remain locked when the jaw is closed?
   a. The instrument needs to be a reliable mechanism of holding the target tissue (e.g., pedicle) or item (e.g., suture needle).
   b. If the ratchets do not remain locked, complications (e.g., hemorrhage) could result.
   c. Ratchets need to be protected by lock and key so that only the surgeon can unlock them when it is appropriate.
   d. Both a and b.

3. Which scissors is finer and more lightweight therefore used on delicate tissues?
   a. Metzenbaum.
   b. Mayo.
   c. Operating.
   d. Suture

4. Of the following needle holders, which have scissors included in the jaws?
   a. Olsen-Hegar.
   b. Mayo-Hegar.
   c. Derf.
   d. Crile-Wood.

5. *True or False:* The Allis tissue forceps is considered a traumatic type of forceps.

6. *True or False:* The Gelpi retractor is a handheld retractor that is frequently used in orthopedic surgery.

7. *True or False:* The Balfour retractor is a self-retaining retractor that is frequently used during abdominal exploratory procedures.

8. What part of the anesthesia machine converts the liquid anesthetic into a gas anesthetic?
   a. Pressure manometer.
   b. Oxygen flowmeter.
   c. Pressure-reducing valve.
   d. Vaporizer.

9. Which valve allows for room air to enter the anesthesia system if negative pressure is detected in the system?
   a. Pop-off valve.
   b. Flowmeter.
   c. Negative-pressure relief valve.
   d. Pressure manometer.

10. When might a situation of negative pressure exist in the anesthesia system?
   a. When the oxygen source is depleted.
   b. During anesthesia induction.
   c. During recovery from anesthesia.
   d. Only during "high-flow" anesthesia.

11. Which part of the anesthesia machine indicates the amount of pressure in the system?
   a. Pressure-reducing valve.
   b. Flowmeter.
   c. Carbon dioxide canister.
   d. Pressure manometer.

12. When the rebreathing bag is being squeezed to ventilate the patient manually, the pop-off valve needs to be:
   a. Open and then closed after giving a breath.
   b. Closed and then opened after giving a breath.
   c. Open and remain open after giving a breath.
   d. Closed and remain closed after giving a breath.

13. Why is it important to confirm that the pop-off valve is completely open after the anesthesia machine and circuit are checked for leaks?
   a. It can only reset if it is open.
   b. When the patient is connected to the anesthesia machine with the pop-off valve closed, the patient will not be able to exhale.
   c. It is not important; the pop-off valve can be open or closed after the system is checked for leaks.
   d. All of the above.

14. Which of the following anesthesia monitoring devices is used primarily to measure the percentage of available hemoglobin that is saturated with oxygen?
   a. Capnometer.
   b. Pulse oximeter
   c. Noninvasive blood pressure monitor.
   d. Direct blood pressure monitor.

15. Which of the following statements best describes the difference between direct and indirect (noninvasive) blood pressure monitoring?
   a. Noninvasive blood pressure monitoring is more accurate.
   b. Direct monitoring requires placing a catheter with a sensor in an artery, and indirect monitoring requires placing a catheter with a sensor in a vein.
   c. Noninvasive pressure monitors can be placed only by veterinarians.
   d. None of the above.

16. Ideally the surgery room is
   a. at least 12 × 12 feet in dimension.
   b. a separate room used only for surgery.
   c. adjacent to the scrub sinks.
   d. has no doors for easy communication.

17. A 27-kg patient would need what size rebreathing bag?
   a. 1.0 L.
   b. 2.0 L.
   c. 3.0 L.
   d. 5.0 L.

18. The suction tip best used to remove large volumes of fluid is the:
   a. Yankauer.
   b. Adson.
   c. Poole.
   d. Plastic connector.

19. Which instrument would be used to collect large amounts of bone graft material intraoperatively?
   a. Jacobs hand chuck.
   b. Periosteal elevator.
   c. Bone curette.
   d. Biopsy needle.

20. Of the procedures listed below, which should be scheduled as the first of the day?
   a. Corneal laceration.
   b. Splenectomy.
   c. OHE.
   d. Knee replacement.

ANSWERS

1. d	6. False	11. d	16. b
2. d	7. True	12. b	17. b
3. a	8. d	13. b	18. c
4. a	9. c	14. b	19. c
5. True	10. a	15. d	20. d

BIBLIOGRAPHY

Association of periOperative Registered Nurses (AORN): Standards, recommended practices, and guidelines: recommended practices for maintaining a sterile field, Denver, 2004, AORN.

Bassert JM, McCurnin DM, editors: McCurnin's clinical textbook for veterinary technicians, ed 7, St Louis, 2010, Saunders.

Centers for Disease Control and Prevention (CDC), Healthcare Infection Control Practices Advisory Committee (HICPAC): Draft guidelines for environmental infection control in healthcare facilities, Atlanta, 2001, CDC.

Copich W: Avoiding the common errors made in the designing of animal hospitals, Vet Clin North Am 2:537, 1972.

Crawford L, Yu ZJ, Keegan E, et al: A comparison of commonly used surface disinfectants. Infect Control Today, Nov 1, 2000. Available at http://www.infectioncontroltoday.com/articles/0b1feat2.html.

Fossum TW, Hedlund CS, Hulse DA, et al: Small animal surgery, ed 3, St Louis, 2007, Mosby.

Kennedy J, Bek J, Griffin D: Selection and use of disinfectants, Institute of Agriculture and Natural Resources, 2000, University of Nebraska-Lincoln. Available at http://ianrpubs.unl.edu/animaldisease/g1410.htm.

Recommended practices for environmental cleaning in the surgical practice setting. AORN J 67:448, 1998.

Recommended practices for environmental cleaning in the surgical practice setting. AORN J 76:1071, 2002.

Sacred cow survey. OR Manager 14:1, 1998.

Sonsthagen, TF: Veterinary instruments and equipment: a pocket guide, ed 2, St Louis, 2011, Mosby.

Thomas JA, Lerche P: Anesthesia and analgesia for veterinary technicians, ed 4, St Louis, 2011, Mosby.

Preoperative Patient Considerations

Marianne Tear

2

KEY TERMS

Agonists
Anticholinergic
Auscultation
Balanced anesthesia
Chief complaint
Nociception
Premedication
Prophylaxis
Signalment

OUTLINE

LEARNING OBJECTIVES

After completion of this chapter, the reader will be able to:
* Understand the importance of and be able to perform a complete physical examination on the day of a scheduled surgery.
* Know the legal significance of a signed surgical consent form.
* Explain to clients the details in a surgical consent form.
* Collect and analyze preanesthesic diagnostic tests.
* Describe what is considered a minimum database for particular patients.
* Bring the veterinarian's attention to any abnormal or invalid results.
* Understand the reasons for premedicating surgical patients.
* Explain the importance of preemptive analgesia.
* Describe the drug options available for preemptive analgesia.
* Explain the mechanisms of action of the different types of analgesics.
* Discuss the indications for placement of an intravenous (IV) catheter.
* Identify appropriate sites for placement of IV catheters.
* List the supplies required for IV catheter placement.
* Discuss the technique for IV catheterization of peripheral vessels.
* Identify the components of an endotracheal (ET) tube.
* Discuss factors considered for determining ET tube size.

- List supplies required for endotracheal intubation.
- Identify the anatomic structures of the larynx.
- Discuss the differences between the one-person technique and the two-person technique of performing endotracheal intubation.
- Discuss methods of assessing proper ET tube placement.
- Describe hair removal protocols for a variety of soft tissue, orthopedic, neurologic, and miscellaneous surgical cases.
- List antiseptic products available for use to prepare patients for surgery.
- Discuss different patterns used in applying materials for the surgical preparation.

- Discuss potential patient reactions from clipper or chemical irritation.
- Secure the patient to the surgery table in a safe, accessible manner.
- Properly position the patient for various surgical procedures, providing access to the (1) surgical site, (2) IV catheter site, (3) ET tube, (4) other venous access sites, and (5) monitoring sites.
- Perform a sterile preparation of the surgical site.
- Describe the final preparation before surgery.
- Use appropriate techniques to conserve body heat.

History Taking

The ability to collect a history that is both concise and chronologically accurate is a skill that takes practice. After the client (owner, guardian) and patient (animal) have been brought into the examination room and introductions have been made, a good starting point for collecting the history is to confirm the patient's signalment. Confirming the patient's age, gender, and breed with the owner, then comparing this information with the patient's medical record, ensures the record's accuracy and clarifies any confusion should a discrepancy be found.

Once the patient's signalment has been established and verified, the client should be asked about the chief complaint (or reason for the visit). This is usually a brief but complete description of the current problem; for example, "HBC [hit by car] 2 days ago and fractured right femur." Once the chief complaint has been established or confirmed, ask the client to explain the sequence of events, starting from the beginning of the particular problem.

While collecting a history, the technician should avoid asking leading questions. Leading questions make the client feel compelled to answer a certain way; for example, "You don't feed your dog anything other than dog food, do you?" The owner feels compelled to answer in the negative because the question is leading toward or encouraging a specific answer. Formatting the question in a different way encourages the owner to answer the question truthfully, without prejudice. "What do you feed your dog?" is a nonleading, nonthreatening question that usually yields more useful information than the first example. Follow-up questions should be asked when appropriate. If there is a concern regarding the dog's nutritional status or body condition, it would be appropriate to ask how much and how often the dog is fed, in addition to what the dog is fed. A concluding question for the specific topic is often revealing as well. A final question about the dog's diet could be asked as follows: "Is there anything else your dog eats?" Again, this is a nonleading question and allows the owner to share information that may be helpful or even significant.

During the history it is important to review what other treatments have been tried to address the current problem, including any attempts by the owner to treat the problem at home. In addition, it is important to establish the nature of the treatment and the patient's response to each treatment. A review of the current medications and supplements that the animal may be given, including both over-the-counter (OTC) and prescription medications, is an important part of the history. Certain medications and supplements may interact with diagnostic tests or premedications and anesthetic drugs.

Once the history of the current problem has been thoroughly investigated, a general question about any previous medical problems is appropriate. If a patient has had surgery or medical treatment in the past, additional follow-up questions may be in order. A good way to conclude the history-taking session is to ask the owner whether there is anything else that would be helpful to know but that was not addressed. Occasionally, this general question reminds clients about something else that is relevant to the situation or that they wanted to ask.

Allowing the animal to explore the examination room at will (e.g., letting the cat out of the carrier) during the history taking helps the technician determine the patient's general attitude and condition without even touching it. In addition, most animals will take this opportunity to familiarize themselves with the scents and sounds of the hospital, and they may even relax if given a chance to explore the exam room on their own terms. An observant technician can establish a first impression of the patient's personality and degree of anxiety during the history.

After the history has been collected, the details need to be recorded in chronologic order in the medical record.

Physical Examination

The veterinary technician should be adept in the performance of the physical examination (PE), even though veterinarians may elect to perform the PE themselves. The veterinary medical team will consult the PE findings when determining the appropriate anesthetic and surgical protocols for the patient. The owner's presence during the PE allows for ongoing communication between the technician or veterinarian and the owner in regard to the findings and provides a historical perspective to unusual findings. This is especially true for any physical findings that might affect the surgical procedure or anesthetic protocols (e.g., retained testicles, pregnancy).

The complete PE should become a routine for the veterinary technician. This routine should be carried out in the same manner every time the PE is performed (e.g., head to tail or by body systems). This approach minimizes the possibility of forgetting to check a vital system and helps ensure patient safety. Being able to perform a complete PE is the first step in being the patient's advocate. The PE reveals the needs of the patient more than any other diagnostic procedure, and knowing their needs is the only way to advocate for patients.

Even if the animal was seen recently, it is imperative that a thorough PE is performed the day of the surgery, ideally with the owner present. The goal of this chapter is not to detail every aspect of a PE, but rather to give an abbreviated overview. Many wonderful textbooks have complete chapters dedicated to performing PEs.

General Body Condition and Mentation

The patient's general body condition (e.g., "strong and healthy" or "weak and emaciated") and mentation (e.g., "bright, alert and responsive" [BAR] or "dull and depressed") should be observed and noted during the history taking. The patient's ability to see and hear is assessed during the history taking as well. If the patient is clearly distressed or aggressive, it is appropriate to request an assistant and to use a restraint device (e.g., muzzle) before the "hands-on" portion of the PE. If the patient is scared and timid, a slow, calm, and soft-spoken approach may sufficiently relax and calm the patient to allow for a thorough PE. Any gait abnormalities (lameness, ataxia), muscle atrophy, or asymmetry should be noted while observing the animal during the history taking and should be examined more closely during the hands-on examination.

The complete exam should include an evaluation of the temperature, pulse, and respiration (TPR).

Thoracic Auscultation

Thoracic auscultation requires using a stethoscope to listen to the chest for both heart and lung sounds (Figure 2-1). The heart and lungs are heard best with the animal standing still on all four legs. A talented veterinary technician will quickly learn how to keep a cooperative animal standing quietly while auscultating the thorax without an assistant (Figure 2-2). Occasionally it is necessary to prevent a dog from panting or a cat from purring. To stop a dog from panting, use the hand with the wristwatch to extend the neck by gently lifting up on the dog's mandible using the top surface of the hand, while the other hand holds the stethoscope to the patient's chest. Clamping the mouth shut to try to prevent a dog from panting (Figure 2-3) frequently results in excessive movement as the dog tries to wriggle out of the technician's grip. Most dogs

FIGURE 2-1 Typical stethoscope, with both diaphragm and bell in chest piece. Swiveling the chest piece determines whether the diaphragm or bell is used for auscultation. Note the curvature in the stems of the ear pieces. The stems should be placed in the examiner's ear canals and pointing toward the nose.

FIGURE 2-2 If the patient is cooperative, one technician can easily restrain the patient in a standing position while auscultating the thorax.

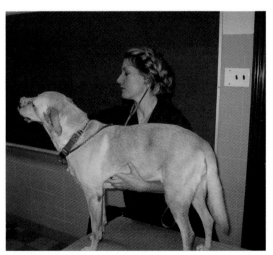

FIGURE 2-3 Preventing a dog from panting by gently closing the mouth while auscultating the thorax helps the examiner hear heart sounds over breath sounds.

tolerate a gentle lift of the mandible with the top of the hand better and stand quietly long enough to count a heart rate. To stop a cat from purring, it may be necessary to restrain the cat firmly near a sink and turn on the water to a slow stream.

Begin auscultating the heart by placing the diaphragm of the stethoscope's chest piece just caudal to the point where the dog's left elbow meets the chest. For cats a more ventral placement of the chest piece may be necessary to hear the heart best. One heartbeat normally has two sounds; that is, the "lub-dub" is two sounds but one heartbeat. Once the distinctive lub-dub heart sounds have been identified, time 15 seconds on a watch and count the number of heart sounds heard. To determine the heart rate, multiply the number of beats heard in 15 seconds by 4; this number is the heart rate in beats per minute. Systolic murmurs are usually heard as a swishing sound between the lub-dub ("lub-shh-dub"). Moving the stethoscope one rib space cranially or caudally may amplify the sound of the murmur. The rib space where the murmur is heard the loudest is the point of maximum intensity (PMI). The rib space can be identified by counting backward from the last (13th) rib. Keep in mind that some murmurs are heard loudest on the right side of the chest. The presence of a murmur and the PMI of the murmur should be noted in the medical record.

The lungs should fill up the pleural space when fully expanded during maximum inhalation. Normal lung sounds should be distinct but soft and free of any wheezing, crackling, and popping sounds. Normal lung sounds should be heard equally well on the left and the right sides of the thorax. Be sure to listen to both sides (cranial and caudal, dorsal and ventral) for lung sounds. One breath is a two-part movement: inhalation and exhalation. To determine the respiratory rate (number of breaths per minute), count the number of breaths in 15 seconds and multiply that number by 4. Any increased effort by the animal to breathe (dyspnea) and any increase or absence of lung sounds must be noted in the medical record and addressed. Usually, addressing respiratory abnormalities includes giving the patient supplemental oxygen. The lungs should be assessed, not only for respiratory rate but also for crackles, wheezes, and any other abnormalities. Any abnormalities or noteworthy findings in the PE need to be recorded in the medical record and brought to the attention of the attending veterinarian.

Taking the Temperature

Ideally the temperature is taken rectally with a well-lubricated thermometer. Some patients strongly resist this part of the PE, and therefore taking the temperature should be saved for the end of the examination so that the patient may be more cooperative for most of the PE. Some states no longer allow the sale or purchase of mercury thermometers, but it is still important that every veterinary technician can read a mercury thermometer (Figure 2-4). Most mercury thermometers require 90 to

FIGURE 2-4 Digital thermometer *(top)* and two mercury thermometers. Note the differing ranges between the lower and upper limits of the two mercury thermometers (94° F to 108° F and 96° F to 106° F).

FIGURE 2-5 Ear thermometer.

120 seconds to record the patient's temperature (check the manufacturer's recommendation). Most digital thermometers emit a series of audible beeps within 60 seconds to indicate that the final temperature has been recorded.

If it is not possible to take the temperature rectally, an aural temperature measurement can be taken. There are several styles of ear thermometers on the market. Ear thermometers read the temperature of the tympanic membrane using infrared technology. The probe sits several millimeters off the ear drum as it records the temperature. This space and the shape of the animal's ear canal can lead to inaccurate readings (Figure 2-5).

Consent Form

A consent form is a piece of paper that identifies the patient (name, signalment, and descriptors such as hair coat color and body weight), the specific procedure(s) to be performed along with the potential risks to the patient, the physician(s) who will perform the procedures, and the signature of the owner consenting to the procedure(s). Frequently, the receptionist merely hands the consent form to the owner to sign when the animal is brought to the hospital on the day of the scheduled procedure. Because the consent form contains such important information, however, the veterinary technician familiar with the surgical procedure should review the form in detail with the owner at completion of the PE. This gives the owner the opportunity to ask any last-minute questions about the procedure before the animal is admitted to the hospital. Open and clear communication is essential to avoid any confusion and to prevent miscommunication that could lead to legal complaints later. Many legal complaints originate with poor or rushed attempts at client communication.

Descriptions of the procedures should be written out and should be all inclusive; that is, everything that will be done to the animal needs to be listed. This form also should document whether or not the patient was fasted appropriately, should include a notation that the owner received an estimate for the procedure(s) to be performed, and should provide a way of contacting the owner during the time the procedure(s) will be performed. It is extremely important that the owner can be contacted during the procedure, should the need arise (Figure 2-6).

Preanesthetic Diagnostic Tests

With the ever-increasing standards of care in veterinary medicine and the owner's expectations for the surgical patient's optimum health care, the minimum preanesthetic diagnostic database, or minimum database (MDB), is continually rising in scope. Information collected in the history and PE will help determine which diagnostic tests should be performed before the patient is anesthetized. What is considered the MDB for an elective surgical procedure on a young, healthy animal will be different from the MDB for a procedure on a geriatric patient with preexisting health problems. The MDB results may suggest additional diagnostics may be indicated, or that the original anesthetic protocol may have to be amended.

Minimum Database

A minimum database for a young, healthy surgical candidate should include a packed cell volume, total solids, blood glucose, blood urea nitrogen (BUN), and alanine aminotransferase. These tests should be considered a starting point, and other diagnostic tests should be performed if any of these four basic parameters cause any concern. These tests are generally easy to run, can usually be performed as "point of care" or "in-house" tests, and require only a small amount of blood. With minimal time and effort, much useful information can be gained from these tests. Several laboratories and in-house analyzer companies sell packaged pre-anesthetic test panels, making the process even easier.

Packed Cell Volume (Hematocrit)
The packed cell volume (PCV), or hematocrit (Hct), is the percentage of whole blood that is made up of red blood cells (RBCs). Low PCVs are found in cases of decreased RBC production (as in chronic renal failure),

decreased RBC life span (as with some autoimmune diseases and parasite infections), and blood loss (secondary to trauma, blood-clotting disorders, or gastric ulcers). Increased PCV may indicate dehydration (common) or absolute polycythemia (rare). Any values outside the normal ranges need to be brought to the attending clinician's attention.

Checking a PCV requires microhematocrit tubes, a tube sealant (e.g., Critoseal), a centrifuge, and a hematocrit card reader (Figure 2-7). If whole blood is collected in a syringe without an anticoagulant, heparinized microhematocrit tubes should be used for this test. If blood is collected into a heparinized syringe or placed in a Vacutainer tube with anticoagulant (ethylenediaminetetraacetic acid [EDTA]) in it, a plain microhematocrit tube should be used. Glass microhematocrit tubes are generally easier to work with than the plastic variety.

After spinning the microhematocrit tube for the appropriate time in the centrifuge (Figure 2-8), the tube is placed on the card reader. Line up the top of the clay with the "0%" line on the card reader. Roll the tube across the card until the top of the plasma lines up with the 100% line on the card. Read the percentage line that crosses the point where the packed RBCs are separated from the plasma, at the "buffy coat"; this percentage is the PCV (Figure 2-9). The buffy coat usually appears as a small column of white between the packed RBCs below it and the clear plasma above it. The buffy coat contains white blood cells (WBCs) and platelets. The area just above the buffy coat can be examined under a microscope to perform a heartworm screening for live microfilaria.

Normal range of packed cell volume
- Canine: 37% to 54%
- Feline: 27% to 48%

Plasma is the liquid (noncellular) component of blood that separates out from the packed RBCs after whole blood is placed in a microhematocrit tube, sealed with the clay, and spun in a centrifuge. Normally, plasma is clear and colorless. If the plasma has any color, the color should be noted next to where the PCV percentage is recorded in the medical record and brought to the attention of the veterinarian.

Total Solids or Proteins
Total solids (TS) or total proteins (TP) provide information on the animal's plasma protein levels. There are three major plasma proteins: albumin, globulin, and fibrinogen. These levels have a direct effect on serum oncotic pressure. The lower the TP value, the lower the serum oncotic pressure. Changes in serum oncotic pressure directly affect changes in the patient's fluid shifts between the interstitium and the vasculature. With a low serum oncotic pressure, fluid tends to accumulate in the interstitium, resulting in edema. On the other hand, with a high serum oncotic pressure, fluid shifts out of the interstitium and back into the vasculature (blood vessels).

DATE_____   CASE NUMBER_____

COMPANION ANIMAL CLIENT/PATIENT INFORMATION FORM

Please provide the following information for our records: **PLEASE PRINT!**

OWNER INFORMATION

OWNER'S NAME	SOCIAL SECURITY NUMBER

STREET ADDRESS

CITY STATE	ZIP CODE	PARISH OR COUNTY

TELEPHONE NUMBER(S) (Area Code, if long distance) →	HOME	BUSINESS

DRIVER'S LICENSE NUMBER	PLACE OF EMPLOYMENT	HOW LONG?

ANIMAL INFORMATION

ANIMAL SPECIES (Dog, Cat, Other)	BREED

ANIMAL'S NAME	SEX	HAS ANIMAL BEEN SEXUALLY ALTERED? ☐ Yes ☐ No

COLOR	BIRTHDATE (Month/year, or approximate)	The undersigned owner or agent certifies that the herein described animal has a maximum value of approximately **$**

REFERRAL INFORMATION

WERE YOU REFERRED BY A VETERINARIAN? ☐ Yes ☐ No	IF YOU WERE REFERRED BY A VETERINARIAN, PLEASE COMPLETE THE FOLLOWING:

VETERINARIAN'S NAME	PHONE

STREET ADDRESS

CITY/STATE	ZIP CODE

You will be advised of estimated cost and anticipated procedures. Please feel free to discuss the proposed treatment and its cost with the veterinarian. A minimum deposit of 50% of the initial estimated charges will be required for hospitalization of an animal patient.

STATEMENT OF OWNERSHIP AND CONSENT: I am the owner of the above described animal, or have authorization from the owner to consent to its treatment.

I hereby authorize the performance of professionally accepted diagnostic, therapeutic, anesthetic, and surgical procedures necessary for its treatment.

I accept financial responsibility for these services.

I have read the above consent and understand why the above procedures may be necessary. I also have been told of the possible complications and alternatives to the listed procedures.

PAYMENT CHOICE: ☐ Cash   ☐ Check   ☐ Bank Card

SIGNATURE (Owner/Agent)	DATE

FIGURE 2-6 Companion Animal Client/Patient Information Form. (From McCurnin DM, Bassert JM, editors: McCurnin's clinical textbook for veterinary technicians, ed 7, St Louis, 2010, Saunders.)

FIGURE 2-7 Heparinized (red) and plain (blue) microhematocrit tubes *(top)*, packed cell volume (PCV) card reader *(bottom)*, and clay to seal blood in microhematocrit tube *(middle)*.

FIGURE 2-8 Place microhematocrit tube in centrifuge with clay plug toward the outside.

FIGURE 2-9 To read packed cell volume (PCV) on a card, line the top of the clay plug on the 0% line and the top of the plasma on the 100% line. PCV is read on the line where plasma and packed red blood cells meet. On this sample, PCV is approximately 40%.

FIGURE 2-10 A refractometer is needed to determine the total solids in plasma.

Elevated plasma protein values are associated with dehydration, malignancies (e.g., lymphosarcoma), and infections. Decreased plasma protein values are associated with inadequate production (albumin is made in the liver), inadequate intake (starvation), increased loss (renal disease, blood loss, parasites), and inadequate absorption from the gastrointestinal tract (pancreatic disease, inflammatory bowel disease).

In addition, plasma protein levels are important because some anesthetics (some barbiturates) are highly bound to proteins. If a patient is hypoproteinemic, more free drug (not bound to plasma proteins) will be available to function as an anesthetic, effectively increasing the dose. Therefore the animal's protein levels should be noted when deciding which anesthetics to use, or the anesthetic dose may need to be adjusted accordingly.

Supplies needed to check plasma proteins include a refractometer (Figure 2-10) and microhematocrit tubes. After the PCV level is checked, snap the glass microhematocrit tube in the area of the plasma column. Take care not to touch or scratch the glass platform of the refractometer with the sharp edges of the microhematocrit tube. Allow the plasma to drip onto the refractometer out of the microhematocrit tube. The TS level is read on the scale seen in the refractometer.

Normal range of total solids
- Canine: 5.5 to 7.5 g/dL
- Feline: 6.5 to 8.2 g/dL

Blood Glucose

Blood glucose (BG) levels indicate carbohydrate metabolism and measure the endocrine function of the pancreas. Eating raises BG levels, and fasting lowers them. Stress will elevate BG levels in cats. In juvenile patients and diabetic patients, BG values may need to be checked intraoperatively and postoperatively if the procedure is especially long.

Glucometers are available at most pharmacies and are easy to use (Figure 2-11). Usually, only a drop of fresh whole blood is required. Some glucometers (e.g., Roche's ACCUCHEK Advantage, Roche Diagnostics,

FIGURE 2-11 A small glucose meter can be purchased at most pharmacies; shown is ACCUCHEK Advantage (Roche Diagnostics, Indianapolis, IN).

FIGURE 2-12 Bottle of reagent strips (Azostix, Siemens Healthcare Diagnostics, Washington, DC) used to estimate blood urea nitrogen (BUN); color scale is used to estimate BUN value.

FIGURE 2-13 Comparing sample reagent strip with color scale on bottle provides estimated BUN level.

Indianapolis, IN) can determine BG levels using blood collected in EDTA or heparin, two types of anticoagulants, but they will not accurately measure BG in serum. It is important to use recently collected blood because glucose values are affected by how long the blood sits before it is analyzed. Likewise, it is important to follow the manufacturer's guidelines and directions. Any invalid results should be addressed (e.g., repeat with another sample) and any abnormal results should be brought to the attending veterinarian's attention and addressed.

Normal range of blood glucose
- Canine: 80 to 130 mg/dL
- Feline: 70 to 180 mg/dL
- For both canine and feline patients, less than 40 mg/dL indicates hypoglycemia.

Blood Urea Nitrogen
Urea is a nitrogenous compound that is a product of amino acid breakdown in the liver. BUN levels are used to evaluate the kidney's ability to remove nitrogenous wastes (urea) from the blood. If the kidneys are not working properly, an insufficient amount of urea is removed from the plasma, resulting in increased BUN levels.

An estimate of the patient's BUN value can be assessed quickly using a reagent strip (e.g., Azostix, Siemens Healthcare Diagnostics, Washington, DC; Figure 2-12). Blood mixed with the anticoagulants EDTA or heparin (as long as it does not contain an ammonium salt) will not affect the estimated BUN of an Azostix; however, neither serum nor plasma should be used for this test. Supplies needed to check BUN on a reagent strip include the reagent strip, fresh blood sample, watch with second hand, and a strong stream of water to rinse the strip. The color change on the reagent strip is compared with the color scale on the bottle for the strips. The corresponding color match between the reagent strip and the bottle indicates the estimated BUN (Figure 2-13).

Some anesthetics are primarily metabolized by the kidneys, and if there is any question of the patient's renal function, choosing a drug that is not primarily metabolized by the kidneys ought to be considered. Further diagnostic tests assessing kidney function (e.g., urinalysis) should be considered as well.

Normal range of blood urea nitrogen
- Canine: 5 to 35 mg/dL
- Feline: 5 to 35 mg/dL

Alanine Aminotransferase
Alanine aminotransferase (ALT) is an enzyme found in high concentration in the liver cells of dogs, cats, and primates. Damage to hepatocytes can elevate blood ALT levels. Certain drugs, such as anticonvulsants and corticosteroids, can also raise blood levels. ALT, while not indicative of specific liver disease, can be used as a general hepatic screen.

Normal range of alanine aminotransferase
- Canine 8.2-109 U/L
- Feline 25-97 U/L

Additional Tests

Other diagnostic tests specific to the patient's history and PE findings should be performed before any surgery. Generally, preanesthetic diagnostics are noninvasive and may eliminate ("rule out") the need for more invasive procedures. However, these diagnostic tests may support the need for additional, more invasive diagnostics or procedures. For example, the logical progression of diagnostic testing for a puppy with vomiting and diarrhea would start with an intestinal parasite test ("fecal") and a parvovirus ("parvo") test, followed by abdominal radiographs, then an abdominal ultrasound, and finally an abdominal exploratory procedure. In addition, the puppy with vomiting and diarrhea should receive a complete blood count (CBC) and serum chemistry panel and electrolyte panel to aid in determining what type of intravenous fluids or additional support (e.g., antibiotics, parenteral nutrition, plasma transfusion) is indicated.

It is important to note that preanesthetic diagnostic tests will not be the same for every patient and that not all preanesthetic diagnostics are limited to blood tests (e.g., CBC; serum chemistry, electrolyte, thyroid, and clotting panels; heartworm and feline leukemia virus tests; blood cultures). For example, intestinal parasite tests, radiographs, diagnostic ultrasounds, urinalyses, and electrocardiograms may need to be performed before surgery on certain patients, depending on the history and PE findings.

Preoperative Medications

Once all the preanesthetic diagnostic tests have been performed and analyzed, if the results still indicate that surgery is necessary and is the appropriate next step, the patient is premedicated for anesthesia.

Surgical patients are routinely premedicated with a combination of agents, including analgesics, sedatives, and at times anticholinergics. The purpose of administering these agents before induction is threefold. First, the patient is more relaxed, allowing a less stressful transition to anesthesia. Second, pain management is provided at the optimum time, before surgical tissue trauma occurs. Third, appropriate premedications ("premeds") ease the transition out of anesthesia, facilitating a smooth recovery. Anticholinergics may be added to prevent some of the undesired effects of the analgesia and sedation, mainly bradycardia.

Balanced Anesthesia

Premedication is an important part of balanced anesthesia. The objective of balanced anesthesia is to combine several agents, in smaller dosages, to maximize the positive effects, such as analgesia and muscle relaxation, while minimizing the negative effects, like cardiac and respiratory depression. The goal is to calm the patient, minimize pain, and reduce the adverse effects of the agents used (Box 2-1).

BOX 2-1 Components of Balanced Anesthesia

Premedication
Induction
Maintenance
Recovery—pain medication

Principles of Pain Management

The basic principles of current pain management involve (1) preemptive (preventive) analgesia, (2) multimodal analgesia (using different classes of drugs simultaneously to interrupt the pain pathway at various points), and (3) appropriate follow-up analgesia. Using this strategy, veterinarians design an analgesic plan for each patient that maximizes pain control, keeps patients on an analgesic plane, and reduces unwanted side effects.

These simple principles have evolved from our current understanding of the pain pathway, or *nociception*. Pain signaling occurs in a distinct pathway that begins at the onset of a noxious stimulus. The stimulus may be tissue trauma, surgical incision, or even heat. When tissue is traumatized, the first phase of the nociceptive pathway is triggered, and the event is converted to a signal that can be sent to the central nervous system (CNS) for processing. This phase is called *transduction*. The second phase, *transmission*, is the propagation of the impulses up toward the spinal cord. Once in the spinal cord, pain signals may undergo a number of different effects. Some signals are handled locally by the release of endogenous opioids, whereas others are sent to the brain for further processing. This sorting process is called *modulation*, the third phase; pain signals are said to be "modulated" in the spinal cord. The fourth and final phase of nociception, *perception*, occurs only in the conscious patient. Perception is "knowing" that pain is present and usually results in such reactions as withdrawal, vocalization, and, in some cases, aggression. Anesthesia interrupts the perception phase only. It is important to remember that interfering with perception alone does not address transduction, transmission, or modulation. Patients who undergo surgery only with anesthesia have essentially no pain management; the spinal cord is continually bombarded by pain signals, which will become evident as soon as the animal wakes.

The four distinct phases of the pain pathway allow pain to be interrupted at more than one juncture. Pain management specialists believe that interrupting nociception or pain perception can be achieved most effectively by targeting multiple points along the pathway. The analgesic drugs currently available target one or more of the nociceptive phases, although each class of agents exerts a major effect on one of the four phases (Figure 2-14). This is the rationale for combining different analgesics as premedications for surgery, a process called *multimodal analgesia*.

Modulation of spinal pathway (inhibit central sensitization)
- Local anesthetics
- Opioids
- α-agonists
- Tricyclic antidepressants
- Cholinesterase inhibitors
- NMDA antagonists
- NSAIDs
- Anticonvulsants

Inhibit perception
- Anesthetics
- Opioids
- α-agonists
- Benzodiazepines
- Phenothiazepines

Inhibit transmission (inhibit impulse conduction)
- Local anesthetics
- α-agonists

Inhibit transduction
(inhibit peripheral sensitization of nociceptors)
- Local anesthetics
- Opioids
- NSAIDs
- Corticosteroids

Pain

FIGURE 2-14 Analgesic drugs work at one or more of the phases of nociception. *NMDA,* N-methyl-D-aspartate; *NSAIDs,* nonsteroidal anti-inflammatory drugs. (From Tranquilli WJ, Grimm KA, Lamont LA: Pain management for the small animal practitioner, Jackson, WY, 2000, Teton New Media.)

Analgesics

Optimum premedication for surgery is likely to include several agents, as just discussed. Four classes of drugs can be effectively used to deliver preemptive analgesia: opioids (e.g., butorphanol, buprenorphine, morphine, fentanyl), nonsteroidal anti-inflammatory drugs (NSAIDs; e.g., carprofen, meloxicam, deracoxib), local anesthetic agents (e.g., bupivacaine, lidocaine), and α_2-adrenergic agonists (e.g., medetomidine, xylazine). (The appendix provides complete dosage information.) The most effective time to administer analgesia is before tissue trauma or damage occurs. Preemptive analgesia, the anticipation of pain and its treatment in advance, is a critical pain management strategy. Most patients require less anesthesia and actually experience less pain on recovery with smaller doses of analgesics when effective preemptive analgesia is administered.

Table 2-1 summarizes the side effects of analgesics. Note that not all the agents described in this table are approved for use in veterinary patients. Some are approved for use in dogs but not cats, and some are approved for use as single agents rather than in combination with other

TABLE 2-1	Side Effects of Analgesics	
Agent	Adverse Effects	Monitoring
Opioids	Sedation, low blood pressure, respiratory depression	Mentation, blood pressure, respiratory rate and quality
Local anesthetics	None unless given by CRI With CRI: nausea, vomiting, neurologic signs, seizures	Observe regularly for muscle tremors and GI upset
Nonsteroidal anti-inflammatory drugs	GI disturbances, GI bleeding, renal disturbances	General observation, hydration status, stool quality, urine production
α_2–agonists	Bradycardia, cardiac arrhythmias, hypertension, peripheral vasoconstriction	Palpate femoral pulse rate and quality; auscultate heart; monitor blood pressure.

CRI, Constant-rate infusion; *GI,* gastrointestinal.

drugs. However, although the U.S. Food and Drug Administration (FDA) has not approved all the previously cited analgesics for use in veterinary medicine, the Animal Medical Drug Use Clarification Act of 1994 (AMDUCA) permits veterinarians to use them on an "extra-label" basis.

Opioids

Opioids, the mainstay of acute pain management, provide analgesia by binding to specific opioid receptors in both the CNS and the peripheral nervous system (PNS). Opioids work at several locations along the pain pathway, affecting nociceptive signal transduction, modulating signals at the spinal level, and inhibiting perception of pain. In addition to providing analgesia, opioids help reduce anxiety and nonpainful distress.

Almost every patient expected to experience pain is a candidate for opioid analgesia. As a class, opioids produce minimal side effects in animals. The only cases in which opioids may be contraindicated are patients with head trauma, because even mild respiratory depression associated with opioids may worsen potential intracranial pressure. Opioids are most effective when administered before the onset of pain. Opioids can be administered through the conventional intravenous (IV), intramuscular (IM), and oral (PO) routes. Other, less common but effective routes of administration are transdermal (e.g., fentanyl), epidural, and intra-articular, as well as by constant-rate infusion. Buccal administration has become a popular route for buprenorphine in the cat, whose unique oral pH allows for excellent absorption by this route. (See the Appendix for an in-depth description of these techniques).

How opioids work. Opioids bind to opioid receptors in the spinal cord. The mu (μ) and kappa (κ) opioid receptors are primarily responsible for producing analgesia, with the μ receptor producing the most profound analgesia. The κ receptors produce much milder analgesia. Both receptor types are also responsible for producing respiratory depression, euphoria, sedation, and miosis. An opioid can interact with one or more types of opioid receptor. Drugs that bind to a receptor and cause expression of activity are called *agonists*. Drugs that bind to receptors and block their action are called *antagonists*. There are further subclassifications into full (pure) agonists, partial agonists, and mixed agonist-antagonists. The opioid drugs are classified by these subdivisions, which describe their potential action and duration.

Pure agonists (e.g., morphine, hydromorphone) bind and stimulate all types of opioid receptors, causing maximum analgesia. They are extremely effective but of only moderate duration, typically about 4 hours. Full agonists are also the most likely to have side effects.

Partial agonists function much the same as full agonists, but the interaction occurs with less than full activity at the receptors. Buprenorphine is a μ partial agonist. Although buprenorphine only partially binds to the μ receptor, it does so with great affinity. Therefore, although it provides analgesia of less intensity than morphine, buprenorphine has a much longer duration of action, up to 8 to 12 hours.

Agonist-antagonist opioids (e.g., butorphanol) bind to more than one type of opioid receptor, having an effect at one type but blocking effects at another receptor. Butorphanol binds and activates κ receptors to produce analgesia and sedation; it also binds with μ opioid receptors, blocking (antagonizing) the receptors. For this reason, butorphanol is considered a mild analgesic with extremely short duration, less than 1 hour in most cases. Butorphanol does produce profound sedation for up to 2 hours, outlasting the analgesia provided. Coadministration with butorphanol may result in reversal of the μ effects of full opioid agonists.

Antagonist opioids fully or partially reverse the effects of opioid agonists. Naloxone is a pure opioid antagonist that completely reverses the effects of all opioid agonists at all receptor sites. Butorphanol can be used as a partial reversing agent, reversing μ activity but not κ effects.

Side effects. Opioids have few clinically significant cardiovascular effects, other than bradycardia, in dogs and cats when administered at recommended doses. However, opioid-induced bradycardia is responsive to anticholinergics and can be reduced if a patient is pretreated with an anticholinergic. Respiratory depression is a common side effect with opioids in humans but rarely is clinically significant in veterinary patients. Emesis (vomiting) is a common side effect of some opioids, particularly morphine and hydromorphone. Vomiting typically occurs once when opioids are used as a premedication rather than when administered to an animal already in pain. Panting is a fairly common side effect of many opioids, especially at higher doses. This potential side effect may not be clinically important, but it can make patient monitoring difficult postoperatively because it is difficult to differentiate between panting as a sign of pain and panting as a reaction to an opioid.

Nonsteroidal Anti-inflammatory Drugs

NSAIDs have been used in human and veterinary medicine for many decades to treat fever, inflammation, and pain. More recently, NSAIDs have been shown to be quite efficacious for treating inflammation and pain associated with surgery, and several NSAIDs have been approved for preoperative use in dogs. NSAIDs can be incorporated into premedication protocols to control mild to moderate pain associated with surgery. For maximum effect, NSAIDs should be administered preoperatively, up to 1 to 2 hours before tissue trauma. When they are used in this way, controlling inflammation before it begins, dramatic results can be observed in the postoperative period. Patients who receive preemptive NSAIDs tend to recover with significantly less pain and often require less postoperative analgesia than those who do not. This class of drugs can be safely combined with opioids to provide excellent multimodal analgesia. NSAIDs are available in several formulations, including oral tablets, chewable forms, liquids, and injectable solutions.

How Nonsteroidal Anti-inflammatory Drugs Work

When cells are damaged as a result of trauma, surgery, or disease, fatty acids such as arachidonic acid (AA) are released from cell membranes. The release of AA triggers a cascade of biochemical activities that ultimately produce prostaglandins, which serve many functions in the body; some prostaglandins are essential for normal homeostasis, and some result in inflammation and pain. The enzyme cyclooxygenase (COX) metabolizes AA to prostaglandin and is the target of NSAIDs. To date, two forms of COX enzymes have been identified. These enzymes are closely related and are now known as COX-1 and COX-2. Each converts AA to prostaglandins, although the prostaglandins produced by each COX enzyme appear to serve very different functions. COX-1 is continuously present in most cells and is important for normal body functions. In the stomach, COX-1 plays a key role in maintaining integrity of gastric mucosa. In platelets, COX-1 is essential for thromboxane A_2 production. In contrast, COX-2 is not readily present in the cells, but it is rapidly synthesized in response to various inflammatory stimuli. Once induced by tissue injury, COX-2 converts AA into prostaglandins that create inflammation and pain. Both COX-1 and COX-2 play a vital role in the kidney as important mediators of salt and water balance, rennin (chymosin) release, and vascular tone. NSAIDs exert their anti-inflammatory effects by inhibiting activity of COX-1, COX-2, or both. This inhibitory activity varies between NSAID compounds and with animal species.

Side effects. As a class, NSAIDs are associated with specific types of potential side effects. Some of these are species specific and drug specific, as in the case of acetaminophen metabolism in cats. Possible side effects associated with NSAIDs include gastrointestinal tract damage, hepatopathy, renal toxicity, impaired platelet function, and cartilage destruction. Administration of NSAIDs should be restricted to well-hydrated, normotensive animals with normal hepatic and renal function, no hemostatic abnormalities, and no evidence of gastric ulceration.

Alpha₂-Adrenergic Agonists

Alpha₂-adrenergic agonists (α_2-agonists) are short-duration sedative-analgesic–muscle relaxants that can be rapidly reversed with α_2-antagonists. This characteristic makes these drugs suitable for procedures requiring short-term restraint and analgesia as well as premedication for longer surgical procedures. Use of α_2-antagonists as premedications may result in substantial reduction in both induction and inhalant anesthetic dosages. α_2-agonists are nonnarcotic and nonscheduled agents. Medetomidine and xylazine are the two α_2-agonists currently approved for use in dogs in the United States.

Medetomidine is a dose-dependent sedative-analgesic often used as a preanesthetic agent in healthy animals. Onset of effect is 5 to 15 minutes depending on route of administration, which can be IV or IM, and sedation can last up to 90 minutes.

How α_2-agonists work. α_2-agonists inhibit release of the excitatory neurotransmitter norepinephrine to produce analgesia and sedation. These agents interrupt the pain pathway by inhibiting nerve impulse transmission, modulating nociceptive signals in the spinal cord, and inhibiting perception within the brain. Because α_2-adrenoceptors are found in various sites throughout the body, α_2-agonists normally induce a number of physiologic changes in addition to sedation, analgesia, and muscle relaxation. Administration results in physiologically normal peripheral vasoconstriction, which creates a transient increase in blood pressure. Because the normal cardiovascular response to these events is a reflexive decrease in heart rate, patients are expected to become bradycardic. All cardiovascular parameters smoothly return to presedation levels on reversal of the agent with atipamezole.

Side effects. α_2-agonists can have profound effects on the CNS and cardiovascular system, but using low dosages can minimize these adverse events. Bradycardia and vomiting are the most common side effects. All α_2-agonists have potential side effects, including hypertension, bradycardia and heart block, respiratory depression, excessive CNS depression, vomiting, increased urine production, and peripheral vasoconstriction.

Candidates for α_2-agonist administration should be healthy, have sound cardiovascular systems, and be exercise tolerant. An α_2-agonist should never be administered to an animal with a compromised cardiovascular or respiratory system.

Local Anesthetics

Local anesthetics are inexpensive to use and quite effective in blocking the transmission of nociceptive signals at the source. Use of local anesthetics offers three major benefits. First, these agents produce true analgesia, that is, a complete absence of pain. Second, they are nonscheduled agents, requiring no cumbersome paperwork. Third, the techniques used to administer local anesthetics are relatively easy to perform. Most blocking techniques are well within the skill level of licensed veterinary technicians. Local anesthetics can and should be used in any surgical patient with an identifiable site for nerve blockade. For example, local anesthetics can be used effectively in patients undergoing thoracotomy, elbow surgery, maxillomandibular procedures, local excisions, feline declawing, and knee or cruciate repair. Anesthetic agents can be administered to create local and regional anesthesia and analgesia (Box 2-2).

In addition, local anesthetics are most often the drugs of choice for epidural anesthesia and analgesia. This technique is a good alternative to general anesthesia or as an

- Field block, such as an incisional line block, produces regional anesthesia.
- Infraorbital nerve block provides anesthesia and analgesia to the upper lip and nose, the dorsal aspect of the nasal cavity, and the skin ventral to the infraorbital foramen.
- Mandibular nerve block provides anesthesia of the teeth, skin and mucosa of the lower lip, and chin.
- Intercostal block provides analgesia after thoracotomy and for desensitizing the area around broken ribs.
- Intra-articular administration of a local anesthetic provides analgesia to a joint before and after a surgical procedure.
- Circumferential ring block provides anesthesia and analgesia around a given area, such as a foot or claw.

TABLE 2-2 Comparison of Local Anesthetic Agents

Drug	Onset	Duration
Lidocaine	5-10 minutes	45-90 minutes
Bupivacaine	15-20 minutes	Up to 6 hours

adjunct to inhalant anesthesia, especially for patients at high risk during general anesthesia and those undergoing painful orthopedic surgeries of the hind limb. Finally, an IV constant-rate infusion of a local anesthetic can provide sustained pain control in a variety of patients undergoing extensive nerve trauma, such as limb amputation. Lidocaine and bupivacaine are the agents most often used for dogs and cats. Lidocaine is characterized by rapid onset (5-10 minutes) but short duration (45-90 minutes). In contrast, bupivacaine has a longer onset (15-20 minutes) but provides up to 6 hours of analgesia (Table 2-2).

How local anesthetics work. Local anesthetics act by inhibiting transduction and transmission of nerve impulses and by modifying the signals at the spinal cord. Local anesthetics inhibit generation and transmission of nerve impulses by blocking sodium channels in the neuron's cell membrane. This effect slows the rate of depolarization of the neuron cell membrane and prevents the threshold potential from being reached.

Side effects. When administered at an appropriate dose, local anesthetics have relatively few, if any, adverse side effects. The potential systemic side effects of local anesthetics involve the CNS and cardiovascular system. Other potential side effects include development of methemoglobinemia, nerve and skeletal muscle toxicities, and allergic reactions, including hypersensitivity and anaphylaxis.

Sedation and Tranquilization

Sedatives alone do not possess any analgesic properties but are an important adjunct to premedication protocols.

Sedation should be incorporated into preoperative regimens to reduce stress, fear, and anxiety, all of which exacerbate pain, and vice versa. However, sedatives alone (with the exception of α_2-agonists) should never be administered to an animal without analgesia when pain is anticipated. Sedation alone may decrease the animal's ability to express pain and give the false impression that the animal is pain free. The most frequently used sedatives for premedication include the tranquilizing agents phenothiazines (acepromazine) and benzodiazepines (diazepam, midazolam).

Anticholinergics

Anticholinergic drugs such as atropine and glycopyrrolate are sometimes added to premedication protocols that are expected to produce profound, sustained bradycardia. For example, anticholinergics are frequently given to patients who receive opioids and are expected to have a long gas inhalation anesthesia time. Anticholinergics are given to reduce bradycardia and to dry oral secretions. Atropine sulfate has a quick onset of action and rapid elimination and can be given subcutaneously (SC), IM, or IV to prevent or to treat bradycardia and to dry oral secretions. Glycopyrrolate can be given SC, IV, or IM, although onset of action is substantially increased when given IV. Glycopyrrolate is typically used to prevent bradycardia rather than treat it once it has occurred. The effects of glycopyrrolate are much longer lasting than those of atropine.

Anticholinergics can increase the incidence of cardiac arrhythmias and sinus tachycardia. Increasing heart rate is not always beneficial to the patient because higher heart rates do not necessarily translate into better perfusion. Whether or not an anticholinergic should be routinely administered in conjunction with drugs that lower heart rate (e.g., α_2-agonists) has been the subject of considerable scientific debate. Initially, treatment of α_2-agonist–induced bradycardia was thought to be beneficial. Currently, however, anticholinergic drugs are not generally recommended to prevent periods of expected transient bradycardia. Bradycardia that is considered life threatening because it is associated with poor perfusion can be rapidly corrected with atropine. The most practical approach may be to avoid "routine" use of anticholinergics, administering them on a case-by-case basis only to patients in need.

Antibiotics

An important consideration is whether or not the surgery patient needs intraoperative antibiotics and, if antibiotics are indicated, which type is appropriate. If the procedure is elective and a possible break in sterility during it is not a concern, antibiotics are generally unnecessary. However, if the surgical procedure is done specifically to treat contaminated or infected wounds, or if possible contamination during an elective procedure is a concern, intraoperative antibiotics may be indicated. Specific guidelines for prophylactic antibiotic use follow this section on wounds.

When determining whether antibiotics are indicated, it is helpful to know what type of wound is present. See Chapter 8 for a discussion on wound classifications.

Prophylaxis refers to the measures taken in the prevention of disease. The administration of antibiotics just before and during surgery is known as *perioperative prophylaxis.* The purpose of this practice is to decrease the chances of postoperative infection of the surgical site. Few surgical cases or circumstances warrant prophylactic antibiotic treatment; one example is an orthopedic procedure involving the placement of implants.

The choice of antibiotic depends on the type of bacterial contamination expected. For example, staphylococci from the skin are of concern in orthopedic procedures. Gram-negative bacteria (e.g., *Escherichia coli*) are of concern in large-bowel procedures. The antibiotic's spectrum of activity should be narrow and limited to the predicted bacterial contaminant.

The antibiotic must be administered by IV injection just before induction. The dose may be repeated during the surgical procedure to ensure adequate serum levels throughout the surgery. The antibiotic administration is usually not continued after the procedure is completed. Antibiotics that cannot be administered IV are not used as prophylactic antibiotics.

If an animal is taken to surgery with an infection that is already established, the clinician may have prescribed antibiotics for a period before the surgery. This situation is not considered "prophylactic" in nature. The antibiotics have been prescribed in response to an already established infection. In this case, it is important to continue the administration perioperatively and postoperatively, during the recuperative period. The antibiotic may need to be administered by injection (SC, IM, or IV) immediately before the surgery. Oral antibiotic administration can be reinstituted as soon as the animal can tolerate ("keep down") food and water after the surgery.

Intravenous Catheters

After the patient has received the appropriate premedication, an IV catheter should be placed. In addition to the analgesic benefits provided by premedicating the surgical patient, premedication makes for a more sedate and cooperative patient when the catheter is placed.

The placement of an IV catheter offers many benefits to the surgical patient. Once an IV catheter has been placed, it is easier for the veterinary technician to administer, as well as less stressful for the patient to receive, multiple IV medications. Puncturing through the skin and vein (venipuncture) for every injection is unnecessary when an IV catheter is in place. Also, the patient with an IV catheter is not poked with a needle every time an IV medication is administered. Likewise, the veterinary technician does not need to find a "good" vein for every drug

administered intravenously. Many drugs needed by a surgical patient are intended to be, and some can only be, administered intravenously, and the IV catheter allows for easier administration of these drugs. For example, induction agents for general anesthesia, analgesics, antibiotics, and fluids may need to be given to the surgical patient at some point during its hospital stay. Having established access to the vascular system through an IV catheter aids in the efficiency of administering these medications. From a safety standpoint, having venous access allows for immediate administration of emergency drugs if necessary.

The type and placement site of the catheter greatly influence its capabilities. Peripheral catheters are completely adequate for short-term use (1-3 days), anesthesia induction, and medication administration. However, for long-term use (>3 days), extended fluid therapy, or systemic monitoring, a jugular catheter (central line) should be placed.

Peripheral Catheters

Peripheral catheters are most often placed in the following sites:

Canine: cephalic and lateral saphenous veins
Feline: cephalic, medial saphenous, and femoral veins

Almost any palpable vessel can be used to place a catheter.

Supplies
Regardless of the site, the basic supplies needed to place the catheter remain the same (Figure 2-15).

Catheter. Many styles of catheters are available for use. The three most common styles are the over-the-needle catheter, the through-the-needle catheter, and the butterfly catheter (Figure 2-16). The choice of catheter style is primarily determined by the site of placement and the intended use. The over-the-needle type is typically used for short-term and surgical catheters and is usually placed

FIGURE 2-15 Supplies required for placement of IV catheter and administration of IV fluids. *From left:* IV fluid bag (1-L bag of lactated Ringer's solution shown), cotton balls and scrub product, IV fluid administration set, IV catheters, gauze squares, tape, and clippers.

FIGURE 2-16 Examples of IV catheters (a) through-the-needle catheter; (b) over-the-needle catheters; (c) butterfly catheter.

FIGURE 2-18 Injection cap (left) and two examples of T-ports or T-sets (right).

FIGURE 2-17 Through-the-needle catheter.

FIGURE 2-19 Buretrol administration set can be attached to bag of IV fluid and the chamber filled with amount of fluid to be administered. These sets are generally used on small (e.g., pediatric) patients when an electric infusion pump is not available.

in a peripheral vein (e.g., cephalic vein). The butterfly catheter is useful when vascular access is required for medications that need to be administered once (as in outpatient treatments) and slowly (i.e., over 1-3 minutes). Butterfly catheters are sharp and rigid and are not intended to remain in a patient that is not being directly monitored (i.e., with hands-on monitoring). Through-the-needle catheters are often placed in the jugular veins of animals that will need intensive nursing care postoperatively (Figure 2-17).

The choice of catheter size is primarily influenced by five factors: (1) site of placement, (2) length of time the catheter will be needed, (3) reason for placement, (4) diameter of the vessel, and (5) length of the vessel working area. Catheter diameter (gauge) should be chosen after evaluation of the vessel's size and the reason for placement. The length of the catheter needs to be considered after the vessel has been chosen so that the length of the working area is known. For example, a 2-inch catheter placed in the cephalic vein of a dachshund is inappropriate, because once completely seated, the catheter would be proximal to the patient's elbow and would be more likely to kink every time the leg was bent. Table 2-3 provides guidance in making appropriate catheter selections based on the factors listed.

Injection caps, T-ports, and fluid administration sets. Injection caps may be placed on the catheter if occasional injections or blood sample collections are anticipated (Figure 2-18). An injection cap allows for repeated punctures through the cap without resulting in damage to or leaking from the cap. Needle-less styles of injection caps are available and are a good option because they reduce accidental needle punctures of workers.

T-ports (or T-sets) serve the same purpose as an injection cap and also allow easier access to the catheter (see Figure 2-18). The short tubing incorporated into the design of the device allows sample collection or medication administration to be done more easily. A fluid administration set of the appropriate size should be used if continuous infusion of fluids or IV medications is anticipated, and the set can be connected to the T-port.

Usually an administration set supplying 15 or 20 drops/ mL (macrodrip set) is used for patients weighing more than 7 kg. Sets supplying 60 drops/mL (microdrip set) are used for patients weighing less than 7 kg for more accurate fluid administration. For extremely small patients, a Buretrol solution administration set (Baxter, Deerfield, IL) can be employed for the most accurate measurement of fluids administered, and it is especially useful if an electric fluid infusion pump is not available (Figure 2-19).

TABLE 2-3   Intravenous Catheter Selection Guidelines

Patient Size (lbs)	Vein	Type of Catheter	Catheter Diameter (Gauge)	Catheter Length (Inches)
CANINE				
0-5	Saphenous/cephalic	Over the needle	24	¾
5-25	Saphenous/cephalic	Over the needle	22	1-1¼
25-80	Saphenous/cephalic	Over the needle	20	1-2
80 and up	Saphenous/cephalic	Over the needle	18	1-2
0-5	Jugular	Through the needle	21	1 1½
5-25	Jugular	Through the needle	18	1 1½
25-80	Jugular	Through the needle	16-18	1 1½
80 and up	Jugular	Through the needle	16	1 1½
0-5	Saphenous/cephalic	Butterfly	24-23	¾-1
5-25	Saphenous/cephalic	Butterfly	22	¾-1
25-80	Saphenous/cephalic	Butterfly	20	¾-1
80 and up	Saphenous/cephalic	Butterfly	18	¾-1
FELINE				
0-4	Femoral/cephalic	Over the needle	24	¾
4 and up	Femoral/cephalic	Over the needle	22	1
0-4	Jugular	Through the needle	21	1 1½
4 and up	Jugular	Through the needle	18	1 1½
0-4	Cephalic	Butterfly	24	¾
4 and up	Cephalic	Butterfly	22	¾

Extension sets. An extension set may be used in conjunction with an administration set to allow for better animal mobility in the cage postoperatively. The administration sets are often not long enough to be practical, so extension sets may be used.

Tape. The tape is one of the most important components of the catheter. Without proper anchoring, even the best placed catheter is useless. The technique for taping can vary from technician to technician, the only constant being that the catheter must be secure without being too tight. A loose tape job would allow the catheter to lose patency, but applying the tape too tightly could occlude blood flow. Typically, 1-inch and ½-inch tape are used in varying orders to secure the catheter. If ½-inch tape is not available, the 1-inch tape can be ripped in half. The first piece of tape should be long enough to encircle the patient's limb or neck, depending on where the catheter is placed. Two additional pieces of tape, the same length as the first, will be needed to secure the catheter further in place.

Catheter "Prep" materials. Clippers with a number 40 (No. 40) blade are required for hair removal from the catheter site (Figure 2-20). The amount of hair to remove depends on the catheter site and the patient's size. In general, for peripheral veins, a margin of 1½ to 2 inches on all sides of the proposed puncture site is appropriate

FIGURE 2-20 Two types of clipper blades, a No. 50 *(left)* and a No. 40 *(right)*, that can be used to clip hair in preparation for surgery or placement of an IV catheter.

(clipping an area of this size often requires clipping the entire circumference of the limb). For catheters placed in the jugular vein, a larger area should be clipped.

Preparation materials include cotton balls saturated with either dilute (50:50) povidone-iodine scrub or chlorhexidine scrub for the cleansing step and cotton balls saturated with 70% isopropyl alcohol for the rinsing step. Jugular catheter sites may be prepared with saturated gauze sponges instead of cotton balls.

Fluids or heparinized saline. Either continuous infusion of IV fluids or regular flushing of the catheter with heparinized saline is necessary to maintain patency of the catheter once it is placed. If fluids are used, 0.9% sodium chloride (NaCl) or lactated Ringer's solution (LRS) is most often used (Box 2-3).

Bandage materials. Bandage materials are needed if the catheter is to remain in place after the surgical procedure is completed. Antibiotic ointment, elastic gauze, and elastic tape (or Vetrap, 3M, St Paul, MN) are the materials of choice. (It should be noted that the benefits of using antibiotic ointment are anecdotal. Research in human medicine has shown that the use of such ointments at the catheter insertion point has actually led to antibiotic resistance and fungal growth.) Usually, 1-inch widths of all materials work best, given the area that will be bandaged on most dogs and cats, but personal preference eventually becomes the determining factor. Tegaderm (3M) is a sterile, transparent, breathable adherent dressing used to cover the insertion site of the catheter. This dressing is impervious to liquids and bacteria and therefore is effective in maintaining a catheter. Other sterile wound dressings may be used, depending on the indication for and placement site of the catheter.

Even with aseptic placement and appropriate bandaging, peripheral catheters should remain in place for only 3 days. Daily evaluation of the catheter and insertion site helps prevent phlebitis and detects any problems early. It is helpful to write the date, time, and initials of the technician placing the catheter on the outer bandage as well as on the inner tape. This information ensures that the catheter is replaced in the appropriate time frame.

Placement Technique

Box 2-4 details the placement of IV catheters in a peripheral vein.

Jugular Catheters

Some surgical patients require intense postoperative critical care. If part of this care requires central venous pressure (CVP) measurements or long-term fluid therapy, a jugular catheter (central line) should be placed.

Supplies

The supplies required for placement of a jugular catheter are similar to those used for a peripheral vein catheter.

Jugular catheters are longer, usually 8 to 12 inches, and can be single lumen or double lumen. The extra length is needed to ensure placement of the catheter close to the right atrium of the heart, which is required to measure CVP. Because they are long-term catheters, jugular catheters should always be secured with a sterile bandage in addition to the tape. Antimicrobial ointment, elastic gauze, and elastic tape can be used for the bandage.

Placement

With the animal in lateral recumbency, a large area is clipped over the ventrolateral neck to reveal the jugular vein. The site is aseptically prepared as done for a peripheral catheter. Because these catheters are generally left in place for a longer time, a final "paint" is applied after the last rinse. The person placing the catheter should wear sterile gloves, and a sterile drape should cover the prepared area. Different catheters need to be inserted with different techniques, so it is best to consult and follow the manufacturer's recommendation for the catheter used.

After the catheter has been placed and is secured, it is essential to maintain the patency of the line. The administration of fluids will aid in ensuring line patency. If fluids are not being administered, heparinized saline should be used to flush the line at regular intervals (e.g., every 6 hours).

Sample Collection

Sample collection from the catheter is easily accomplished and much less stressful on the patient than performing a venipuncture each time a sample is needed. The clinician must keep in mind that residues from medications administered through the catheter could interfere with test results. A three-syringe technique can be used to help decrease the incidence of contaminants in a blood sample collected from an IV catheter. A three-mL syringe is half-filled with heparinized saline, and blood is withdrawn into the syringe from the catheter. This helps clean any contaminants from the catheter. The second syringe is used to withdraw the appropriate sample and place it in the desired collection tubes. Lastly, the original syringe is used to replace the withdrawn blood and flush the catheter with the remaining heparinized saline.

Central Venous Pressure

CVP monitoring is done to assess how well blood is returning to the heart as well as how effectively blood is pumped from the heart. This procedure is helpful in monitoring a patient with right-sided heart failure because blood backs up into the vena cava in such a patient. CVP monitoring also helps to assess overhydration with fluids because as blood volume increases, CVP rises. A water manometer is connected to the catheter to determine the measurement. A normal reading for cats and dogs is less than 8 cm H_2O.

BOX 2-4   Technique for Placement of a Peripheral Intravenous Catheter

1. Before beginning the placement of the catheter, be sure all supplies are available and readily accessible.
2. Clip an ample amount from the area where the catheter is to be placed. Bear in mind that no component of the catheter and no accessories (e.g., injection cap, end of fluid line) should be resting in hair once the catheter has been placed. When in doubt, shave more than would seem necessary.
3. After clipping, remove all loose hair from the tabletops and dispose of it in the waste can.
4. To begin, the restrainer should occlude the vessel to be catheterized. Proper restraint must be used to prevent contamination of the prepped catheter site (Figure 2-21).
5. Cleanse the area using a surgical scrub product and rinsing agent combination, either povidone-iodine/70% isopropyl alcohol or chlorhexidine/70% isopropyl alcohol (Figure 2-22). Cotton balls are best used to help prevent depositing excessive amounts of fluid on the area. The target pattern should be used when preparing the area. Begin at the proposed puncture site and move in a circle progressively toward the hair margins. Cotton balls that have left the center of the area must never return to the center. A rinsing agent should be used in the same manner to remove the scrub from the skin. A minimum of three "cycles" of scrub/rinse should be performed. If, however, after the third rinse the skin is still dirty, continue cleansing until the skin is clean. No final prep solution is necessary unless

the catheter will be left in place after the surgery is completed. In this case, apply the solution using the target pattern as previously described.
6. Open the catheter using aseptic technique. Remove both the injection plug at the end of the catheter and the cover on the catheter. If the cap at the end of the catheter has a paper filter, the cap may be left in place as the catheter is placed. The filter will allow the blood to "flash back" while preventing excessive bleeding. Take care to avoid touching the exposed catheter.
7. Place the thumb of the nondominant hand parallel to, but not touching, the prepared vessel. The same hand should be holding the leg in extension as well.
8. Hold the catheter at the junction of the catheter and stylet with the thumb and index finger of the dominant hand (Figure 2-23).
9. Ensure that the bevel of the stylet is facing up.
10. Using a 10- to 20-degree angle, quickly penetrate the skin with the catheter and then insert it into the vessel.
11. Check the stylet for blood flow (Figure 2-24). If flow is present, advance both the catheter and the stylet 1 to 2 mm. Check the stylet again. If blood flow is still present, grasp the stylet with the hand that is holding the leg. Using the other hand, advance only the catheter into the vessel (Figure 2-25). (*It is possible to use one hand to hold the stylet and advance the catheter; grasp the stylet with the*

FIGURE 2-21 Scrubbing clipped area before catheter placement.

FIGURE 2-23 Proper holding of catheter and appropriate approach to vessel.

FIGURE 2-22 Aseptically prepared and properly restrained catheter site.

FIGURE 2-24 "Flash" of blood in stylet of catheter ensures proper placement in vessel.

FIGURE 2-25   Advancing catheter into vessel.

FIGURE 2-26   Attachment of injection port, T-port, or fluid administration set to catheter hub. Note hand placement to stabilize hub.

FIGURE 2-27   Attached fluid line.

middle and ring fingers while using the index finger to advance the catheter.) Be sure to advance the catheter all the way to the hub. If blood flow is not present, redirect the catheter until blood flow is established.

12. Using the other hand, quickly remove the stylet and connect either an injection cap, a T-port, or a fluid administration set to the catheter hub (Figures 2-26 and 2-27).

13. If using a fluid administration set, be sure to turn on the fluids to maintain a patent line. If using an injection cap or a T-port, flush the catheter with 2 mL of heparinized saline.

FIGURE 2-28   Placement of ½-inch piece of tape, sticky side up, under hub of catheter.

FIGURE 2-29   A long piece of tape is brought over hub and around leg.

(It may be easier to insert an injection cap, secure the catheter with the first piece of tape, and then hook up the fluid line. The weight of the fluid line may otherwise pull the catheter out.)

14. Use a dry gauze sponge to remove any blood on the clipped area or hair near the catheter.

15. Begin securing the catheter by using a ½-inch-wide piece of tape long enough to encircle the limb at least once. Place the tape, sticky side up (Figure 2-28), under the hub of the catheter all the way up to the puncture site. Bring the long side of the tape over the hub (Figure 2-29) and tape all the way around the leg, leaving a tab of tape folded over (Figure 2-30) to aid in removal of the tape when the catheter is removed later. This piece should be snug, but not occlusive, because it is the "anchor" for keeping the catheter in place.

16. Place a 1-inch-wide piece of tape, sticky side down, under the catheter all the way up to the first piece of tape (Figure 2-31). Bring the long side of the tape over the catheter hub and around the leg, securing the hub of the catheter. Be sure the connection of the fluid line and the catheter is not covered.

17. The final step in securing the catheter is to use the piece of tape to secure the fluid line with a stress loop (Figure 2-32). When making the stress loop, be sure not to kink

BOX 2-4   Technique for Placement of a Peripheral Intravenous Catheter—Cont'd

FIGURE 2-30 Anchor piece of tape properly placed.

FIGURE 2-31 1-inch piece of tape, sticky side down, is placed under catheter.

FIGURE 2-32 A stress loop is made by carefully folding a length of the IV fluid line and taping it securely to patient's leg. The stress loop relieves direct pressure at the connection between catheter (or T-port) and fluid administration set should patient exert tension on administration set, making it less likely that patient will pull the catheter out while shifting positions and moving about the cage.

the line to impair or obstruct the flow of fluid. Tape the loop to one of the other pieces of tape to ensure that it is secure.

18. Ensure that the catheter is still patent by checking the limb for any swelling or "blebs." Generally the fluids will not run if the catheter is not in the vessel. The drip chamber of the fluid administration set can also be observed to see that the fluid is flowing. Another trick to check catheter placement is to place the bag of fluid lower than the patient's heart and see whether blood flows back into the catheter.

FIGURE 2-33 Endotracheal tube; *a*, hose connector; *b*, body; *c*, cuff indicator; *d*, cuff; *e*, Murphy eye.

Endotracheal Intubation

Endotracheal (ET) tubes are an important piece of anesthetic equipment. They are used for two main reasons: administration of oxygen and inhalation anesthetics and assistance with resuscitative needs.

Components of Tube

All ET tubes have several components (Figure 2-33). It is important to know each of these components in order to

use the tubes properly and evaluate the integrity of each tube before use.

- The hose connector is found at one end of the ET tube. It connects the tube to the Y-piece, non-rebreathing system, or Ambu bag.
- The body is the major portion of the ET tube. Several numbers may be found on the tube body. The length measurements are in 2-mm increments and identify the length of the tube. The manufacturer's name may also be seen on the body. The large bold number is the size of the internal diameter in millimeters. The most common tubes are available in sizes ranging from 3.0 to 12.0 mm in 0.5-mm increments.
- The cuff indicator is used to determine the pressure of the cuff on the trachea once air has been infused into the cuff.
- The cuff is present to permit the creation of a leakproof system. Air is infused into the cuff, via the cuff indicator, to ensure a seal between the ET tube and the lumen of the trachea. The cuff prevents the patient from inhaling room air, which would dilute the gas delivered to the patient during anesthesia. The cuff also prevents the patient from exhaling anesthetic gas into the

How to "Leak Check" an Endotracheal Tube

The ET tube must be checked for leaks each time it is used, as follows:
1. Completely submerse the tube in a pan of clean water.
2. Attach a syringe to the cuff indicator.
3. Fully inflate the cuff and observe for any bubbles. Bubbles in the water, seen coming from any spot on the tube, indicate a leak in the tube.

The ET tube may be thrown away, or it may be kept and identified as a leaky tube if that type of equipment would be needed (e.g., as a tracheostomy tube).

TABLE 2-4 Approximate Sizes for Endotracheal Tubes Based on Body Weight

Body Weight (kg)	Internal Diameter (mm)
CANINE	
2	3-4
5	5-6
10-12	7-8
14-16	8-9
18-20	9-10
>20	11 and up
FELINE	
2	3.0-3.5
4-5	3.5-4.0
>5	4.0-4.5

operating room and from aspirating any vomitus while intubated.
• The Murphy eye is found at the tip of the ET tube. It allows airflow in the event that the end of the tube becomes occluded with respiratory secretions (mucous plugs).

Box 2-5 explains how to check an ET tube for leaks before using it in a patient.

Selection of Proper Tube Size

The largest size ET tube possible, without being traumatic, should be used. Generally, tube size is based on a patient's weight, although palpation of the trachea and experience will aid in this decision. Table 2-4 is provided as a reference. Because of the variability in patient size, multiple tubes should be set aside for possible use and checked for leaks with every patient. An acceptable practice is to choose the size thought to be needed, in addition to a tube 0.5 mm smaller and a tube 0.5 mm larger.

Supplies

Using the proper supplies in the proper manner will significantly increase the success rate of intubation (Figure 2-34).

FIGURE 2-34 Supplies needed for endotracheal intubation.

Endotracheal Tube

Both clear and colored ET tubes are available. Although the two types work equally well, the clear tubes have two distinct advantages. First, any type of occlusion in the tube (e.g., blood, mucus) is more easily identified in a clear tube than in a colored or nonclear tube. Second, clear tubes allow visualization of the fog that moves along the lumen of the ET tube as the patient breathes. This is another useful means of quickly confirming that the patient is breathing.

Securing the Tube

A method of securing the tube in place is necessary. Rolled gauze is most commonly used to secure the ET tube to the patient once proper placement has been established. Any width can be used, although 2-inch gauze is most often employed. The gauze should be a nonstretch type, like muzzle gauze. Kling gauze can stretch, leading to tube slippage. The gauze is placed on the tube to indicate the depth of placement of the ET tube in the patient. Another method of securing the tube is using pieces of IV lines or plastic ties. The plastic can be cleaned and used with many different patients; it can also be less "messy" for performing dental procedures. The plastic or tubing is placed in a similar fashion to the gauze. Proper depth of insertion is determined by measuring the tube before placement. Box 2-6 describes the procedure for measuring the tube for proper placement in the patient.

Sterile Lubricant

Sterile lubricant is needed to lubricate the tip and cuff of the ET tube to permit easier passage of the tube through the larynx. The lubricant should be placed on a clean gauze sponge or clean paper towel and then applied to the tube. Water can also be used to lubricate the tube.

Cuff Syringe

The cuff syringe, or "puffer cuffer," is needed to inflate the cuff of the ET tube. Generally, a 6- or 12-mL syringe is

FIGURE 2-35 Laryngoscope handle and various blades.

used. It should be readily available throughout the procedure, but the syringe should not be placed in a pocket, out of sight. Securing a syringe case to an accessible area of the anesthesia machine provides reliable storage for constant availability.

Laryngoscope or Light Source

The use of some type of light source significantly enhances the process of intubation. Easy visualization of the larynx permits greater success of first attempts to intubate. Laryngoscopes are composed of two major parts: the blade and the handle (Figure 2-35). The blade houses the light bulb and can be curved or straight. Curved blades are commonly identified as Miller blades, and straight blades are often called Wisconsin blades. The numbers

included in the identification process refer to the length of the blade. The higher the number, the longer the blade. Often, "0" blades work well with cats, No. 1 blades for small dogs, No. 2 for medium-sized dogs, and No. 3 blades for large dogs. The handle houses the batteries that power the laryngoscope. Alternative light sources include floor lamps and overhead lights.

Mouth Speculum

The use of a mouth speculum is not necessary, but its use can be advantageous to some. First, the mouth can be opened wider to allow better visualization, therefore increasing success rates for endotracheal intubation. Second, the speculum prevents the patient from biting the ET tube if the patient transitions into a lighter stage of anesthesia. Third, the speculum helps the restrainer keep the mouth open.

Tube Placement

Patient Anatomy

Proper knowledge of the anatomy of the throat is critical to placement of the ET tube. Proper recognition of structures assists in the detection of abnormalities and helps ensure proper placement of the tube. Figure 2-36 displays the anatomy of the throat. When one is viewing the throat, the following structures can be seen: vocal folds, epiglottis, and glottis. The *vocal folds* are the most lateral structures, located on the lateral edges of the glottis. The *epiglottis* is a triangular flap of tissue that covers (or protects) the glottis when in the "up" or most dorsal position. The epiglottis must be lying down for intubation to be accomplished. The vocal folds are located on the lateral edges of the glottis. The *glottis* is the most ventral opening in the throat. The esophagus runs along the dorsal surface of the trachea, just left of center.

One-Person Technique

Box 2-7 describes the technique for performing single-person endotracheal intubation.

Two-Person Technique

Box 2-8 describes the technique for performing two-person endotracheal intubation.

Laryngospasms

Certain species, most often cats and rabbits, experience the phenomenon of laryngospasm during endotracheal intubation. If excessively stimulated, the muscles of the larynx spasm, and the vocal folds clamp shut. Application of 0.05 mL of 2% lidocaine to each vocal fold (dripping the lidocaine out of a tuberculin syringe onto the vocal folds with the needle removed) just before attempting intubation will significantly decrease the occurrence of laryngospasm. Care must be taken with this step because laryngeal paralysis can occur. A safer tactic to avoid laryngospasm is good technique. Repeated stimulation of the area may cause the muscles to spasm, so avoiding

Hard palate

Soft palate

Epiglottis

Tongue

Glottis

Epiglottis

Laryngoscope

FIGURE 2-36 Anatomy of the throat. (From McKelvey D, Hollingshead KW: Veterinary anesthesia and analgesia, ed 3, St Louis, 2003, Mosby.)

BOX 2-7   Single-Person Endotracheal Intubation

1. Place the animal in sternal recumbency.
2. Place the mouth speculum in the mouth.
3. Position a floor lamp or overhead light if being used.
4. Holding the mandible with the nondominant hand, fully extend the tongue and hold it in place with the thumb. The thumb should be caudal to the canine tooth, and the rest of the hand should be on the ventral surface of the mandible.
5. Visualize the glottis. If the epiglottis is lying dorsally, it will need to be pulled down with the ET tube to ensure visualization of the glottis.
6. Pass the lubricated tube through the glottis to the predetermined length, as indicated by the gauze tie placed on the tube.
7. Secure the tube to the patient.
   a. For dogs, tie the gauze tie in a bow on the muzzle, just caudal to the canine teeth.
   b. For cats or brachycephalic dogs, tie the gauze in a bow behind the ears at the base of the skull.
8. Leave the mouth speculum in place until the patient has reached a surgical plane of anesthesia, to avoid accidental biting of the tube.
   Alternatively, a blind technique can be utilized, as follows:
1. Place patient in lateral or dorsal recumbency.
2. Place the mouth speculum in the mouth.
3. Insert the nondominant hand into the mouth and feel for the epiglottis with the index finger.
4. With the dominant hand, pass the lubricated ET tube through the glottis using the index finger of the nondominant hand as a guide.
5. Follow steps 7 and 8 from above.

BOX 2-8   *Two-Person Endotracheal Intubation*

1. The restrainer holds the patient in sternal recumbency.
2. The restrainer opens the mouth by holding the maxilla in one hand and the mandible in the other hand.
   a. In a dog, the maxilla should be held caudal to the canine teeth.
   b. In a cat, the maxilla should be held just caudal to the ear pinna so that the skull is in the palm of the restrainer's hand.
3. The hand holding the mandible grasps the tongue and fully extends it over the mandibular incisors (Figure 2-37).
4. The restrainer lifts the head and extends the neck to aid the intubator's visualization.

5. Using the laryngoscope, the intubator illuminates the larynx for proper visualization (Figure 2-38).
6. The intubator visualizes the glottis and passes the tube between the vocal folds into the glottis (Figure 2-39).
7. The intubator advances the tube to the predetermined depth as indicated by the preplaced gauze tie.
8. The intubator secures the tube to the patient:
   a. For a dog, tie the gauze in a bow on the muzzle (Figure 2-40). The gauze should be snug but should not constrict circulation.
   b. For a cat or brachycephalic dog, tie the gauze in a bow caudal to the ears at the base of the skull.

FIGURE 2-37 Proper positioning for endotracheal intubation.

FIGURE 2-39 Passing endotracheal tube.

FIGURE 2-38 Placement of laryngoscope.

FIGURE 2-40 Endotracheal tube tied in place.

unnecessary touching of the area until the tube is actually passed is beneficial.

Confirmation of Proper Tube Placement
The following methods are used to confirm proper placement of the ET tube:

Cough: Many animals cough as the tube is passed into the trachea. Although fairly accurate, this method can be deceiving because as the animal coughs, the ET tube

may move off the glottis and into the esophagus as it is advanced.

Fogging in the tube: When an ET tube has been properly placed in the trachea, there should be fogging of the lumen of the tube with each expiration. This method can be employed only if a clear tube is used.

Blowing of gauze or hair: A few strands of gauze or hair placed at the connector end of the ET tube blow away with each expiration if the tube is correctly placed. A disadvantage is that the hair may move from the tube because of excessive movement of room air rather than expiration.

Air movement: If the ET tube is in the trachea, forced air should be felt at the connector end of the tube with each expiration. Bilateral chest compressions can be used with this method to ensure placement. Care must be taken to avoid compressing the abdomen, because an incorrectly placed tube may provide a false-positive assessment.

Palpation: Palpation of the ventral neck should result in the identification of one "tube." If the ET tube is in the trachea, only one firm, tubelike structure should be felt. If the ET tube is in the esophagus, however, two firm, tubelike structures are palpated.

Whatever method is used to ascertain correct tube placement, it should be performed before the patient is connected to the anesthesia machine. Once the patient is connected to the machine, a double check of placement can be done. Movement of the flutter valves and the rebreathing bag with each inspiration and expiration confirm proper placement. A stethoscope can also be used to auscultate bilateral lung sounds, the presence of which ensures that the tube has not migrated too far down in the trachea.

Once the patient is successfully intubated, the intended surgical site can be prepared.

Patient Preparation

Proper preparation ("prepping") of the surgical patient is a critical part of the surgical process. The veterinary technician should be the primary staff member responsible for this task. Proper prepping should include the following steps:

- Extremely dirty patients may require a bath before surgery. The bath decreases overall body soil and aids in reducing the risk of postoperative complications from iatrogenic contamination. However, the patient's hair coat must be completely dry before general anesthesia is induced. Wet animals are at an increased risk of hypothermia while under anesthesia.
- A double check (with the neck ID band, cage card, and medical record) and triple check (with the surgeon) of the patient's correct identity and exact procedure are made. Cross-check that the consent form has been signed by the client for the correct procedures. If the procedure is an amputation, double-check (with the record and consent form) and triple-check (with the surgeon) that the correct limb is being prepared. Any radiographs taken before anesthesia should be in the surgery room and hung on the view boxes.
- Ensure that the anesthesia form has been started.

Anesthesia Form

The anesthesia form "tells the story" of the anesthesia event from beginning to end. It is an important piece of the patient's medical record and can serve as a legal document. It can help guide the choice of anesthetic protocols to follow in the future. The anesthesia form documents vital signs and their trends intraoperatively. For example, a graph of the patient's blood pressure may be a line that goes down over time, with an occasional spike as the procedure proceeds, indicating that the trend for the overall blood pressure is dropping, which is a cause for concern.

The anesthesia form should be filled out completely and accurately, starting the minute the patient is given any premedications. The following paragraphs entail the information typically found in each section of the form.

Demographics

The demographics section records the owner's name and the patient's signalment, with date of birth (DOB). The technician should fill in the blanks using the information from the medical record.

Preanesthetic Values and Disposition

The preanesthetic values and disposition section of the anesthesia form records the date and patient's weight, identifies the clinician, and lists the surgical procedure(s) to be performed, as follows:

Weight: Be sure to enter both pounds (lb) and kilograms (kg).

Procedures: More than one procedure may be done. List the procedures in the order they will be performed.

Preanesthetic values (Pre-anes. values): Temperature (Temp), heart rate (HR), respiratory rate (RR), mucous membrane color and capillary refill time (MM/CRT), packed cell volume (PCV), total protein (TP), renal function, and hydration are the values obtained just before premedication is given.

ASA status: The American Society of Anesthesiologists (ASA) rating system is used to assess a particular patient's risk for an anesthetic procedure, helping to define the patient's anesthetic risk category (Table 2-5).

Preanesthetic disposition (Pre-anes. disposition): Circle the descriptive term that best describes how the patient appears before any premedication is given.

Preanesthetic Drugs

Preanesthetic drugs are usually given IM or SC to relax and sedate the patient. This relaxed state generally allows for a more willing patient when it is time to place the IV catheter and induce anesthesia. The following information should be entered in the preanesthetic drug section:

Drug: Write out full name of drug.

Dose: Write in a weight unit, such as mg. It is important here to avoid units of volume, such as mL, because one drug may be available in different concentrations. Depending on which concentration of the drug is used, the amount of mg in 1 mL of the same drug varies. The important amount to know is how many milligrams of

TABLE 2-5 | **American Society of Anesthesiologists (ASA) Rating System for Anesthetic Risk (ASA Status)***

Category	Physical Condition	Examples Of Possible Situations
Class I: Minimal risk	Normal healthy patient with no underlying disease	Ovariohysterectomy; castration; declawing procedure; hip dysplasia radiographs
Class II: Slight risk	Patient with slight to mild systemic disturbances Patient able to compensate; no clinical signs of disease	Neonatal or geriatric patients; obese patients; fracture without shock; mild diabetes; compensated heart or kidney disease; full-blown estrus
Class III: Moderate risk	Patient with moderate systemic disease or mild clinical signs	Anemia; anorexia; moderate dehydration; low-grade kidney disease; low-grade heart disturbances, heart murmur, or cardiac disease; moderate fever
Class IV: High risk	Patient with preexisting systemic disease or severe disturbances	Severe dehydration; shock; anemia; uremia or toxemia; high fever; uncompensated heart disease; diabetes; pulmonary disease
Class V: Grave risk	Surgery often performed in desperation on patients with life-threatening systemic disease or disturbances not correctable by surgery; includes all moribund patients not expected to survive 24 hours	Advanced cases of heart, kidney, liver, lung, or endocrine disease; profound shock; major head injury; severe trauma; pulmonary embolus

*ASA recommends that every patient with ASA status of III, IV, or V have a responsible person solely dedicated to managing the patient during the anesthetic period. However, more veterinarians are finding it advantageous to have an anesthetist assigned to all patients under anesthesia.

the drug the patient received, not how many milliliters, which depends on the concentration.

Route: IM, IV, or SC.

Time: Note the time when the drugs are administered.

Anesthetic Induction

Anesthetic induction drugs are generally given IV and have a rapid onset and short duration. Anesthesia induction should be a rapid and smooth event that brings the patient to a level of anesthesia that allows the patient to be quickly and safely intubated with an ET tube. The following information about anesthetic induction should be noted on the anesthesia form:

Drug: Full name of drug.

Dose: Use a weight unit (e.g., mg) only. Remember that this information cannot be filled in before the drug is given. IV induction agents are given to effect. The desired effect is sufficient muscle relaxation of the jaw and diminished gag reflex such that the patient can be intubated. For example, the calculated IV dose may be 2 mL, but the patient may require only 1 mL for sufficient relaxation to be intubated. The amount of milligrams of induction drug in the 1 mL administered is what needs to be recorded here. This underscores the importance of filling out the dose box *after* the induction drug is administered. Induction agents given by the IM or PO route are based on the calculated dosage rate.

Route: This is the route of administration of the induction drug.

Time: Note the time the drug was administered. In the case of gas induction, note the time the anesthetic gas was first turned on.

Premedication Results

Sedation: Record results after administration of premedication. How well did the patient seem to be sedated?

Resistance: How much did the patient resist manipulation, such as catheter placement?

Breathing System

Breathing system: Check that appropriate breathing system is used (non-rebreathing system).

Size of tube: Record size of ET tube used. The size is stamped on the side of the ET tube. If a patient's medical history includes recent general anesthesia, the anesthesia form for that procedure may help in tube selection for this procedure.

Recumbency: Enter the position in which the patient is placed for the procedure. For example, "LL" may be entered here for "left lateral" recumbency (patient's left side is in contact with surgery table). Recumbency is important to note, especially if a complication occurs (e.g., nerve paralysis in a limb, burn from heating pads). If more than one procedure is performed, the patient may be in more than one position during this anesthetic period.

Postoperative Values

Measure the postoperative values after extubation, as follows:

1. Temperature.
2. Pulse.
3. Respiration.
4. Total fluids: Total volume administered and type of fluids given.

FIGURE 2-41   Graph component of the anesthesia form.

Time: Each block (or small square) represents 5 minutes. If "start anesthesia" time is 9:15, start recording all the parameters at the 15-minute mark (see graph).

Percentage of anesthetic: A record of the percentage of anesthetic gas being delivered to the patient. It corresponds to the settings on the vaporizer (%).

Oxygen flow rate: A record of the flow of oxygen throughout the procedure. This corresponds to the rate of flow at which the flowmeter is set on the anesthesia machine.

Heart and respiratory rates: Record every 5 minutes. See "Code" at far left.

Anesthetic depth: Subjective assessment of the patient's depth of anesthesia graphed over time reveals whether the patient may be "getting light" or "getting too deep" for the specific procedure. Assessment is affected by trends in heart and respiratory rate, pupil position, and presence or absence of reflexes.

Fluids given: A record of how many milliliters (mL) of fluid the patient received throughout the procedure. *Top number* is the number of mL give over 15 minutes (mL/hour divided by 4). *Bottom number* is a running total of how much the patient has received at that particular point in the procedure, again in 15-minute blocks. First box is usually written as "start," but "0/0" is also acceptable.

Temperature: Is measured every 15 minutes; however, you may not be able to obtain a body temperature measurement once the procedure has started and the patient has been draped.

Intraoperative Updates

It is important to keep the anesthesia form as current as possible throughout the surgical procedure. Record all information every 5 minutes (heart and respiratory rates, level of anesthetic, oxygen flow rate, patient's depth of anesthesia); fluids need to be updated every 15 minutes.

Figure 2-41 describes the graph component of the anesthesia form.

Hair Removal

Once the patient has been stabilized under anesthesia, the process of clipping may begin. It is ideal to have the patient positioned for the preparation in the same way as for the procedure (Figure 2-42). Although this may be easily accomplished (for an exploratory laparotomy) or

may be more of a challenge (perineal surgery), it is an important step to ensure an appropriate "prep" of the surgical area can be accomplished. Except in an emergency, it is recommended that the anesthetist be comfortable with the patient's level of anesthesia before any manipulation begins. Emergency procedures are more critical and time is of the essence; therefore the anesthetist may not have the patient at the ideal anesthetic depth before the prep begins. While waiting for the nonemergency patient to stabilize at the appropriate anesthetic level, the surgery technician (frequently the circulating nurse) can complete some of the prep tasks, such as securing the leg ties to the patient and manually expressing the bladder.

The area of hair clipped needs to be neat, tidy, and symmetric (Figure 2-43). The client's impression of the

FIGURE 2-42 Patient positioned for ovariohysterectomy (OHE, "spay").

FIGURE 2-43 Holding clipper at 90-degree angle to skin creates an even, neat margin for clipped area.

FIGURE 2-44 Clipper should be held like a pencil for best control.

FIGURE 2-45 Proper hand position for clipping.

clip's appearance may influence the client's impression of the entire clinic and staff. Clipping should be done only with a surgical clipper blade. This design has close-set teeth to achieve the closest possible shave. When clipping, the person performing the clip needs to hold the clippers in a pencil grip (Figure 2-44). This grip permits the greatest amount of control and maneuverability. Other grips will prove to be cumbersome and may strain the wrist and arm. The clipper should be held flat against the patient's

skin for the closest shave. The hand not holding the clipper can tense the skin to encourage as easy a movement as possible for the clipper (Figure 2-45).

Alternative hair removal products are not routinely used in veterinary surgery. Depilatories generally are not effective given the length of the hair. Using a razor after the initial clipping may provide a close shave, but there is a high risk that it will cause skin trauma.

The amount of hair to be removed depends entirely on the surgery being performed. For general soft tissue surgery, a good rule of thumb is to clip two (2) clipper-blade widths in every direction from the proposed incision site. However, depending on the size of the animal, its length of hair, and the procedure being done, the clip may be altered. For example, a gastrotomy will require a very different clip than a prostatic biopsy. The technician should be sure to check with the surgeon for any special circumstances or anticipated additional procedures. Preoperative clipping and prepping need to include preparations for any ancillary procedures that may be done (e.g., chest tube placement, drain placement, feeding tube placement). Table 2-6 provides clipping guidelines for specific procedures.

Orthopedic preps use the rule of thumb of clipping the limb from the joint distal to and the joint proximal to the surgical incision. The limb needs to be clipped circumferentially to allow complete limb draping and manipulation. As with soft tissue procedures, the rule for clipping may need to be adjusted according to the patient's size, the surgeon's preference, and additional procedures to be performed (e.g., bone graft harvest, drain placement). Tables 2-7 (forelimb) and 2-8 (hind limb) provide clipping guidelines for most orthopedic procedures.

Neurologic surgical patients are usually quite easy to clip, especially when the surgical site is a caudal thoracic or lumbar vertebral space. Clipping two vertebral spaces cranial and two vertebral spaces caudal to the affected site is usually adequate. As with other surgical procedures, communication with the surgeon is critical to ensure adequate prepping of the neurologic surgical patient. Particularly in the event of a cervical vertebral procedure, the

TABLE 2-6 **Clipping Guidelines for Selected Soft Tissue Surgical Procedures**

Soft Tissue Procedure/Area	Guidelines
Exploratory laparotomy	Mid-sternum to pubis; laterally to edge of ribs
Gastric, liver, splenic	Mid-sternum to pubis; laterally to edge of ribs
Urinary bladder	Umbilicus to caudal pelvis; laterally to edge of ribs
Kidney	Mid-sternum to pubis; laterally to edge of ribs
Prostate	Umbilicus to caudal pelvis, including prepuce; laterally to edge of ribs
Uterine, ovarian	Xiphoid to pubis; laterally to edge of ribs
Ventral neck	Cranially to mid-mandible; caudally to thoracic inlet; laterally to commissure of lips

TABLE 2-7 **Clipping Guidelines for Selected Forelimb Orthopedic Procedures**

Forelimb Area	Guidelines
Digit	Nails to mid-humerus; use towel clamp through nail to suspend limb
Metacarpal	Nails to mid-humerus; use towel clamp through nail to suspend limb
Carpus	Second metacarpal to mid-humerus
Radius, ulna	Mid-metacarpals to shoulder; ventrally to midline; cranially to thoracic inlet; caudally to seventh rib
Elbow	Carpus to dorsal midline; ventrally to ventral midline; cranially to thoracic inlet; caudally to seventh rib
Humerus	Carpus to dorsal midline; ventrally to ventral midline; cranially to base of neck; caudally to seventh rib
Scapula	Mid-radius to 2 clipper-widths past dorsal midline; cranially to base of neck; caudally to tenth rib

TABLE 2-8 **Clipping Guidelines for Selected Hind Limb Orthopedic Procedures**

Hind Limb Area	Guidelines
Digit	Nails to mid-femur; use towel clamp through nail to suspend limb
Metatarsal	Nails to mid-femur; use towel clamp through nail to suspend limb
Tarsus	Second metatarsus to mid-femur
Tibia, fibula	Mid-metatarsals to hip; ventrally to midline; cranially to last rib
Stifle	Tarsus to hip; cranially to last rib; caudally to tuber ischii
Femur	Tarsus to dorsal midline; cranially to last rib; caudally to tuber ischii
Hip	Tarsus to 2 clipper-widths past dorsal midline; cranially to last rib; caudally to tail head
Pelvis	Depends on area of pelvis to have surgery (ilium vs. pubis vs. ischium); consult surgeon

TABLE 2-9 **Clipping Guidelines for Selected Neurologic Procedures**

Vertebrae	Guidelines
Cervical: ventral approach	Mid-ventral mandible to mid-sternum; laterally to halfway between dorsal and ventral midline
Cervical: dorsal approach	Mid-skull to two vertebral spaces caudal to affected space; laterally to halfway between dorsal and ventral midline
Thoracic	Two vertebral spaces cranial and caudal to affected space; laterally to edge of transverse process
Lumbar	Two vertebral spaces cranial and caudal to affected space; laterally to edge of transverse process

technician should be sure to ascertain whether the surgeon will make a ventral or dorsal incision. If multiple intervertebral spaces are affected, clipping should extend from the most cranial to the most caudal space affected. Table 2-9 provides clipping guidelines for neurologic surgical procedures.

Some procedures may fall into either the soft tissue category or the orthopedic category, depending on the reason for surgery. For example, aural surgeries are generally considered soft tissue, but if a bulla osteotomy is done, it is more of an orthopedic procedure. Likewise, facial surgery is soft tissue surgery if it is a tumor removal or nasal procedure, but if there is maxillary or mandibular involvement, the procedure is considered orthopedic. Table 2-10 provides guidelines for clipping for these types of surgical procedures.

After clipping, the patient and the area must be thoroughly vacuumed (Figure 2-46). The hair removed from the animal must be cleared from the surgical site as well as from the work area. Loose hair can be a source of contamination in the surgery room, so it is important to avoid transporting any hair into the surgical suite. Brushing away loose hair from the clipped site with a hand is not as effective as vacuuming (Figure 2-47).

TABLE 2-10 | **Clipping Guidelines for Miscellaneous Surgical Procedures**

Procedure/Area	Guidelines
Aural	Lateral canthus of eye; dorsal midline on head and neck; ventrally to ventral midline
Ophthalmic: intraocular	Trimming of eyelashes; limited skin clip because of potential irritation
Ophthalmic: extraocular	Entropion, ectropion: one clipper-width past lateral canthus, lower lid, and medial canthus
Enucleation: midline of muzzle to cranial edge of ear pinna; dorsally to midline; ventrally to commissure of lip
Facial	Procedures vary widely among nasal, maxillary, and mandibular; best to consult surgeon
Perineal	Dorsally to tail head; laterally to tuber ischii (bilaterally); ventrally to mid-thigh (caudal aspect)

FIGURE 2-46 The area should be thoroughly vacuumed after clipping.

FIGURE 2-47 Clipped abdomen ready to be prepared.

Urination

The urinary bladder should be emptied independently by the animal or manually by the technician before the surgical prep. Caution should be used if the abdomen has been traumatized or if the procedure will involve the urinary bladder. Expression of the bladder may be contraindicated and may do more damage to the bladder in these situations. The technician may contact the surgeon either to request permission to attempt manual expression or to state that the bladder was not expressed. The patient undergoing nonabdominal surgery must also undergo bladder emptying if possible. Otherwise, the patient may urinate during the surgical procedure, soaking the table linens as well as the patient's hair coat and skin. Lying in urine for any period exposes the patient to the risk of "urine scald" (the moist, irritating effect of urine in contact with the skin). Even if the animal does not urinate during the surgery, it will probably do so during recovery. The patient soaked in urine is at increased risk not only of urine scald but also of contamination of the surgical wound with urine. For patients that will require critical care nursing postoperatively, a urinary catheter may be placed to prevent these problems.

The bladder can be expressed with the patient either in dorsal or in lateral recumbency. Some type of receptacle should be used to collect the expressed urine to avoid saturating the fur with urine or having the urine pool under the animal. During expression of the bladder, care is taken to use gentle, constant pressure rather than a pulsating action.

Surgical Site Preparation

The skin of a patient cannot be "sterilized," in the true definition of the word, but reducing the contaminants on the skin can greatly reduce the risk of wound infection. Multiple options exist for the products used to prep the patient as well as for the applicators used to apply these products. The use of the particular cleansing products, in a particular fashion and in a particular order, is done to render the skin as clean as possible by eliminating or decreasing as many of the skin flora as possible.

Antiseptics

The first product used in the preparation of the patient is a "scrub" product. This solution has a soap or detergent base and therefore creates a sudsy appearance when used. Some properties of the scrub product are desired for maximum effect. Although no available scrub product has all the desired qualities to achieve maximum effect, the choice of product should contain as many of these qualities as possible.

One product available for use as a patient scrub is povidone-iodine. This scrub is an iodine-based product that has a detergent and a wide spectrum of antimicrobial activity. Povidone-iodine is bactericidal, virucidal, fungistatic, and fungicidal. Its toxicity to tissues is relatively low, and it is inexpensive and readily available. Because of the iodine base, it does stain clothing and discolor the white hair of animals. Povidone-iodine has a better residual activity level than hexachlorophene but is not as effective as chlorhexidine. The povidone-iodine scrub is generally diluted 50:50 with tap water when used.

Chlorhexidine gluconate is another scrub product available. Its residual effect is the best of any available product, and it works well in the presence of organic material. Chlorhexidine has shown bactericidal action against 30 bacterial genera, including *E. coli* and *Pseudomonas* species. It also has demonstrated virucidal and fungicidal properties. Chlorhexidine scrub has relatively low tissue toxicity, except for mucous membranes. Although it is more expensive than other products, it does have the advantage of not staining. Chlorhexidine is generally used in a 60:40 dilution with tap water.

Rinsing Agents

After the application of a scrub product, a rinsing agent is needed to remove the detergent. A common rinsing product is 70% isopropyl alcohol, which is effective against most gram-negative bacteria. Alcohol coagulates protein, contraindicating its use on open wounds and mucous membranes. Isopropyl alcohol is generally well tolerated by patients, and it is inexpensive and readily available. Alcohol can be used with either povidone-iodine or chlorhexidine scrub. Residual properties of the chlorhexidine seem to be enhanced when it is used with 70% isopropyl alcohol, whereas povidone-iodine does not show any increase in residual activity.

Alcohol's tendency to evaporate rapidly is both an advantage and a disadvantage. The advantage of rapid evaporation is the ability to move quickly through the prepping process without diluting subsequent products. The extreme cooling effect that results from rapid evaporation is a disadvantage. Use of excessive amounts of alcohol to prepare the patient can significantly contribute to the hypothermia experienced by the anesthetized patient. Alcohol that is allowed to pool under an animal or saturate the fur can contribute to the risk of thermal burn if electrocautery is used. Therefore, alcohol should not be used as a rinsing agent if electrocautery will be used intraoperatively.

Another rinsing agent available is bottled sterile water or sterile saline. Sterile water or saline is effective at removing the detergent product, although it has no antimicrobial properties itself. For prepping of open wounds, compound fractures, or mucous membranes, this is the rinsing agent used. Because 70% isopropyl alcohol is not appropriate in certain situations, sterile water or sterile saline is a practical and reasonable alternative.

Applicators

Regardless of the prepping products used, applicators used can vary widely depending on the site being prepared. The most common applicator used is a gauze sponge. Sponges can be used individually as needed and saturated with the product by squirting the liquid from a bottle onto a dry sponge, or sponges can be mass-produced and stored in jars or plastic containers. If mass-produced, the prep sponges and the containers need to be dumped and cleaned weekly to inhibit the growth of contaminants. It is best to place the sponges needed in a separate, smaller container (e.g., "weigh boat") to avoid reaching into the large storage container with dirty hands.

As applicators, cotton balls usually are practical only when prepping small areas, so their use is limited. Cotton balls would be indicated for IV catheter sites and perhaps ophthalmic procedures.

Similarly, a cotton-tipped applicator is usually chosen only for intraocular procedures. The limited amount of preparation needed for the eye can be best accomplished with the delicate control provided by a cotton-tipped applicator.

A spray bottle is an appropriate "applicator" only for application of the final "paint" solution (e.g., povidone-iodine). This is an efficient method of application but can be messy. The mist from the spray bottle can easily be deposited on the patient's skin as well as other areas. Monitoring devices, table linens, and even the rest of the animal may be covered with a mist of paint solution.

Special Male Dog Preparation

In preparation of the abdomen of a male dog, one task must be done before the surgical site prep is started. After all the hair has been removed from the prepuce, the sheath must be flushed to remove potential contaminants, as follows:

1. Combine 1 mL of povidone-iodine solution with 9 mL of tap water.
2. Insert the syringe tip into the prepuce and inject 5 mL of solution (Figure 2-48). Pinch the prepuce around the syringe tip before removing the syringe.
3. While still pinching the prepuce closed, gently massage the solution in the prepuce.

FIGURE 2-48 Prepuce of a male dog should be flushed before surgical site is prepared for abdominal procedure. (From Fossum TW, Hedlund CS, Hulse DA, et al: Small animal surgery, ed 3, St Louis, 2007, Mosby.)

FIGURE 2-49 Target pattern for preparing surgical site begins at proposed incision site.

FIGURE 2-50 Target pattern moves progressively outward from proposed incision site.

FIGURE 2-51 Rinsing agent is applied with the same target pattern.

FIGURE 2-52 Clipping of a forelimb.

4. Place a towel over the end of the prepuce to absorb the solution.
5. Release the pinch hold on the prepuce.
6. Repeat the process with the remaining 5 mL of solution. This step is required only for intra-abdominal procedures when the prepuce will be in the draped surgical field.

Patterns for Scrubbing

Depending on the area of the body that is undergoing surgery, one of three patterns of action should be used to prepare the site: target, orthopedic, or perineal.

Target Pattern

The most common pattern is the target pattern, which resembles a target or bull's-eye. This pattern is primarily used to prepare surgical sites for abdominal, thoracic, and neurologic procedures. The prep begins after the hair has been removed by the clipper and vacuumed from the area. The first step is to take one of the rinsing sponges and wipe around the periphery of the clipped margin. This action moistens the hair and flattens it down, helping to keep the hair from flying onto the clipped area once the prep begins.

To begin preparation of the surgical site, pick up one scrub sponge and fold it in half and then in half again, or bring all four corners to the center and hold the sponge by the corners. Either method produces a smaller contact surface that will be easier to control. Always start at the proposed incision site (Figure 2-49), and then move the sponge progressively outward in a circle until the hair is reached (Figure 2-50). Excessive pressure is not encouraged because it may abrade the skin; the wound may be more prone to healing complications if the dermal layer is compromised. Once the hair or any other dirty or contaminated area has been touched with the sponge, the sponge must never return to the incision site.

The surgical site should be rinsed with 70% isopropyl alcohol. The same target pattern should be used with the alcohol rinsing sponges as with the scrub sponges (Figure 2-51). The process of scrub, then rinse should be performed a minimum of three times. If dirt is still present

with the last rinse, repeat the process until the last rinse gauze is clean.

Orthopedic Pattern

The second prep pattern is used with orthopedic procedures. After the hair has been removed from the surgical site (Figure 2-52), any hair remaining on the foot must be covered. An inverted examination glove is placed over the foot (Figure 2-53) and secured with tape (Figure 2-54). To avoid a tourniquet effect, be sure the tape is not applied too tightly. Cover with tape (or Vetrap), again not too tightly. Also, make a stirrup to allow suspension of the limb for preparing and draping; take a long piece of white

FIGURE 2-53   Inverted glove placed over an unshaven foot.

FIGURE 2-55   Stirrup is secured to the foot.

FIGURE 2-54   Tape covering an examination glove.

tape (≈2-3 feet), leaving 2 to 3 inches at either end, then fold the remainder of the tape on itself to make it ½ inch wide. Place the ends of the stirrup on either the medial and lateral or the anterior and posterior sides of the gloved foot. Secure the stirrup to the foot with tape (Figure 2-55). The limb should be suspended for the preparation to allow access to all surfaces of the limb. Place the stirrup over the hook of an IV pole and then fully extend the pole to elevate the limb (Figure 2-56). In the event of a fracture, it is imperative that the limb and bones be supported as the pole is extended. With fractures, the extension of the limb may actually provide some distraction and traction to fatigue the muscles, which will aid in reduction of the fracture. Once the limb is suspended, clipping can be completed (Figure 2-57), and the scrub prep can begin.

FIGURE 2-56 Suspension of the limb.

FIGURE 2-57 Completion of clipping after suspension of the limb.

FIGURE 2-58 Completed orthopedic preparation.

FIGURE 2-59 Patient ready to be transported to surgery room.

With a scrub sponge in hand, begin the prep at the tape edge of the suspended limb. Scrub the limb from distal to proximal, moving circumferentially around the limb. As the sponge dries out, discard it and continue with a new sponge. As with the target pattern, the wrist must be kept moving to provide the scrubbing action. Repeat the scrub a minimum of three times before rinsing to achieve the best antimicrobial efficacy. The rinsing agent is applied in the same pattern, starting at the taped foot and moving

proximally to the dorsal midline (Figure 2-58). Generally a final solution is not applied because another prep will be done once the patient is positioned on the surgery table.

After the final rinse, place a clean towel over the medial surface of the "down" limb. This provides a clean surface on which the prepped limb can lie. The final prep is performed in the surgery room, so the towel only needs to be clean, not sterile. Carefully lower the limb, supporting any broken bones, to the towel (Figure 2-59). The patient is now ready to be transported to the surgical suite.

Perineal Pattern
The third pattern that can be used is that for perineal surgery. It is important that a purse-string suture be placed in the anus before the preparation is begun. This

suture prevents the evacuation of fecal material onto the surgical site during the procedure. The purse-string suture needs to be placed carefully to avoid puncturing the anal glands. It is the technician's responsibility to ensure that the suture is removed after the procedure; a reminder note on the anesthetic monitoring sheet helps the technician remember this task.

The perineal pattern is basically three separate target patterns performed in a particular sequence. The first step is to do a target pattern on the clipped area to the right of the anus. The second step is to perform another to the left of the anus, and the third pattern is done on the anus itself. The "dirty" area should always be prepared last to minimize contamination. As with other patterns, the scrub is followed by a rinsing agent.

Potential Reactions

Clipper-Related Reactions

If dull clipper blades are used or the technique is harsh, clipper burn can occur. Clipper blades should be checked before use for chipped or missing teeth, rust, and other inhibitors of performance. Such inhibitors will pull on the skin and can cause clipper burn. Using excessive pressure with the clippers can also cause clipper burn. Irritation of the skin can inhibit wound healing if the irritation is over the proposed incision site. Irritation can also promote bacterial growth, which could cause an infection. Clipper burns on the peri-incisional skin can be an irritation to the animal, promoting excessive licking, which can also compromise the healing process.

Chemical-Related Reactions

Reactions to prepping products generally manifest as plaques or wheals. Certain breeds (Labrador, Shar Pei) seem more prone to these reactions, although any breed may be affected. Povidone-iodine tends to cause more reactions than chlorhexidine. If a patient has a chemical-related reaction, a notation should be made in the medical record so that an alternative product can be used the next time.

Initial Preparations And Positioning

Finishing Preparation of Surgical Site

The final sterile scrub is performed in the surgical suite after the patient has been positioned appropriately on the surgery table. It is difficult, if not impossible, to maintain asepsis of the intended site when moving the patient from the prep area into the surgical suite. Contaminated clothing or personnel will likely have some contact with the intended surgical site during transfer and positioning of the patient, so the final sterile scrub is performed after the patient is positioned. Details for the final sterile scrub are covered later in this chapter. The patient needs to be positioned and secured appropriately to provide adequate exposure of the surgical site and sufficient access to the patient for monitoring vital signs.

Securing Patient in Position on Surgery Table

Properly securing the animal to the table aids in the aseptic preparation of the surgical site and ensures that the surgeon has an immobile subject with adequate room for working. The techniques used are dictated by the surgical procedure. The animal's limbs may be tied to the table. The body may be braced in position by a V-trough or sandbags. The head, neck, or abdomen may need to be elevated through the use of a foam rubber tube or rolled towels. The patient's legs should not be forced to bend or extend beyond their natural anatomic limitations. Bony prominences should be cushioned to protect against excessive compression.

The use of a sturdy, flexible cord is common practice for securing the animal's limbs in position to the table. Most surgery tables are fitted with four stays (supports) located near the corners of the table. Some tables have adjustable stays that are capable of sliding and thus accommodating patients of various sizes. The end of the cord can be wrapped in a figure-eight fashion around the stay with a half-hitch loop to secure the cord in place. It is important to tie the cord to the table with a quick-release method because the patient may need to be untied quickly. The cord should be wrapped around the stays only two or three times, and then locked with a half-hitch loop at the end (Figure 2-60). If the surgery table does not have stays to secure the cords, they can be tied to each other under the tabletop. The knot used should be a quick-release knot such as a bow tie (Figure 2-61).

It is best to spread out the distribution of pressure around the limb by placing two half-hitch loops, one proximal to and the other distal to the elbow, carpus, or hock (Figure 2-62). If the animal has a catheter in its leg, both loops should be placed distal to the catheter. The tie may prevent the administration of fluid to the animal during the procedure if the cord loop is placed proximal to the catheter. The paws should be checked throughout the surgical procedure. If the paw becomes swollen or the toes feel unusually cold compared with the opposite paw,

FIGURE 2-60 Figure-8 wrap with a half-hitch as the last loop.

FIGURE 2-61 Two half-hitch loops are placed on each foreleg; then the end of each rope is extended underneath the tabletop and tied with a bow tie.

FIGURE 2-62 Two half-hitch loops are tied around the limb. This technique distributes the pressure on the limb evenly between the two hitches. Care is taken to keep all the joints of the leg in anatomic alignment; that is, the limb is not forced into an unnatural position that may strain or torque the joints.

the ties are too tight and are cutting off circulation to the paw. In this situation the cord needs to be loosened and repositioned.

Positioning for Specific Procedures

Abdominal Surgery

For abdominal procedures the patient is placed in dorsal recumbency and secured by all four legs to the table. Keeping the patient in perfect dorsal recumbency is a challenge in the animal with a deep-chested conformation. Deep-chested dogs need to be placed in a V-trough or braced up by sandbags (Figures 2-63 and 2-64). Some surgery tables are designed with built-in adjustability to form a V-trough (Figure 2-65). Another technique to keep the patient balanced on the table involves tying the forelegs crossed over the chest (Figure 2-66).

Castration

For canine castration, the veterinary surgeon may prefer dorsal recumbency or a modified version of this position.

FIGURE 2-63 Plastic V-trough.

FIGURE 2-64 Sandbags for supporting the sides of the patient.

FIGURE 2-65 Surgery table capable of forming a V-surface to help stabilize the patient in position.

For modified dorsal recumbency, the hind legs are secured to the table. The forelegs are not tied, and the cranial half of the dog rolls toward the side on which the surgeon stands (Figure 2-67).

For feline castration, the cat is placed in dorsal recumbency with the hind legs pulled toward the head. The legs may be taped into position, held by the assistant, or tied to the surgery table (Figure 2-68).

CHAPTER 2 Preoperative Patient Considerations   77

FIGURE 2-66 Tying the legs in a crossed position across the chest helps stabilize the patient in dorsal recumbency. Care must be taken when this technique is used to avoid restricting chest excursions as the patient breathes.

FIGURE 2-67 Canine patient in position for castration procedure.

FIGURE 2-68 Feline patient in position and surgically prepared for castration. The legs are secured to the table with two half-hitches on each leg and then carefully pulled in the cranial direction.

Orthopedic and Extremity Surgery

The patient is placed in lateral recumbency for procedures involving the extremities. If the left limb is the focus, the patient is positioned in right lateral recumbency. If the right limb is the surgical site, the patient is placed in left lateral recumbency. The paw is wrapped in gauze and tape. The limb is suspended from above by tying the tape

FIGURE 2-69 Patient's leg is suspended by a piece of tape secured to an IV stand. This patient has a skin mass on the medial aspect of the thigh, so suspending the leg from the IV pole facilitates the preparation process.

around the paw and tying the tape to an IV pole. The leg is clipped and scrubbed in this position. All sides of the leg are prepared (Figure 2-69).

Tail and Perianal Surgery

The patient is placed in ventral recumbency for procedures involving the tail or perianal area. The forelegs are secured to the table, with the hind legs hanging over the edge at the end of the table. A rolled towel is placed under the caudal abdomen for extra padding. A piece of adhesive tape is placed in a spiral on the tail, with a long extension of the tape attached above to an IV pole or other object (Figure 2-70).

Back Surgery

The patient having back surgery is placed in ventral recumbency. Positioning in a V-trough or placing sandbags on both sides helps brace the patient and prevents listing to one side. The forelegs are extended cranially. The hind legs are bent in a natural sitting or squatting position. A strip of adhesive tape may provide additional stabilization across the shoulders (Figure 2-71).

FIGURE 2-70 Positioning patient for surgery of the tail or perineal area. Note the rolled towel placed under the abdomen for extra cushioning.

FIGURE 2-71 Use of tape helps to stabilize patient in ventral recumbency.

Thoracic Surgery

The patient undergoing thoracic surgery is placed in lateral or dorsal recumbency, depending on the surgeon's intended approach. The forelegs are extended cranially as much as possible and secured to the table.

Final (Sterile) Surgical Site Preparation

Once the patient has been transported and appropriately positioned on and secured to the surgery table, the final surgical prep is performed in the surgical room. The area is scrubbed and rinsed as described early in the chapter. In some university or specialty clinic settings, the doctor may wish the final prep to be performed sterilely (i.e., applied by the sterile surgical assistant); however, in most small animal settings this is not the case. Box 2-9 lists the procedure for a sterile final prep.

Solutions ("Paint")

The final step in the surgical site preparation is the application of the solution product, or "paint." Povidone-iodine solution is in the same chemical family as the scrub, but the paint does not contain a detergent. The solution

| BOX 2-9 | Sterile Final Prep |

1. Open the sterilized surgical bowl containing gauze sponges.
2. Pour off a small amount of surgical scrub solution into a trash can to cleanse the lip of the container, then pour the soap on the gauze sponges.
3. Open the container of sterile water and pour off a small amount into trash can to cleanse the lip of the container, then dilute the scrub soap in the bowl with sterile water.
4. Open a second sterile bowl containing sterile gauze.
5. After pouring a small amount of "rinse" (70% rubbing alcohol or sterile water) into the trash can, carefully pour the rinse on the sterile sponges until they appear soaked.
6. Aseptically perform the open-gloving technique (see Chapter 2).
7. Once you have put on surgical gloves, grasp a gauze sponge filled with scrub using your designated "clean hand," then squeeze out the excess liquid.
8. Transfer this sponge to your other hand, designated your "dirty hand," and start scrubbing. Use the same (clean) hand to retrieve each new sponge then transfer it to the other (dirty) hand to do the scrubbing; thus the term "clean hand, dirty hand" technique. Only the clean hand goes into the sterile bowl, and only the dirty hand touches the patient. (Rather than clean and dirty, both hands are actually sterile because they are covered with sterile gloves.)
9. The surgical site is scrubbed for the appropriate length of time recommended by the manufacturer of the scrub product, usually about 5 minutes. Scrubbing is done in a target pattern starting from the intended incision site and working outward to the edge of the shaved area. The time can be adjusted according to the duration of the initial surgical scrub performed in the surgery prep area.
10. Begin at the center of the clipped area over the proposed surgical incision.
11. Without touching the hairline, scrub the length of the incision with long, straight strokes. Scrub outward toward the periphery while slightly overlapping the previously scrubbed line in a circular fashion.
12. Never go back to the center of the area with the same gauze sponge.
13. After scrubbing the skin at the margin of the clipped area, discard the used gauze sponges and start again.
14. The skin should be cleansed thoroughly but gently. Excessive friction can result in hyperemia and bleeding of the skin and subcutaneous tissues.
15. The surgical scrub must have an overall contact time as recommended by the manufacturer. After the appropriate duration has elapsed, wipe the scrub away by using the "rinse"-soaked gauze.

also has a stronger concentration of iodine, therefore increasing its potential for staining. It is corrosive when it contacts metal. The full-strength solution is applied to the patient and remains on the surgical site. It has much better efficacy when allowed to dry on the patient's skin before the drapes are applied or the incision is made.

A second current option for a final solution is chlorhexidine gluconate. As with povidone-iodine, chlorhexidine as a solution contains no detergent. This product is diluted to a 0.2% solution (30 mL/gallon of distilled water) when used as a final paint. Chlorhexidine also has better efficacy when allowed to dry on the patient's skin before the incision is made.

It is important to remember that only povidone-iodine scrub should be followed by povidone-iodine solution. Likewise, only chlorhexidine scrub should be followed by chlorhexidine solution. Using a povidone-iodine scrub with a chlorhexidine solution, or vice versa, is counterproductive and strongly discouraged.

Regardless of which product is used, the same method of application is utilized. The first squirt from the spray bottle should be directed into the kick bucket. This removes any debris and bacteria from the nozzle. Then, using a swiping motion, the technician applies a light mist from the spray bottle to the center of the proposed surgical site, and allows it to dry.

Techniques For Maintaining Body Temperature

Ideally, if the surgical suite has been thoroughly prepared for the day's procedures, any devices available to help maintain the surgical patient's body temperature will have been turned on and allowed to warm up before the patient is moved into the surgery room. It is preferable to place a patient on a warming device rather than arrange a warming element underneath a patient already positioned on the surgery table.

Several factors contribute to hypothermia in the surgical patient (see Chapter 5). The following devices and techniques should be used as available and appropriate to prevent hypothermia:

- A pad with circulating warm water is placed under the patient as soon as the animal is under anesthesia. Electric heating pads can become too hot and can burn the patient's skin and therefore should not be used. The circulating warm-water pad avoids the risk inherent with electric heating pads because the water is constantly circulating between the pad under the patient and the warming unit (see Figures 2-72 and 2-73). Water bottles do not provide a constantly renewable source of heat and also carry the risk of leaking. A wet patient can quickly become a cold patient.
- Warm-air convection blankets consist of an electrical unit that warms air and pumps it through a tube to a pad. The pad has a series of holes that allows the warm air to escape slowly. The pad is laid on top of the patient, or the patient rests on top of the pad; this creates a warm microenvironment. When used for the surgical patient, the unit is not activated until the surgeon has completed draping the patient (Figure 2-74).

FIGURE 2-72 Circulating warm-water blanket.

FIGURE 2-73 Hard pad for circulating warm water.

FIGURE 2-74 Convection-current patient-warming system (Gaymar Industries, Inc., Orchard Park, NY). The disposable blanket is lying on top of the patient. Air is warmed and pumped into the blanket, through which the warmed air slowly diffuses around the patient.

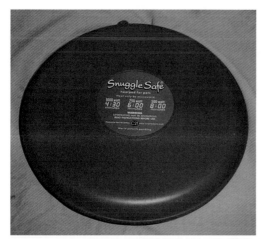

FIGURE 2-75 SnuggleSafe Microwave Heat Pad (SnuggleSafe, Lenric C21 Ltd., Littlehampton, West Sussex, UK).

FIGURE 2-76 Plastic bubble wrap around the extremities, head, and thorax helps to maintain the body heat as this cat is being prepared for a spay procedure.

- Some stainless steel surgery tables are fitted with heating coils that warm the entire surface of the table to approximate body temperature. The need for warm-water blankets and bottles is eliminated while the patient is on the heated surgery table.
- The SnuggleSafe Microwave Heat Pad (SnuggleSafe, Lenric C21 Ltd., Littlehampton, West Sussex, UK) is a flat plastic disc that is placed in a microwave oven for a set number of minutes. This disc retains heat much longer than warm water bottles (Figure 2-75).
- A plastic bottle (e.g., soda bottle) can be filled with dry, uncooked rice and heated in a microwave oven. The bottle with rice holds heat longer than a water bottle and eliminates the risk of leaking water on the patient.
- The bag of IV fluids can be warmed in a microwave oven to approximately the same temperature as body temperature. The line for the IV administration set can run through a bowl of warm water to make the fluid warmer before going into the patient.

FIGURE 2-77 Plastic bubble wrap and latex gloves filled with warm water laid across the pinnas help retain the body heat in the upper portion of this Chihuahua undergoing a spay procedure.

- Plastic bubble wrap can be wrapped around the patient's extremities, including the head. The plastic wrap is light but provides warmth by retaining the body heat that would be lost through the extremities (Figures 2-76 and 2-77).

KEY POINTS

1. Taking an accurate history and recording it in a concise, chronologic order create the foundation for the treatment plan for each surgical patient.
2. During the interview of the history taking, the technician needs to confirm the patient's signalment (age, gender, breed) and chief complaint (reason for the visit to the surgical hospital).
3. While the client is being interviewed, the patient should be allowed to explore the examination room at will, and the technician should make a mental note of the patient's overall condition and mentation (mental status, attitude).

4. The physical examination needs to be thorough and systematic and performed on the day of the scheduled surgery with the owner present.
5. Any abnormalities found on the physical examination need to be brought to the attention of the attending veterinarian and recorded in the medical record.
6. The consent form should identify the patient, the procedures to be performed on the patient, the potential risks involved with those procedures, the name of the veterinarian who will perform the procedures, and a place for the owner to sign indicating consent.

7. The consent form should provide confirmation that the patient was fasted appropriately before admission, that the owner was given an estimate for the costs of the procedures, and that the owner's phone number is readily available so he or she can be contacted during the procedure if necessary.

8. Selection of preanesthetic diagnostic tests depends on the patient's age and health status, type of surgery, and results of initial diagnostic screening tests.

9. Preoperative medications should provide preemptive analgesia and tranquilization and allow for easier anesthesia induction and smoother recovery from anesthesia.

10. To provide the most effective pain prevention and relief, different types of analgesics with different mechanisms of action (multimodal analgesia) need to be administered to surgical patients.

11. The benefits of placing an IV catheter for every anesthetic procedure outweigh any risks.

12. The five factors that should be considered in the choice of a catheter are site of placement, length of time the catheter will be needed, reason for placement, diameter of vessel, and length of vessel.

13. Catheter sites must be aseptically prepared to avoid complications.

14. Having all supplies readily available will aid in the success of the placement procedure.

15. Some surgical patients may require intensive care after surgery and may be better served by placement of a jugular catheter.

16. Successful ET tube placement depends on using the appropriate equipment and minimizing irritation to the patient.

17. Most patients can be intubated using the one-person technique, although the two-person technique is generally the more common practice.

18. Multiple options are available for checking the ET tube for proper placement in the trachea.

19. Clean, neat, symmetric clipping is an important skill to master for the patient's well-being as well as good client relations.

20. Appropriate hair removal helps to prevent contamination of the surgical site.

21. Rather than pressure, contact time is the important consideration when one is using skin preparation materials.

22. When preparing a surgical site, the technician should always move the applicator from clean to dirty surfaces to avoid introducing contaminants to the proposed incision site.

23. It is important to position the animal on the surgery table in the most natural position possible that does not put excess stress on joints, severely compress blood vessels and nerves, or compromise the well-being of the patient in any way.

24. Quick-release knots are tied in the cords securing the patient to the table so that the patient can be easily and efficiently untied.

25. The cords securing the animal to the table can cause problems if wrapped around the legs too tightly. Check the paws repeatedly throughout the procedure.

REVIEW QUESTIONS

1. What information is included in the patient's signalment?
   a. Age, gender, breed.
   b. "Proceed with caution" signals (e.g., "will bite").
   c. Previous surgery.
   d. All of the above.

2. Why is it important to review all medications and supplements that a patient is taking before beginning the surgery?
   a. To avoid possible drug interactions.
   b. To know whether other diagnostic tests are indicated.
   c. To make any necessary adjustments to the anesthesia protocol.
   d. All of the above.

3. Why are leading questions inappropriate to ask during the history taking?
   a. They make the owner feel compelled to answer a certain way.
   b. They may encourage the owner to answer inaccurately.
   c. They are appropriate and should be asked.
   d. Both a and b.
   e. None of the above.

4. Which of the following should be assessed during the history taking?
   a. Patient's attitude and mental status.
   b. Patient's previous medical problems and treatments.
   c. Patient's ability to see and hear.
   d. Patient's gait and body condition.
   e. All of the above.

5. Why should taking the patient's temperature be saved for the end of the physical examination (PE)?
   a. It is the least important part of the PE.
   b. Most animals dislike having their temperature taken, and it is easier to perform a PE on a cooperative patient; taking the temperature early during the PE may make the patient uncooperative for the rest of the examination.
   c. By the end of the PE, the examiner should have already ascertained whether the patient is febrile, and only then does the temperature need to be taken.
   d. None of the above.
   e. All of the above.

6. Which of the following should be performed on the day of the surgery?
   a. Thorough physical examination.
   b. Review of the patient's medical history with the owner.
   c. Verbal review of the consent form and obtaining of the owner's signed consent for anesthesia and surgery.
   d. All of the above.
   e. None of the above.

7. Which tactic(s) may stop a cat from purring during thoracic auscultation?
   a. Gently squeezing the thorax with one hand while the other holds the stethoscope on the chest wall.
   b. Massaging under the cat's chin.
   c. Holding the cat near a sink or faucet, with or without the water running.
   d. All of the above.
   e. None of the above.

8. The minimum database (MDB) for a young, healthy feline patient having elective surgery would most likely include which of the following diagnostic tests?
   a. CBC, parvovirus test, electrolytes, and blood typing.
   b. CBC, serum chemistry panel, FeLV/FIV test, intestinal parasite test, and urinalysis.
   c. FeLV/FIV test, abdominal radiographs, and ECG.
   d. PCV/TS, estimate of BUN, BG, and ALT.
   e. PCV/TS, thyroid panel, and FeLV/FIV test.

9. What is the purpose of premedicating a patient before inducing anesthesia for surgery?
   a. To provide a smooth transition to anesthesia.
   b. To provide preemptive analgesia.
   c. To facilitate a smooth recovery from anesthesia.
   d. All of the above.
   e. None of the above.

10. *True or False:* Anesthesia (as provided by gas anesthetics) provides multimodal analgesia.

11. Which of the following provide multimodal analgesia?
    a. Gas anesthetics, morphine, butorphanol, and fentanyl.
    b. Nonsteroidal anti-inflammatory drugs (NSAIDs), carprofen, and meloxicam.
    c. Xylazine and medetomidine.
    d. Opioids, NSAIDs, local anesthetic agents, and α2-adrenergic agonists.
    e. None of the above.

12. *True or False:* Anticholinergics, such as glycopyrrolate and atropine, increase the heart rate and provide purely beneficial effects for the patient.

13. All of the following are goals of balanced anesthesia except:
    a. Maximize the effects of certain drugs.
    b. Minimize the side effects of certain drugs.
    c. Minimize the likelihood of allergic reactions.
    d. Maximize cardiac depression.

14. *True or False:* Peripheral catheters generally suffice for short-term use (1-3 days), and central lines are more appropriate for long-term vascular access (>3 days).

15. *True or False:* Central venous pressure measurements require that a central line be placed.

16. How can the patient's correct identity be verified?

17. Why should the patient's identity be verified before the animal is anesthetized for surgery?
    a. To avoid anesthetizing the wrong patient.
    b. To avoid performing surgery on the wrong patient.
    c. It is not necessary to cross-check the patient's correct identity because any good technician should be able to distinguish all black cats in the hospital on any given day on the basis of physical appearance alone.
    d. Both a and b.
    e. None of the above.

18. What is the primary purpose of the anesthesia form?

19. Why does an orthopedic "clip and prep" of an extremity need to include a circumferential clip around the entire limb?
    a. If the incision goes all the way through the limb and out the other side, the other side will already be prepared for this scenario.
    b. If the surgeon mistakenly incises the wrong side of the limb with the first incision, and if the leg is clipped circumferentially, the mistake is easily corrected.
    c. For patient comfort.
    d. All of the above.
    e. None of the above.

20. What needs to be done to the patient after the hair clip and before the patient is moved into the surgery suite?
    a. Vacuum the clipped hair and clipped area of skin.
    b. Check to see whether the bladder needs expressing.
    c. Perform initial skin scrub.
    d. All of the above.
    e. None of the above.

21. *True or False:* It is accepted practice to scrub a patient initially with a povidone-iodine product.

22. Which of the following contributes to hypothermia in the anesthetized patient?
    a. Anesthetic-induced muscle relaxation.
    b. The surgical prep using water and alcohol.
    c. Administering room-temperature IV fluids.
    d. Breathing cold gases from compressed cylinders.
    e. All of the above.

23. *True or False:* The first spray of the final prep should be directly over the incision site.

24. *True or False:* Prophylaxis antibiotic therapy should be administered to all surgical candidates.

25. What are some safe techniques for preventing hypothermia in small animal surgical patients?
    a. Circulating warm-water pads.
    b. Electric heating pads.
    c. Snuggle Safe discs.
    d. All of the above.
    e. Both a and c.

26. Which of the following is the next step after the patient has been induced with anesthesia and the intended surgical site has been clipped and had initial prep?
    a. The patient is moved to the surgery room, positioned on and secured to the table, then draped, and the surgeon begins surgery by making an incision.
    b. The final prep is applied, and the patient is moved to the surgery room and positioned on and secured to the table.
    c. The patient is moved to the surgery room, the final prep is performed, and the patient is positioned on and secured to the table.
    d. The patient is moved to the surgery room and is positioned on and secured to the surgery table, and the final prep is performed.
    e. None of the above.

27. Which of the following is true regarding positioning patients on the surgery table?
    a. The particular position of the limbs is insignificant because the patient is anesthetized and cannot feel any pain that might be associated with awkward positioning.
    b. Bony prominences should be cushioned to protect against excessive compression.
    c. The patient's legs should not be forced into unnatural anatomic alignment.
    d. All of the above.
    e. Both b and c.

28. What position is the patient placed in for abdominal exploratory surgery?
    a. Sternal recumbency.
    b. Dorsal recumbency.
    c. Right or left lateral recumbency depending on which side of the abdomen needs to be accessed.

29. What can be done to help prevent a deep-chested dog from tilting to the side while in dorsal recumbency?
    a. Using a V-trough.
    b. Bracing the chest with sandbags.
    c. Tying the forelegs crossed over the chest.
    d. All of the above.
    e. Both a and c.

30. *True or False:* For orthopedic surgeries of the extremity, only the side of the limb to be incised needs to be clipped and prepped.

31. What position is the patient placed in on the surgery table for thoracic surgery?
    a. Dorsal recumbency.
    b. Right lateral recumbency.
    c. Left lateral recumbency.
    d. Any of the above may be appropriate.
    e. None of the above.

32. *True or False:* When scrubbing the skin of the intended surgical site, sufficient friction should be generated to cause hyperemia.

33. *True or False:* Chlorhexidine scrub or solution can be used as the final, sterile surgical paint.

ANSWERS

1. a
2. d
3. d
4. e
5. b
6. d

7. c
8. d
9. d
10. False
11. d
12. False
13. c
14. True
15. True
16. Cross-check the signalment and description in the medical record, cross-check the neck ID band or cage card, and ask a coworker (e.g., surgeon) to confirm the patient's identity.
17. d
18. The anesthesia form "tells the story" of the anesthesia event from beginning to end. It is an important piece of the patient's medical record and can serve as a legal document. It can help guide the choice of anesthetic protocols to follow in the future.

19. e. The entire circumference of the extremity needs to be clipped and prepped so that the surgeon can move and manipulate the leg without contaminating the sterile field.
20. d
21. True
22. e
24. False
25. e
26. d
27. e
28. b
29. d
30. False
31. d
32. False
33. False

BIBLIOGRAPHY

Bassert JM, McCurnin DM, editors: McCurnin's clinical textbook for veterinary technicians, ed 7, St Louis, 2010, Saunders.

Cunningham JG: Textbook of veterinary physiology, ed 4, St Louis, 2008, Saunders.

Fossum TW, Hedlund CS, Hulse DA, et al: Small animal surgery, ed 3, St Louis, 2007, Mosby.

Romich JA: An illustrated guide to veterinary medical terminology, Albany, NY, 2000, Delmar.

Stoeberl TA: Preparing the small animal patient for surgery. AHT 4:271, 1983.

Thomas JA, Lerche P: Anesthesia and analgesia for veterinary technicians, ed 4, St Louis, 2011, Mosby.

Operating Room Personnel

Paige A. Allen

3

KEY TERMS

Endogenous
  contamination
Exogenous
  contamination
Surgical hand rub
Surgical hand scrub
Surgical nurse

OUTLINE

LEARNING OBJECTIVES

After studying this chapter, the reader will be able to:
- Discuss personal preparation for duties as a surgical nurse.
- Describe proper attire in the surgical area.
- Define endogenous and exogenous threats to asepsis.
- Explain the general guidelines for personal hygiene of veterinary surgical personnel.
- Describe and perform a surgical hand scrub.
- Explain and perform a surgical hand rub.
- Describe the different types of surgical hand prep solutions.
- Explain and demonstrate the process to aseptically dry hands and arms after performing a surgical hand scrub or rub.
- Describe and demonstrate the procedure for donning a surgical gown.
- Describe and perform open and closed gloving.
- Define and perform assisted surgical gloving.

For the veterinary technician with a passion for surgery, performing duties as the surgical nurse (or "scrubbing-in") is a coveted job. The technician performs a critical service for the surgeon in providing retraction of tissue, lavaging the surgical field with sterile fluid, and managing ("running") the instrument table. For the surgeon, having a skilled, qualified surgical nurse can significantly affect the duration and outcome of the surgical procedure.

Nutrition, Hygiene, and Appearance

Before scrubbing-in, the technician must review some personal considerations. If personnel know in advance that they will be assisting on a surgical case, they should consume a meal of substance. Complex carbohydrates (e.g., bagel, bread) and protein (e.g., peanut butter, meats) will sustain a person longer than a candy bar or other sugar food. The technician should also consume plenty of fluids to combat dehydration, as well as be sure to visit the restroom before the case begins.

The closeness of the surgical team and the risk of patient infection require consideration of personal hygiene and appearance. Fingernails need to be kept shorter than the fingertips and free of nail polish. The use of perfume or cologne should be avoided. When working in close quarters, it is respectful to remember that people are becoming increasingly sensitive to smells. More importantly, the smell from perfume or cologne may mask odors from the inhalation gas. It is critical that the anesthetist be able to detect any leaks in the system through odors.

Proper Attire in Surgical Area

There are two sources for contamination in the operating room. The first is *endogenous contamination*. This is contamination from the patient itself. It can occur from the patient's skin or if the patient has an underlying, asymptomatic infection. The second source is *exogenous contamination* and comes from the surgical team and from the environment in which the surgery occurs. This is the source that can be more closely controlled by the veterinary technician, and proper attire can assist with this task.

The surgical area should be a restricted clean area, separate from the rest of the hospital. This area should not be used for clipping patients or any other procedures except for sterile surgery. This restricted surgical environment should be kept as free of microorganisms as possible.

The physical and emotional stress associated with surgery can compromise the immune system during surgery and during the convalescent period and make surgical patients vulnerable to infections and disease. Proper surgery room attire reduces microbial shedding, which occurs when microorganisms are released into the environment from the body of surgical personnel. These microorganisms are present in sebaceous and sweat glands around the hair follicles of the entire body. Proper surgical attire of surgery room personnel helps decrease the risk of infection for the patient by providing barriers against microorganisms. In the surgery room, proper surgical attire, for the whole team, should include freshly laundered scrub suits, head covers, masks, and possibly shoe covers.

A dress code should be written and posted so that it can be easily followed and enforced. This dress code should include the definition of areas where surgical attire must be worn, appropriate attire within those defined areas, and the choice of cover apparel outside the surgical suite. The scrub suit should be covered with clean cover apparel at all times when outside the surgical area and must be removed upon entry into the surgical area. It is important that a dress code for the use of cover apparel in the surgical preparation area be written and posted to avoid

---

BOX 3-1　Surgical Dress Code

- A surgical dress code should be written and posted so that it can be easily followed and enforced.
- A dress code should include the defined areas where surgical attire must be worn, appropriate attire within those defined areas, and the acceptable options for cover apparel outside the surgical area.
- The scrub suit should be covered with a clean laboratory coat at all times when outside the surgical area.
- Personnel are not allowed to wear laboratory coats in the surgery room.
- Scrub suits worn in the surgery room should not be worn home.
- Clean, freshly laundered scrub suits should be donned just before entry into the surgery room and should not be worn from home into the hospital.
- Proper surgical attire includes wearing a head cover that completely covers all head and facial hair, surgical masks that effectively cover the mouth and nose, and clean shoes with or without shoe covers.
- Head covers and masks need to be donned before the surgical hand scrub or hand rub is begun.
- Masks must fit properly so that a cough or sneeze is not vented out the side of the mask.

---

contamination of the scrub suit while personnel are working in this area. It is important that the scrub suit covering should be considered when personnel are restraining and clipping the patient for surgery. Guidelines should also be provided for general personal cleanliness, including care of fingernails and the wearing of jewelry when participating in surgical procedures (Box 3-1).

Scrub Suit

Street clothes should never be worn in surgery because they carry dirt, debris, and microorganisms. Instead, all personnel should don clean, freshly laundered scrub suits (scrubs) at the veterinary hospital. Ideally, all scrubs should be laundered in the hospital laundry. Scrubs should not be worn from home to the hospital, nor should they be worn home from the hospital. The scrub suits could bring microorganisms into the hospital and home to infect the surgery personnel's own pets. Only clean scrub suits should be worn in the surgical area. Scrubs should be changed if they become visibly dirty or wet.

The scrub top should fit the body snugly and be tucked into the scrub pants (Figure 3-1). This prevents body scurf (epidermal scales) from being shed as a result of friction produced by the body rubbing against the scrub top. The scrub top should be short sleeved so personnel can scrub hands and arms for surgery. Personnel should not wear the surgical room attire outside the surgical area because microorganisms could be transferred onto the scrub suit. Therefore, when personnel are leaving the surgical area, the scrub suit should be covered by a clean laboratory coat, which is removed when they reenter the restricted area.

FIGURE 3-1 Proper surgical attire includes a clean scrub suit. The scrub top is tucked into the pants. All jewelry and name tags are removed. A head cover, mask, and clean shoes are worn.

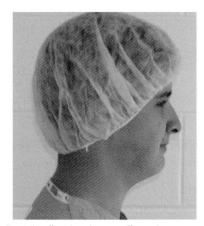

FIGURE 3-2 A bouffant head cover effectively covers all hair on the head and prevents hair from falling into the surgical site.

FIGURE 3-3 This skullcap does not effectively contain all hair on the head and should not be worn; it cannot effectively prevent hair from falling into the surgical site and contaminating the site.

Head Covers

Everyone in the surgical area should wear head covers. All hair on the head and facial hair should be covered because hair collects bacteria when left uncovered. The head cover prevents bacteria, dandruff, and other contaminants from falling either onto the scrub suits or into the surgical environment. Several types of head covers are available, including the bouffant, the hood, and the skullcap. The head cover chosen should fit well and should cover all hair. The bouffant covers the hair on the head adequately and is preferred over the skullcap (Figure 3-2). The hood should be worn if there is facial hair that is not covered by the mask. Skullcaps should be worn only if the hair is very short and there is no hair outside the cap at the side or the nape of the neck. Figure 3-3 is an example of a poor choice of head covering; this person should not wear a skullcap.

Masks

The mask should be worn in the surgery room when open sterile supplies or scrubbed personnel are present. The mask should be worn over the mouth and nose. Because the mask functions to filter droplets containing microorganisms that come from the mouth and nose, it should

be changed frequently. The strings should be tied tightly, and the mask should conform to the face so that no air escapes without being filtered by the mask.

If a sneeze or cough is imminent, without turning the head, the person should step back from the sterile field. If the mask is secured properly, the cough or sneeze should be filtered. If the mask is not secured properly, or if the head is turned, the cough or sneeze will be vented out of the side of the mask directly onto the sterile field.

Shoes and Shoe Covers

Shoes worn in the surgery room should be comfortable and cleaned frequently (whether or not shoe covers are worn). Shoes should have enclosed toes and heels to protect personnel from injury if heavy or sharp objects are dropped onto their feet. Shoe covers are optional. If worn, shoe covers should be changed if they become torn, wet, or soiled and when personnel reenter the surgical area. Although it is not imperative that special shoes be worn only in the surgery area, it is common sense to make sure shoes are clean and are not carrying feces or hair into the surgical area. Foot attire has no proven significance in reducing the incidence of postoperative wound infections, and the primary reason for its use is to decrease floor contamination.

Jewelry

It is recommended that all jewelry and watches be removed, although some hospitals allow jewelry if it is confined within the scrub suit or bouffant. Rings, bracelets, and watches must be removed for scrubbed personnel and should be removed by all surgical personnel. Jewelry may harbor microorganisms that routine handwashing cannot remove, and earrings, necklaces, and body-piercing objects could fall into the surgical field.

Fingernails

Fingernails should be well manicured. They should be short, clean, and healthy. Healthy nails are desired because any small cuts or torn cuticles can harbor microorganisms. Fingernails should not extend past the fingertips because they could cause tears in the surgical gloves, which could be a source of infection to the patient. Artificial nails are unacceptable because they harbor microorganisms, especially fungi. Nail polish should not be worn because polished nails, if chipped, harbor more microorganisms than unpolished nails.

Surgical Hand Scrub and Hand Rub

The *surgical hand scrub* is defined as the process of removing as many microorganisms as possible from nails, hands, and arms by mechanical washing and chemical antisepsis before a person participates in a surgical procedure. The surgical hand scrub is also designed to maintain the lowest possible microbial counts throughout the surgical procedure.

When performing the surgical hand scrub, it is important to remember that the skin is never made "sterile." Skin becomes surgically clean; if there are any holes (detected or undetected) in the surgical gloves or gown, the probability of introducing microbes into the surgical field is reduced. The use of prophylactic antibiotics should never be considered a substitute for a proper hand scrub.

The scrub procedure consists of a mechanical part and a chemical part. The mechanical part is the removal of bacteria and debris by producing friction when rubbing or brushing. This removes dirt, oil, and transient organisms that are loosely attached to the skin. During the chemical part of the scrub, the antiseptic, antimicrobial skin-cleansing agents are used. These agents inactivate or inhibit the growth of microorganisms found on the surface of the skin and in hair follicles, sebaceous glands, and sweat glands.

Two methods of scrubbing procedures can be used. The first is the "timed" method, and the second is the "stroke count" method. Both methods should take a minimum of 5 minutes to perform correctly. The surgical hand scrub should always begin with a brief, general hand and arm wash to loosen surface debris and "transient" microorganisms (organisms that are loosely attached to

the skin surface.) This wash is not included in the 5-minute minimum.

The method chosen is not as important as using the same method consistently so that the lowest number of microorganisms remain on the surface of the skin. As a part of either method, it is important to follow an anatomical pattern each time. Fingers have four sides and the tip, hands, and arms have four sides. Before either method, a nail-cleaning pick should always be used to remove debris from the subungual area of each finger. Stiff brushes are not recommended on the skin because they can cause skin abrasions and may release more resident microbes from the deep layers of the skin, which is counterproductive. Many scrub agents come with disposable, antiseptic-impregnated scrub brushes that have soft brushes, sponge, and nail-cleaning pick included.

The antimicrobial scrub agent or an alcohol-based hand rub should be chosen from the U.S. Food and Drug Administration (FDA) product category defined as "hand scrubs" or "alcohol-based rubs." Avagard (3M, St Paul, MN) is an example of a scrubless, brushless, waterless antiseptic hand preparation product referred to as a "rub." The agent selected should be nonirritating and fast-acting and should have a prolonged depressant effect on residual bacteria. It should cover a broad spectrum of bacteria. The length of scrub time varies according to the manufacturer's recommendations and written directions for use.

The new brushless technique (alcohol rub), with or without water, consists of rubbing an antimicrobial agent on the hands and arms. Brushless rubbing agents typically are alcohol based, with the addition of moisturizing emollients and surfactants that help clean the skin. Some agents are combinations of alcohol and other antimicrobial agents, such as chlorhexidine gluconate or alcohol with preservatives.

Whichever FDA-approved antimicrobial scrub agent or alcohol-based rub is chosen, a standardized protocol should be established and written for each surgical hand procedure according to the manufacturer's recommendations for the particular scrub or rub agent used. A copy should be posted in the scrub room. Every person scrubbing for a procedure should be familiar with these instructions.

Before the surgical hand scrub (or rub) is performed (Box 3-2), the animal should be properly clipped, prepped, moved into the surgery room, and positioned on the table correctly for the surgical procedure. The surgery room should be set up with the proper pack and instrumentation (Figure 3-4).

Types of Scrub Solutions

In the choice of an antimicrobial (antiseptic) detergent, several desirable characteristics are recommended for the surgical scrub product: (1) FDA compliant, (2) broad spectrum of activity, (3) fast acting and effective, (4) nonirritating, and (5) with persistent effects and cumulative

FIGURE 3-4 The operating room is arranged with the appropriate surgical packs before the surgical hand preparation is performed. Note the circulating warm-water pad on the surgery table and the kick buckets with plastic liners. Also note that the surgery room is free of clutter. Only those items needed for the specific procedure to be performed are in the surgery room.

BOX 3-2 Surgical Hand Scrub Guidelines

- All jewelry, name tags, and pens need to be removed before the surgical hand scrub or hand rub is begun.
- The purpose of the surgical hand scrub or hand rub is to remove as many microorganisms as possible from the nails, hands, and arms.
- When an antimicrobial detergent is used, it is important to follow the manufacturer's directions regarding the scrub time and whether or not a scrub brush should be used.

BOX 3-3 Ideal Antiseptic Properties

- Nonirritating to skin
- Fast-acting
- Broad-spectrum
- Has good residual effect

activity. Whatever type of scrub agent is chosen, it is important to follow the manufacturer's written directions for use. These include the scrub time, whether the use of a brush is recommended, and whether it is a brushless, alcohol-based surgical rub.

Several types of antimicrobial skin-cleansing agents are available. The following agents are discussed: chlorhexidine gluconate, iodophors, alcohol, parachlorometaxylenol (Table 3-1), and the brushless rub.

Chlorhexidine gluconate (4%) is a broad-spectrum antimicrobial agent. It is more effective against gram-positive bacteria than gram-negative organisms. Chlorhexidine gluconate is a fair inhibitor of fungi. It is active against enveloped viruses and has minimal action against tubercle bacillus. Organic matter minimally affects it. Most importantly, chlorhexidine gluconate 4% is persistent (has the ability to stop microbial regrowth with repeated use). The residual effect is maintained for more than 6 days.

Iodophors (7.5%) are complexes consisting of iodine and a carrier. Iodophors have a wide range of activity against gram-positive and gram-negative bacteria,

tubercle bacilli, fungi, viruses, and some spores. Iodophors are neutralized rapidly in the presence of organic materials. These agents have minimal residual effect and can cause skin irritation and damage.

Alcohol (60%-90%) is an agent with rapid antimicrobial properties against organisms, but it does not have residual activity. It has excellent bactericidal activity against gram-positive and gram-negative bacteria and good activity against tubercle bacillus as well as many fungi and viruses. It is not sporicidal. It aids in removing oils from the skin. The disadvantages of alcohol are its drying effect on the skin and its flammability, so it needs to be stored carefully.

Parachlorometaxylenol (PCMX) has good activity against gram-positive bacteria and less activity against gram-negative bacteria. It has fair activity against some fungi, viruses, and tubercle bacilli. PCMX has a persistent effect of a few hours and is minimally affected by organic matter. Its antimicrobial effect can be altered by the composition of the antiseptic product. Efficacy data should be reviewed before these products are used for surgical scrubs.

A brushless rub (with or without water) is now available (e.g., Avagard). This brushless technique has an alcohol base with an antimicrobial ingredient such as chlorhexidine gluconate or triclosan. These agents reduce bacterial counts on hands more rapidly than antimicrobial soaps or detergents. Combining alcohol (for rapid reduction of microbial growth) and chlorhexidine (for persistent and cumulative effect) prevents microbial regrowth. The advantages of the brushless rub are that the scrub time is shorter than with other agents and techniques and damage to the skin from brushes is avoided (Box 3-3).

Prescrubbing Guidelines

In preparation for scrubbing, the technician should remove all rings, watches, and jewelry. Pens, name tags, and other items should be removed from scrub top pockets. Fingernails need to be well maintained and should not be longer than the fingertips. Artificial nails or nail polish should not be worn. If eyeglasses are worn, they must be clean and thoroughly dry. Elastic bands are recommended to hold eyeglasses in place, thus preventing them from falling into the surgical field. The cap and mask should be applied, making sure all hair is covered by headgear and that the mask is snug and comfortable. To prevent eyeglasses from fogging up because of the mask, tape can be put over the upper edge of the mask,

TABLE 3-1   Characteristics of Selected Antimicrobials Used in Surgical Scrub Solutions

Spectrum of Activity*	Fungi	Viruses	Tubercle Bacilli	Affected by Organic Matter	Speed of Action	Disadvantages	Advantages
CHLORHEXIDINE GLUCONATE 4%							
Broad spectrum (more effective against gram-positive than gram-negative)	Fair	Enveloped viruses	Minimal	Minimal	Intermediate Significant immediate antimicrobial effect	Eye irritant	Persistent; ability to stop microbial growth with repeated use Residual effect maintained for more than 6 days
IODOPHORS 7.5% (COMPLEXES THAT CONSIST OF IODINE AND CARRIER)							
Broad spectrum (some spores)	Yes	Yes	Yes	Neutralized rapidly	Significant immediate antimicrobial effect	Odor, staining, tissue irritation	Persistent for 4-6 hours
ALCOHOL							
Broad spectrum (not sporicidal)	Many	Many	Yes	Conflicting evidence No residual activity	Rapid	Drying effect Volatile and flammable	Lacks persistence
PARACHLORMETA-XYLENOL (PCMX)							
Broad spectrum (good activity against gram positive, less activity against gram-negative)	Some	Some	Yes	Minimal	Intermediate	Highly formula dependent; does not sustain residual activity	Persistence limited to a few hours Skin sensitivity low

*Including against gram-positive and gram-negative bacteria.

or specially designed masks can be purchased. Hands should be thoroughly washed with an antimicrobial soap and water and towel-dried. Sterile gown and gloves, as well as any other sterile equipment that needs to be opened, should be opened in the surgery area if the circulating nurse is not available.

Surgical Hand Scrub Using Antimicrobial Scrub Agent

A traditional, standardized, surgical hand scrub procedure is important and should become second nature to the surgical nurse. It is important to follow the guidelines from the manufacturer and should include, but may not be limited to, the following actions.

Wash hands and forearms within 2 inches of elbows with antimicrobial scrub and running water immediately before beginning the surgical scrub (Figure 3-5). Make sure to thoroughly cover all areas with the scrub, as contact time is important for most agents to work properly. Clean the subungual areas of both hands under running water using a disposable nail-cleaning pick (Figure 3-6). Rinse hands and forearms under running water. Keep the hands above the elbows, and allow water to run off at the elbows. Remember to always hold the hands higher than the elbows and away from surgical attire.

Dispense the approved antimicrobial scrub agent according to the manufacturer's written directions. Do

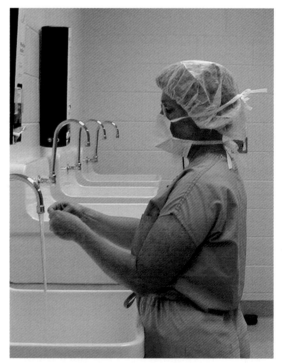

FIGURE 3-5 The hands and forearms are washed with soap and water before the official surgical hand preparation is performed. Note that the head cover and mask are already on before the hand prep begins. The gown and glove pack should be opened before the hand prep is started.

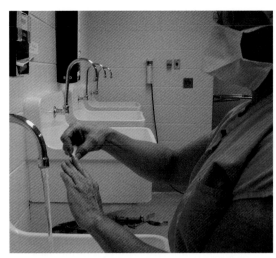

FIGURE 3-6 A nail pick is used to clean under the fingernails as part of the surgical hand prep.

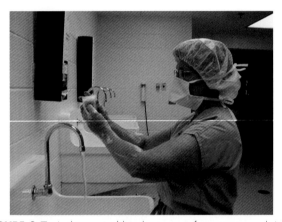

FIGURE 3-7 In this surgical hand prep, a soft sponge is used. Note that the hands are held above the elbows throughout the scrub.

FIGURE 3-8 Begin by brushing the fingertips of the first hand ten times, making sure the brush also goes under the fingernails.

FIGURE 3-9 Move to the lateral side of the index finger and scrub from the tip to the base of the finger 10 times.

not touch anything with your hands. Apply the antimicrobial agent to wet hands and forearms. Some manufacturers may recommend using a soft, nonabrasive sponge (Figure 3-7).

Visualize the surfaces of the fingers, hand, and arm as having four sides with the additional tip of the fingers. Begin by brushing the fingertips of the first hand 10 times, making sure the brush also goes under the fingernails (Figure 3-8). Move to the lateral side of the index finger and scrub from the tip to the base of the finger 10 times (Figure 3-9). Repeat the 10 time scrubbing process on the other three sides of the index finger. Make sure that the brush and antimicrobial scrub also contact the webbing between fingers. Move to the other four fingers and repeat the process on all sides of each finger. When scrubbing the lateral side of the last finger, make sure to scrub the lateral side of the hand in the same motion (Figure 3-10).

Move the brush to the palm of the hand and scrub 10 times (Figure 3-11). Move to the thumb side of the hand and scrub the outside of the thumb and the side of the hand in one motion (Figure 3-12). Complete the three

remaining sides of the thumb. Move to the back of the hand and scrub from the base of the fingers to the wrist using 10 strokes (Figure 3-13). Scrub the arm from the wrist to the elbow in the same manner, using 10 strokes on each of the four sides of the arm (Figure 3-14). Leaving the antimicrobial scrub on the first arm, proceed to the second arm and follow the same process.

When the scrub on both arms is complete, rinse, beginning at the fingertips. Make sure to keep the hands above the elbows and allow water to run off the elbow. Do not allow the any part of the hands or arms to touch anything (sink, scrub top, etc.) (Figure 3-15). Repeat this process on each hand/arm to make sure that manufacturer contact time requirements are met. It is important to avoid splashing surgical attire.

FIGURE 3-10 When scrubbing the lateral side of the last finger; make sure to scrub the lateral side of the hand in the same motion.

FIGURE 3-12 Move to the thumb side of the hand and scrub the outside of the thumb and the side of the hand in one motion.

FIGURE 3-11 Move the brush to the palm of the hand and scrub ten times.

FIGURE 3-13 Move to the back of the hand and scrub from the base of the fingers to the wrist using 10 strokes.

Surgical Hand Rub Using Antimicrobial Rub Agent

A standardized protocol for alcohol-based surgical hand rubs should follow manufacturers' written instructions. The rub should always start with the fingers, proceed to the hands, and continue up the arms to the elbow. It is important to follow the guidelines from the manufacturer, and the rub should include, but may not be limited to, the following activities.

Wash hands and forearms with soap and running water immediately before beginning the surgical hand antisepsis procedure. Clean the subungual areas of both hands under running water using a nail-cleaning pick. Rinse the hands and forearms under running water. Dry

FIGURE 3-14 Scrub the arm from the wrist to the elbow in the same manner, using 10 strokes on the four sides of the arm.

FIGURE 3-15 When the scrub on both arms is complete, rinse, beginning at the fingertips. Make sure to keep the hands above the elbows and to allow water to run off the elbow. Do not allow any part of the hands or arms to touch anything (sink, scrub top, etc.).

FIGURE 3-16 A hand towel is usually found on the top of a sterilized gown pack. Note the distance between the nonsterile scrub top and the sterile, open gown pack.

FIGURE 3-17 The hand towel is used to dry the hand first, then the wrist, then the forearm. Once the towel leaves the hand, it cannot go back up to the hand. Note the bend at the waist and the extended arms required to prevent the sterile towel from touching the nonsterile scrub top.

FIGURE 3-18 Use the opposite end/side of the hand towel to dry the second hand/arm.

the hands and forearms thoroughly with a paper towel. Dispense the manufacturer-recommended amount of surgical hand rub product. Apply the product to the hands and forearms, following the manufacturer's written directions. Some manufacturers may require the use of water as part of the process. Rub thoroughly until dry. Repeat the product application process as indicated in the manufacturer's written directions.

Gowning and Gloving

The purpose of gowning and gloving is to create a barrier between the sterile and nonsterile areas. Gowns and gloves cover the surgical team members' skin to prevent it from being a possible contaminant.

Gowns and gloves should be opened on a dry, flat surface away from other sterile supplies so that dripping water from the scrub person's arms will not contaminate them.

Drying the Hands

After completing the surgical hand scrub (or rub), the hands and arms need to be thoroughly dried with a sterile towel. From the sterile gown and towel pack, pick up the towel by the corner (Figure 3-16). Be careful not to drip water on the gown pack. Step back from the sterile table, always being aware of the sterile items in the environment to prevent contamination. Open the towel full length, using one end of the towel to gently rub the fingers, hand, and arms (in that order) of the first hand and arm (Figure 3-17). Do not rub back and forth; instead, rub circumferentially beginning at the wrist and moving to the elbow. Bend at the waist slightly so that the towel does not brush against the scrub suit. When ready to dry the second hand and arm, bring the first, dry hand to the opposite end of the towel and repeat (Figure 3-18). When drying is

FIGURE 3-19 As the gown is removed from the table, the person steps back away from the table to prevent the gown from touching any nonsterile items as it unfolds.

FIGURE 3-20 The neckline is identified and held while the armholes are found, and the gown is allowed to open.

completed, drop the towel onto the floor with the hand that is currently holding it, without allowing either hand to fall below waist level.

Gowning

Gowns are folded inside out in the packs. Grasp the whole gown, and lift the folded gown out of the package. Step away from the table, making sure there is adequate space to gown without contaminating anything (Figure 3-19). After locating the neckline and armholes, hold the gown by the neckline (Figure 3-20) and allow it to unfold (do not shake it). Keep the inside toward the body and the hands in the armholes. Slide both arms into the sleeves of the gown by reaching and extending both arms at the same time (Figure 3-21). The circulating nurse (nonsterile assistant) will continue to pull the gown onto the scrubbed-in person, carefully bringing the gown over the shoulders, fastening the neck of the gown, and tying the waistline, all while standing behind the person gowning and touching only the hem of the collar and back of the gown. If the gown is not fitting comfortably, the circulating nurse may grasp the gown by the hem at the bottom of the gown and pull downward. This may help the gown fit more comfortably. The scrubbed

FIGURE 3-21 Both arms are advanced into the sleeves simultaneously, but the hands are not allowed to pass all the way through the cuffs in order to allow for closed gloving.

person's hands remain inside the cuffs and must not be exposed outside the gown to perform the closed-gloving technique.

If the surgical gowns used are the "wraparound style," the front tie should not be touched until sterile gloves have been donned by the surgical nurse. On reusable gowns the wraparound ties are tied in the front of the gown by a single bow-tie knot. Another sterile team member must assist in this process to properly finish the donning of the gown.

On disposable gowns, a disposable paper tag covers the end of the ties. This gown can be properly donned with the help of a nonsterile circulator. Both these gowns cover the back of the body, thereby reducing the chance of contamination because most of the body is covered. The back of the gown or the body is never considered sterile. If either tie drops on the reusable gown or the disposable gown, the circulating nurse retrieves both ties and fastens them behind the scrubbed person's back.

Gloving

There are three methods of gloving: (1) closed gloving, (2) open gloving, and (3) assisted gloving. Both open gloving and closed gloving enable the scrubbed personnel to glove themselves. Closed gloving is the preferred method for surgery. Assisted gloving requires the assistance of another scrubbed-in team member.

Closed Gloving

Closed gloving provides assurance against contamination because no bare skin is exposed in the process. The following technique is used for the closed gloving technique. Remember to always keep the hands within the cuffs of the gown.

With the left hand, pick up the right glove from the inner wrapper of the glove package by the folded cuff (Figure 3-22). Extend the right hand (still within the cuff) with the palm facing upward. Place the palm of the glove palm down against the palm of the hand with the thumb

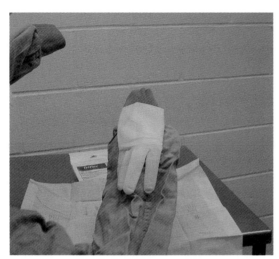

FIGURE 3-22 When performing the closed-gloving technique, "palm to palm, thumb to thumb, and fingers face the elbows" means that the palm of the hand covered by the cuff of the gown is facing up, and the palm side of the glove is facing down toward the palm of the hand. The thumb of the hand covered by the cuff of the gown is directly beneath the thumb of the glove. The fingers of the glove are lying over the wrist of the gown-covered hand, facing toward the elbow of the gown-covered arm.

FIGURE 3-23 During closed gloving, the hands remain within the cuffs of the gown until the gloves are secured over the cuffs of the gown, and then the hand can be extended out of the gown and into the glove. This requires manipulating the gloves through the material of the gown.

FIGURE 3-24 The cuff of the glove is extended over the cuff of the gown to perform closed gloving.

FIGURE 3-25 The cuff of this glove needs to be unfolded and pulled down to cover the entire cuff of the gown; this will assist placement of the fingers and thumb into the glove.

FIGURE 3-26 Once the first hand is gloved, that hand is used to place the second glove palm down onto the extended left hand covered by the cuff of the gown. Note that the palm of the left hand covered by the cuff of the gown is facing up.

and fingers of the glove facing the body. (The thumb side should be underneath on the same side as the thumb of the right hand facing upward.) When performing closed gloving, remember the saying, "Palm to palm, thumb to thumb, fingers of glove facing the elbow."

Through the gown cuff, grasp the back of the glove cuff with the right hand (Figure 3-23). With the left hand, pull and lift the cuff up and over the gown cuff and the right hand (Figure 3-24). The hand is still inside the sleeve. With the left hand, grasp both the top of the right glove cuff and the gown cuff, and pull toward the elbow while pushing the hand through the gown cuff and into the glove. Be sure the cuff of the glove completely covers the cuff of the gown (Figure 3-25). Glove the left hand using the same technique (Figures 3-26 to 3-28).

FIGURE 3-27 The thumb of the glove is directly above the thumb of the left hand covered by the cuff of the gown, and the fingers of the glove are facing the elbow of the left arm. "Palm to palm, thumb to thumb, and fingers facing the elbow."

FIGURE 3-28 Once the hand is extended into the glove, the cuff of the glove needs to be unfolded and to cover the entire cuff of the gown.

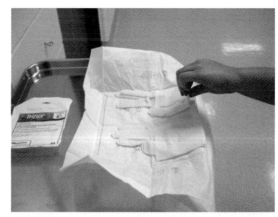

FIGURE 3-29 Only the "skin surface" of the glove being put on during open gloving can be touched. This means that only the folded cuff of the first glove can be touched.

FIGURE 3-30 The hand is extended into the glove, and the cuff is pulled up the wrist.

FIGURE 3-31 Even when the fingers are all the way into the glove, the cuff is not unfolded yet.

Open Gloving

Open gloving is another method that enables the scrubbed personnel to glove themselves. The open-gloving method should not be used routinely for surgical gowning and gloving. The closed or assisted technique is preferred, but the open method is used if one glove becomes contaminated in surgery and an assistant is not available to perform assisted gloving. Open gloving is also used when only the hands need to be sterile and no gown is needed, such as for minor surgical procedures, bone marrow biopsies, or catheterizations. For open gloving in surgery, instead of leaving the hands in the sleeves of the surgical gown, the hands are extended all the way through the cuff and the sleeves. The hands are entirely exposed. The following technique is used for the open gloving technique.

With the left hand, pick up the right glove by grasping the cuff on the "future" inside surface ("nonsterile" surface) of the fold only (Figure 3-29). Gently guide the fingers into the glove, leaving the cuff well turned over the hand. Keep the thumb in the palm of the hand until it is well inside the glove. Do not adjust the cuff (Figures 3-30

and 3-31). Place the gloved fingers of the right hand under the everted left glove cuff, on the sterile side of the left glove (Figure 3-32). Slide the fingers of the left hand into the glove, keeping the thumb inside the palm of the hand, until inside the glove. Pull the glove on all the way (Figures 3-33 and 3-34). With the left hand, slide the fingers under the outside edge of the right cuff and unfold it by stretching it up the wrist. Avoid touching any bare, exposed skin (Figure 3-35).

FIGURE 3-32 The gloved hand carefully reaches under the folded cuff of the second glove to pick it up. The second glove is put on before the cuff of the first glove is unfolded up the wrist.

FIGURE 3-33 Care is taken not to touch the exposed skin of the hand being gloved with the sterile glove already donned. This would contaminate the first glove.

FIGURE 3-34 Pulling the cuff of the second glove up the arm and away from the wrist prevents the gloved hand from touching the exposed skin and assists in finishing the step of pulling on the second glove.

FIGURE 3-35 Once the second glove is all the way on, the cuff of the first glove can be unfolded and extended up the arm. Only the fingers (not the thumb) of the second hand to be gloved are used to unfold the cuff. This prevents the thumb from touching the exposed skin on the arm.

FIGURE 3-36 Assisted gloving requires the help of another scrubbed-in and gloved person. The palm of the glove being placed is held toward the person needing the glove.

Assisted Gloving

Assisted gloving is used when a sterile team member helps another scrubbed-in team member glove. If a glove is contaminated during surgery, it needs to be changed. The contaminated person should step away, or at least keep the contaminated hand away from the sterile field. The circulating nurse grasps the outside of the glove cuff, but below the top of the glove, to ensure the sterile gown is not touched. The glove is pulled off inside out. The cuff of the gown should not be pulled over the hand because the cuff is contaminated with skin cells and scurf. The hands are extended all the way through the cuffs and sleeves. Assisted gloving is the best method to use to reglove. If this is not possible, open gloving away from the sterile field is necessary.

The following technique is used for the assisted gloving technique. The already gloved, sterile team member picks up the sterile glove, then places fingers from both hands under the cuff on the sterile sides of the glove. The palm of the glove is held toward the person being gloved (Figure 3-36). The cuff of the glove should be stretched widely open so that the hand can be placed in the glove without

FIGURE 3-37 The cuff of the glove is stretched wide, and the thumbs of the assistant are not used to hold the glove. This prevents the assistant from accidentally touching the exposed hand of the person needing the glove.

FIGURE 3-38 The assistant pulls the cuff of the glove over the cuff of the gown as the hand is pushed into the glove. Note that the assistant's thumbs are still held away from the glove.

touching the surgical nurse. The surgical nurse can avoid touching the hand to be gloved by holding the thumbs out (Figure 3-37). As the person slips into the glove, pull up on the glove to assist with the entrance of the hand into the glove (Figure 3-38). Make sure to bring the cuff of the glove over the cuff of the sleeve. Repeat for the other hand. The person being gloved can assist by using the one gloved hand to hold open the cuff of the other sterile glove being donned, while the surgical nurse's thumbs are kept under the glove's cuff until the glove is donned.

Contaminated Gown

If a gown becomes contaminated during surgery, it must be removed. The contaminated person steps away from the sterile field. The circulating nurse opens new sterile gloves and gown. The circulating nurse unfastens the gown and pulls it off inside out. The contaminated person then removes the gloves by grabbing the cuff of the glove (not the gown) and pulling the glove off inside out.

Rescrubbing is not required to regown and reglove. If only a sleeve has been contaminated, sterile sleeves may be used to cover the contaminated area.

Responsibilities

Once the surgical nurse is scrubbed-in, maintaining sterility and assisting the surgeon are the primary concerns. In addition, the surgical nurse needs to manage the instrument table (i.e., arrange the instruments on the table, count instruments and gauze squares [sponges] before opening and closing a body cavity), pass instruments to the surgeon, retract and moisten tissues, and maintain hemostasis. With all these duties, it is easy to forget to be considerate of the nurse's own body. To avoid becoming weak in the knees or nauseated during surgery, it is important to avoid locking the knee joints while assisting and to eat before scrubbing-in. Slowly shifting the weight from leg to leg and slightly bending the knees helps surgery personnel to prevent blood from pooling and to stay alert.

KEY POINTS

1. A surgical dress code should be written and posted so that it can be easily followed and enforced.
2. The dress code should include the defined areas where surgical attire must be worn, appropriate attire within those defined areas, and the acceptable options for cover apparel outside the surgical area.
3. The scrub suit should be covered with a clean laboratory coat at all times when outside the surgical area.
4. Personnel are not allowed to wear laboratory coats in the surgery room.
5. Scrub suits worn in the surgery room should not be worn home from the hospital.
6. Clean, freshly laundered scrub suits should be donned just before going into the surgery room and should not be worn from home into the hospital.
7. Proper surgical attire includes wearing a head cover that completely covers all head and facial hair, surgical masks that effectively cover the mouth and nose, and clean shoes with or without shoe covers.
8. Proper surgical attire requires the removal of all jewelry; this includes wedding bands, body-piercing objects, and watches.
9. Fingernails need to be well manicured and cannot extend beyond the tips of the fingers. Fingernails cannot be covered with nail polish.

10. The purpose of the surgical hand scrub or hand rub is to remove as many microorganisms as possible from the nails, hands, and arms.
11. All jewelry, name tags, and pens need to be removed before beginning the surgical hand scrub or hand rub.
12. Head covers and masks need to be donned before beginning the surgical hand scrub or rub.
13. Sterilized gown and glove packs need to be opened before beginning the surgical hand scrub or rub.

14. When using an antimicrobial detergent, it is important to follow the manufacturer's directions regarding the scrub time and whether or not a scrub brush should be used.
15. Closed gloving is the best gloving technique to guard against contamination because no bare skin is exposed in the process.

REVIEW QUESTIONS

1. *True or False:* Going into surgery with an empty stomach is the best way for the surgical nurse to avoid experiencing nausea and hypoglycemia if the procedure is unexpectedly long.

2. For which of the following is the surgical assistant responsible?
   a. Monitoring the patient.
   b. Maintaining sterility.
   c. Maintaining hemostasis.
   d. All of the above.
   e. Both b and c.

3. Which of the following is true?
   a. Proper surgical attire includes wearing freshly laundered scrub top and pants, head cover, and mask.
   b. Each surgical facility should have its own posted surgery dress code.
   c. Proper surgical attire decreases the risk of infection associated with surgery.
   d. All of the above.
   e. None of the above.

4. What should the surgical nurse don on leaving the surgery suite?
   a. Street clothes.
   b. Laboratory coat.
   c. Shoe covers.
   d. Cap and mask.
   e. None of the above.

5. Why should scrub suits not be worn from home to the hospital?

6. Why should scrub suits not be worn home from the hospital?

7. *True or False:* The surgical nurse's scrub top should be tucked into the scrub pants.

8. Why should scrub tops be short sleeve?

9. *True or False:* It is recommended that all nonscrubbed personnel wear long-sleeve laboratory coats in the surgery room.

10. *True or False:* Jewelry and long fingernails are protected by the sterile gloves worn by scrubbed-in surgical personnel and therefore do not need to be removed (jewelry) or cut (nails).

11. Which of the following is false regarding the surgical hand preparation?
   a. The preparation should begin with a quick, general hand and arm wash.
   b. The purpose of the prep is to sterilize the skin on the surgeon's hands and arms.
   c. Stiff scrub brushes should not be used to scrub the hands and arms.
   d. The product manufacturer determines the recommended length of time the product should be scrubbed on the hands and arms during the surgical hand prep.

12. Which of the following is the correct order of events associated with performing the surgical hand prep and donning the surgical gown and gloves?
   a. Confirm removal of or remove all jewelry→open gown and glove packs→don cap and mask→perform hand prep→dry hands using sterile hand towel→gown→perform closed gloving.
   b. Perform hand prep→open gown and glove packs→don cap and mask→don gown and perform open gloving.
   c. Perform hand prep→open gown and glove packs→don cap and mask→don gown and gloves.
   d. Remove all jewelry→gown and glove→perform hand prep.
   e. None of the above.

13. What does managing the instrument table involve?
   a. Keeping the instruments organized for quick retrieval.
   b. Counting instruments and gauze squares at the beginning and end of the procedure.
   c. Loading the needle holders with suture needle.
   d. All of the above.
   e. Only a and c.

ANSWERS

1. False
2. e
3. d
4. b
5. Scrub suits can carry microorganisms into the hospital
6. Scrub suits can bring microorganisms home and infect the personnel's own pets
7. True
8. To allow for scrubbing above the elbows
9. False
10. False
11. b
12. a
13. d

BIBLIOGRAPHY

Association of periOperative Registered Nurses (AORN): Standards, recommended practices, and guidelines, Denver, 2004, AORN.

Fairchild S: Perioperative nursing principles and practice, ed 3, Philadelphia, 1996, Lippincott.

Fossum T, Hedlund CS, Hulse DA, et al: Small animal surgery, ed 3, St Louis, 2007, Mosby.

Gruendemann BJ, Bjerke N: Is it time for brushless scrubbing with an alcohol based agent? AORN J 74:859, 2001.

Paulson D: Comparative evaluation of five surgical hand scrub preparations. AORN J 60:246, 1994.

Phillips N: Berry & Kohn's operating room technique, ed 10, St Louis, 2004, Mosby.

Slatter D: Textbook of small animal surgery, ed 3, Philadelphia, 2003, Saunders.

Spry C: Essentials of perioperative nursing, ed 2, Boston, 2004, Jones & Bartlett.

Asepsis

Paige A. Allen

LEARNING OBJECTIVES

After completion of this chapter, the reader will be able to:
- Define asepsis, sterile field, and surgical conscience.
- Maintain asepsis.
- Maintain a sterile field.
- Open sterile packs without contaminating their contents or the sterile field.
- Discuss the correct method of loading and passing a scalpel blade and handle.
- Discuss the techniques used to pass various types of surgical instruments safely to the surgeon.

Asepsis

The surgical area is a restricted area because it needs to be as free of microorganisms as possible. A surgical wound could easily become infected if the proper techniques are not used. Infections acquired due to lack of attention to aseptic technique can be serious and even fatal. *Asepsis* (absence of pathogenic microorganisms that cause infection) makes the environment surgically clean, but not sterile (absence of all living microorganisms, including spores).

Keeping the surgical area as aseptic as possible, by properly cleaning and disinfecting it, adhering to the written dress code, preparing the patient correctly, and performing proper handwashing and hand scrubbing, helps prevent pathogenic microorganisms from contaminating the environment and entering the surgical wound. Aseptic techniques, along with sterile techniques, are the most important practices to prevent infection in the patient.

Surgical conscience is the commitment of the surgical personnel to adhere strictly to aseptic technique, because anything less could increase the potential risk of infection, resulting in harm to the patient. Any break in aseptic technique is immediately reported and addressed or corrected, whether or not anyone else is present to observe the violation.

Maintaining Asepsis

Maintaining asepsis in the surgical area is accomplished by practicing aseptic and sterile techniques. The Association of periOperative Registered Nurses (AORN) has listed several "Recommended Practices for Maintaining a Sterile Field." These recommendations should also be followed in the veterinary surgery area (Box 4-1).

- Aseptic technique is used to maintain the absence of disease-causing organisms in the surgical environment.
- Asepsis does not guarantee sterility.
- A surgical conscience requires acknowledging when a breach in asepsis or sterility has occurred and taking the necessary steps to address and correct it, even if no one else witnesses the breach.

- The space above and surrounding an open sterile pack is considered part of the sterile field.
- The sterile field cannot be entered or touched by non–scrubbed-in personnel.
- If non–scrubbed-in personnel enter or touch the sterile field, it is no longer sterile and is considered contaminated.

Sterile Field

Scrubbed personnel function within a sterile field. The scrubbed personnel's gowns are sterile in front from the chest to the level of the sterile field. The sleeves of the sterile gown are sterile from 2 inches above the elbow to the top of the edge of the cuff. The neckline, shoulders, and cuffed portion of the gown sleeves may become contaminated by perspiration and therefore are not considered sterile. The back of the gown is never considered sterile because a member of the surgical team cannot observe it constantly. The cuffs of the gown are considered contaminated because hands have passed through them.

Sterile drapes should be used to establish a sterile field. Drapes are barriers that help to prevent microorganisms from passing between sterile and nonsterile areas. The drapes should cover the entire animal, the furniture, and the equipment that is part of the sterile field. The circulating nurse, or any other non–scrubbed-in personnel, should never reach over the draped, sterile areas. Also, if any drapes become wet, they are considered contaminated because strike-through will occur. *Strike-through* occurs when liquids soak through a drape from a sterile area to an unsterile area, and vice versa. A sterile field should be maintained and monitored continuously. The sterile field should never be left unattended (Box 4-2).

Opening Items for Use in the Sterile Field

All items used within a sterile field should be sterile. Before opening any sterile items for the surgeon to be placed on the sterile field, make sure the packages are inspected for sterility. Make sure that (1) there are no tears or holes in the outer package and (2) the items have gone through the proper sterilization by checking the sterile indicators. Indicators are located on the outside of the package, or there may be indicator tape on the front of the package (Figure 4-1). Check the seal of the package to

FIGURE 4-1 Sterilization indicator tape. *Top left,* Steam sterilization indicator tape before being exposed to steam. *Bottom left,* Steam sterilization indicator tape after being exposed to steam. *Top right,* Ethylene oxide gas sterilization indicator tape before being exposed to ethylene oxide gas. *Bottom right,* Ethylene oxide gas sterilization tape being exposed to ethylene oxide.

FIGURE 4-2 Circulating nurse opens a peel-away pouch to expose the contents for removal by surgical nurse.

ensure it is secure and not broken at any point. Check the package itself, and if it looks worn by being handled too much, it should be considered contaminated. A larger surgical pack should have a sterile indicator inside to ensure that the sterilizing agent has penetrated to the center of a thick pack. The expiration date should be checked, although AORN maintains that the sterility of the item is event related and not time related (see Chapter 9). This means that if all the above features have been checked on the package, the time and expiration date of sterilization are not significant.

All items introduced onto a sterile field should be opened, dispensed, and transferred by methods that maintain sterility and integrity. Edges of all sterile wrappers and packages are considered nonsterile. Therefore, when opening an item, be sure all edges are secured so that they do not contaminate the field or the sterile packaged item.

The surgical nurse may lift the item straight out of the package, without touching any of the edges of the package (Figure 4-2). Heavy, sharp, or large items may be opened on a separate table near the sterile field for retrieval by the

FIGURE 4-3 Sterile water being poured into a sterile bowl. Note that the bowl is set in the corner of an empty table to avoid possible contamination if splashing occurs.

surgical nurse. Sterile supplies are opened by unwrapping the flap farthest away first, the sides next, and the nearest flap last.

Opening Fluids for Use in the Sterile Field

Irrigation fluids should be poured carefully to prevent any spills onto the sterile field and to avoid splash-back. Therefore, it is best to have the scrubbed-in person hold the basin away from the field or to place it at the edge of the sterile table. Once the fluids have been opened, the cap is considered contaminated and cannot be replaced onto the bottle, so the remaining fluids must be discarded (Figure 4-3).

Moving Around the Sterile Field

All personnel moving within or around a sterile field should do so in a manner to maintain the integrity of the sterile field. The surgical team must be aware of the sterile and nonsterile areas in the surgery room at all times. Movement creates air currents, which can be a source of contamination in the surgical room. Minimal movement is required.

Scrubbed personnel should not walk away from the sterile field by wandering around the room or leaving it. When scrubbed-in personnel must change positions around the sterile field, they should be a safe distance apart so as not to touch. When they pass each other, they should pass face to face (sterile to sterile) or back to back (unsterile to unsterile).

Unscrubbed (non–scrubbed-in) personnel should always face the surgical field. Unscrubbed persons should not walk between two sterile fields. For example, unscrubbed personnel should not walk between the sterile, draped patient and the sterile equipment table.

The surgical scrub team should not change levels of position—from sitting to standing, and vice versa—during a procedure. The lower portion of the gown is considered contaminated, and when the scrubbed person sits, this portion of the gown is closer to the hands,

arms, and the sterile field and therefore could cause contamination.

There should be minimal talking in the surgery room and the surgery room doors should remain closed as much as possible. All non–scrubbed-in persons should be a safe distance from the sterile field. A limited number of non–scrubbed-in observers should be allowed in the surgery room at one time. The more congested the surgery room, the more difficult it is to monitor the sterile field, and the sterile team has less room to move adequately around the sterile field. The surgical conscience is followed to report any breaks in aseptic or sterile technique.

Duties of the Circulating Nurse

The *circulating nurse* is the person who opens packs and is a runner for the surgical team. Proper opening of sterile packs is important to maintain a sterile field. All packages have to be checked thoroughly for any damage or inadvertent break in the material. Speed should not be a top priority. Although opening items in a timely way is necessary, rushing can cause unnecessary mistakes. Timing is also a factor. If the scrubbed-in person is not ready to receive the item, or if the equipment table is not properly prepared, the circulating nurse should consider delaying opening the item until a later, more convenient time.

Wraps and packages can be sterilized at the hospital or by the manufacturer. Wraps and packages sterilized by the manufacturer are usually disposable items. Packages sterilized at the hospital often do not come with directions on how to open them. This skill comes with knowledge and practice. The manufacturer often supplies directions explaining which end to open first.

Opening Peel-Away Pouches

Many paper or plastic pouches for packaging individual sterile instruments have a side sealed with an arrow (↑) indicating which end to open. Holding the packet at the end with the arrow allows easy opening of this type of seal; with both hands, grasp the package with the thumbs and slowly peel the package open by adducting the thumbs (Figure 4-4). Do not roll the wrists, as doing so may cause the package to not open properly. While peeling the package open, hold the item firmly so that the item is stabilized and does not slide across the nonsterile edges of the package.

The plastic or paper tubing or pouches with a straight seal are opened similarly, except that a constant pull must be maintained on both sides. Instruments and sutures can be either handed to the surgeon or unwrapped to make them available for the surgical team. If necessary, small, sterile items can be opened on a clean, dry, flat, nonsterile surface. Place the item, paper side down, hold onto the top sealed edge with a thumb and finger of one hand, and pull the plastic side with the other hand. The scrubbed-in assistant can carefully pick the item off the sterile paper

FIGURE 4-4   Opening a peel-away pouch by touching only the outer edge of the separated ends, then carefully pulling them apart by adducting the thumbs.

FIGURE 4-5   Opening a pack with one hand. The thumb of one hand is slid under the tab of the taped edge, and the pack is held between that thumb and the fingers of that hand while the other hand unwraps the pack.

and transfer it to the sterile table. Suture can be given directly to a scrubbed-in person by opening the package and allowing the scrubbed-in person to retrieve the inner suture package.

Opening Wrapped Packs

Wrapped sterile packs are opened on a clean, flat, dry surface in the surgery room. Place the sterile pack on a flat surface so that the wrapped edges are uppermost. Remove the indicator tape and open the distant flap first, taking care not to reach over the sterile contents of the pack. Open the side flaps one at a time, taking care to touch only the exposed tabbed corners and no other part of the wrap. Open the nearest flap last. For especially large packs, the circulating nurse may need to walk around the table to avoid reaching over the sterile field. If the package is double wrapped, the scrubbed-in team member can open the inner wrap.

Some wrapped items are small enough to be opened with one hand by the circulating nurse. Opening a pack correctly with one hand allows the circulating nurse to hand the item to the scrubbed-in team member for its removal from the wrap without contaminating the scrubbed-in person. To open a sterile pack with one hand, start by holding the pack in one hand (hand A), then insert thumb of hand A under the taped fold (Figure 4-5). Then, using hand B, remove the tape and lift the top fold back, tucking the top flap into the grasp of hand A by folding the top flap under the pack. Using hand B, unwrap the two side folds, one at a time, tucking each one into the grasp of hand A underneath the pack. Using hand B, grasp the last corner tab, and pull it back to be held by hand A, as the item is carefully removed from the wrap by the scrubbed-in personnel (Figure 4-6).

Opening Gowns and Gloves

Gowns are opened much like packs. There needs to be a clean, flat, dry surface for both gown and gloves. Remove

FIGURE 4-6   Circulating nurse holds the outer wrap of an opened pack in an extended hand to allow the scrubbed-in person to reach in to remove the pack's contents without breaking sterility.

the gown from the package (if a disposable, sterile gown) and place the gown on a flat surface so that the wrapped edges are uppermost. If a resterilized cloth gown is used, remove the tape from the outer wrap.

Open the distant flap first, taking care not to reach over the sterile contents of the pack. Open the side flaps one at a time, taking care to touch only the exposed tabbed corners and no other part of the wrap. Open the nearest flap last. For especially large packs, the circulating nurse may need to walk around the table to avoid reaching over the sterile field. If the gown is double wrapped, the scrubbed-in team member can open the inner wrap.

Sterile gloves are removed from the outer package and placed on the table. At the top and bottom of the package are folds. Unfold these ends, taking care to over-fold slightly to decrease the memory of the paper. Place hands under the flaps of the side and pull toward the outside. Take care that the top and bottom folds do not come back in and contaminate the gloves. If possible, fold the cuff end of the paper wrap over the edge of the counter.

KEY POINTS

1. The surgical environment needs to be thoroughly cleaned on a daily basis to prevent contamination of the surgical site and to prevent hospital-acquired patient infection.
2. Aseptic technique is used to maintain the absence of disease-causing organisms in the surgical environment.
3. Asepsis does not guarantee sterility.
4. Sterile items are used in surgery and are free of all microorganisms, including spores.
5. A surgical conscience requires acknowledging when a breach in asepsis or sterility has occurred and taking the necessary steps to address and correct it, even if no one else witnesses the breach.
6. The space above and surrounding an open sterile pack is considered part of the sterile field.
7. The sterile field cannot be entered or touched by non–scrubbed-in personnel.
8. If non–scrubbed-in personnel enter or touch the sterile field, it is no longer sterile and is considered contaminated.

REVIEW QUESTIONS

1. What are the two most important practices used to prevent surgical infections?
   a. Aseptic and septic technique.
   b. Sterile and septic technique.
   c. Septic and antiseptic technique.
   d. Aseptic and sterile technique.
   e. Sterile and antiseptic technique.

2. What areas of the scrubbed-in personnel's gown are part of the sterile field?
   a. Back of the gown.
   b. Front from chest to the level of sterile field.
   c. Cuffs of the sleeves.
   d. All of the above if the gown was autoclaved.
   e. None of the above.

3. *True or False:* Strike-through renders surgical drapes "sterile proof," and therefore drapes affected by strike-through cannot become contaminated under any circumstance.

4. *True or False:* The edges of all sterile packages are considered nonsterile.

5. *True or False:* It is acceptable practice for the circulating nurse to reach over the sterile field if required to assist the surgeon or surgical assistant.

6. Which of the following statements is true regarding the sterile field?
   a. Only scrubbed-in personnel need to know what is sterile and nonsterile.
   b. Only the circulating nurse needs to keep track of what is sterile and nonsterile.
   c. Excessive talking and movement among scrubbed-in personnel are acceptable, but not among non–scrubbed-in personnel.
   d. All of the above.
   e. None of the above.

7. Which of the following statements is false regarding the sterile field?
   a. Unscrubbed personnel should not walk between two sterile fields.
   b. Unscrubbed personnel should never face the sterile field.
   c. All unscrubbed personnel should keep a safe distance from the sterile field.
   d. Only sterile items should be in the sterile field.
   e. The sterile field should never be left unattended.

8. *True or False:* If unscrubbed personnel enter or touch the sterile field, it is no longer considered sterile.

9. *True or False:* The space above and surrounding an open sterile pack is considered part of the sterile field.

ANSWERS

1. d	4. True	7. b
2. b	5. False	8. True
3. False	6. e	9. True

BIBLIOGRAPHY

Association of periOperative Registered Nurses (AORN): Standards, recommended practices, and guidelines: recommended practices for maintaining a sterile field, Denver, 2004, AORN.

Bassert JM, McCurnin DM, editors: McCurnin's Clinical textbook for veterinary technicians, ed 7, St Louis, 2010, Saunders.

Fairchild S: Perioperative nursing: principles and practice, ed 2, Philadelphia, 1996, Lippincott.

Fossum TW, Hedlund CS, Hulse DA, et al: Small animal surgery, ed 3, St Louis, 2007, Mosby.

Spry C: Essentials of perioperative nursing, ed 2, Boston, 2004, Jones & Bartlett.

Tobias KM, Johnston SA: Veterinary surgery: small animal, St Louis, 2012, Saunders.

Patient Monitoring

5

Teri Raffel

LEARNING OBJECTIVES

After completion of this chapter, the reader should be able to:
- Perform complete monitoring of the patient under anesthesia, assessing cardiovascular, respiratory, and neurologic parameters.
- Discuss the special anesthetic considerations regarding monitoring of various surgical procedures and patient positions.
- List examples of anesthesia monitoring devices.
- Describe the functions of anesthesia monitoring devices.
- Discuss cause and effect of various physiologic changes that may occur during anesthesia.

Role of the Veterinary Technician Anesthetist

For surgical procedures it is desirable to have a veterinary technician anesthetist, whose sole responsibility is to monitor the patient under anesthesia, as well as a circulating nurse to help transport the patient from the surgery prep area to the surgical suite. This team approach allows the surgeon and surgical assistant to be scrubbing while the anesthetist and circulating nurse arrange the patient, anesthesia machine, and monitoring devices in the surgery room. When the circulating nurse takes responsibility for positioning the patient on the surgery table, attaching the monitoring devices to the patient, and performing the final skin prep and paint in the surgery room, the anesthetist is able to focus on the most important task, monitoring the patient. Without the help of a circulating nurse, the veterinary technician would need to perform all these tasks alone in rapid succession. If the technician is working alone, the primary task is careful and constant monitoring of the surgical patient. This may mean delaying the final surgical scrub (or other, less critical tasks) until the veterinary technician is confident that the patient is stable.

Monitoring

Constant monitoring of the animal under general anesthesia or sedation is an extremely important responsibility. The patient that is monitored closely is the patient that is safely anesthetized. Close and constant monitoring allows the anesthetist to detect dangerous trends and to make appropriate adjustments. If the patient is showing signs of waking up, the anesthetist can increase the concentration of anesthetic. If the patient is showing signs of becoming too deeply anesthetized, the anesthetist can decrease the concentration of gas delivered. Table 5-1 summarizes the stages of anesthesia.

Constant monitoring by a technician responsible solely for that patient is the preferred situation. Recommendations include checking the patient every 5 minutes and recording the findings on an anesthesia form. When gas anesthetic agents that provide quick induction and recovery are used, such as sevoflurane, more frequent monitoring may be needed. The observant surgeon and surgical assistant can supplement intermittent and frequent monitoring by nonsterile personnel.

Several patient parameters should be monitored every 5 minutes, including heart rate and rhythm, respiratory rate and rhythm, capillary refill time, color of mucous membranes, eye position, muscle tone, and reflexes. The patient's temperature should be monitored at least every 15 minutes if possible. Several anesthetic and treatment parameters should be tabulated every 5 to 15 minutes, including volume of fluid administered, oxygen flow rate, oxygen tank pressure, and anesthetic gas concentration.

The most reliable way to monitor the patient is through personal, direct contact. The technician can listen for the heart rate and respiratory rate through the stethoscope. The pulse can be palpated to obtain a general impression of pulse strength and therefore of blood pressure (Figures 5-1 to 5-5). The reservoir bag can be observed for frequency and extent of movement. The color of the mucous membranes can be visually assessed, and the capillary refill time is directly measured. The technician's sense of smell can detect possible anesthetic leakage problems.

Heart Rate and Rhythm

The heart rate can be monitored through direct palpation of the thoracic wall or by listening through a stethoscope. The stethoscope can be the conventional type that is placed on the thoracic wall. However, the location of the surgical site may prevent the use of a conventional stethoscope. An esophageal stethoscope is a more convenient and less intrusive means of monitoring heart rate intraoperatively.

FIGURE 5-2   Checking the digital pulse.

FIGURE 5-3   Checking the femoral pulse.

FIGURE 5-1   Checking the lingual pulse.

FIGURE 5-4   Direct palpation of the heart through the chest wall.

TABLE 5-1 Stages of Anesthesia

Behavior	Respiration	Cardiovascular Function	Response to Surgery	Depth	Eye Position	Pupil Size	Pupil Response to Light	Muscle Tone	Reflex Response
STAGE I Disoriented	Normal, may be panting: respiration rate 20-30 breaths/min	Heart rate unchanged	Struggle	Not anesthetized	Central, may be nystagmus	Normal	Yes	Good	All present
STAGE II: "EXCITEMENT STAGE" Excitement: struggling, vocalization, paddling, chewing, yawning	Irregular, may hold breath or hyperventilate	Heart rate may increase	Struggle	Not anesthetized	Central, may be nystagmus	May be dilated	Yes	Good	All present, may be exaggerated
STAGE III—PLANE 1: LIGHT ANESTHESIA Anesthetized	Regular; rate 12-20 breaths/min	Pulse strong: Heart rate >90 beats/min	May respond with movement	Light	Central or rotated, may be nystagmus	Normal	Yes	Good	Swallowing poor or absent, others present but diminished
STAGE III—PLANE 2: MEDIUM SURGICAL ANESTHESIA	Regular (may be shallow): rate 12-16 breaths/min	Heart rate >90 beats/min	Heart and respiration rates may increase	Moderate	Often rotated ventrally	Slightly dilated	Sluggish	Relaxed	Patellar, ear flick, palpebral, and corneal may be present; others absent
STAGE III—PLANE 3: DEEP ANESTHESIA	Shallow: rate <12 breaths/min	Heart rate 60-90 beats/min; CRT increased; pulse less strong	None	Deep	Usually central, may rotate ventrally	Moderately dilated	Very sluggish or absent	Greatly reduced	All reflexes diminished or absent
STAGE III—PLANE 4	Jerky	Heart rate <60 beats/min; prolonged CRT; pale mucous membranes	None	Overdose	Central	Widely dilated	Unresponsive	Flaccid	No reflex activity
STAGE IV Moribund	Apnea	Cardiovascular collapse	None	Dying	Central	Widely dilated	Unresponsive	Flaccid	No reflex activity

CRT, capillary refill time; min, minute.
From McKelvey D, Hollingshead KW: Veterinary anesthesia and analgesia, ed 3, St Louis, 2003, Mosby.

FIGURE 5-5 Auscultating the heart and monitoring the femoral pulse simultaneously.

FIGURE 5-7 Esophageal stethoscope with amplifier.

FIGURE 5-6 Esophageal stethoscope with ear pieces.

In positioning the esophageal stethoscope, special sensory plastic tubing is placed in the esophagus next to the heart. The tubing is passed through the mouth into the esophagus. The endotracheal (ET) tube prevents the esophageal stethoscope tubing from entering the trachea. The heart sounds can be heard through ear pieces, or an amplifier can be attached to broadcast the sound (Figures 5-6 and 5-7). If the end of the tubing is adjacent to the lung fields, breath sounds will be heard.

The heart rate of an anesthetized dog or cat is expected to be slower than the animal's rate when awake and excited about being examined by a stranger. Most anesthetic drugs have cardiac depressant effects. Hypothermia can also cause a decreased heart rate. When the heart rate falls below an acceptable limit, the surgeon should be notified. Suggested guidelines for acceptable lower limits are 50 beats per minute (beats/min) for a large dog, 70 beats/min for a small dog, and 100 beats/min for a cat. Rates lower than these warrant notifying the surgeon immediately.

Anticholinergic drugs such as atropine sulfate and glycopyrrolate are administered to help maintain the heart rate above the acceptable lower limits (see Chapter 2). Dissociative anesthetics such as ketamine and tiletamine can also elevate the heart rate. When an animal is in shock or pain, the heart rate is usually rapid. Regardless of the reason, once the heart rate exceeds the acceptable limits, the surgeon should be notified. Suggested guidelines for acceptable upper limits are 180 beats/min for a large dog, 200 beats/min for a small dog, and 220 beats/min for a cat.

An irregular heart rhythm may be detected through auscultation of the thorax or on an electrocardiogram (ECG). Some anesthetic agents sensitize the heart muscle to arrhythmias. When the heart beats arrhythmically, the heart is inefficient at pumping the blood through the body. This inefficiency leads to poor tissue perfusion, acidosis, poor oxygen delivery to the tissues, and buildup of waste products in the body tissues. These irregular beats may spontaneously disappear. If the arrhythmic beats are frequent or continuous, the veterinarian should be alerted.

Detection of a pulse deficit is cause for concern. A *pulse deficit* occurs when the heart contracts (beats) but does not generate enough push to produce a palpable peripheral pulse. Pulse deficits are detected when the heartbeat is arrhythmic; tissue perfusion is poor, and the patient may quickly go into shock. The veterinarian should be alerted immediately. "Skipped" beats are detected when one is listening to the heartbeat with a stethoscope but is unable to palpate that individual beat simultaneously as a peripheral pulse. In this case the single skipped beat is a result of a single premature depolarization of the heart muscle.

Tissue Perfusion

To maintain healthy and functioning tissues and organs, adequate tissue perfusion must be maintained. If not,

FIGURE 5-8 Cat with pale mucous membranes.

adverse long-term effects may be sustained. The kidneys are particularly sensitive to states of low perfusion. During inadequate perfusion states, waste products from cellular metabolism are not removed, and nutrients such as oxygen and glucose are not delivered to the cells.

Mucous Membranes

The color of the mucous membranes is a general indicator of tissue perfusion. The pink color of the mucous membranes results from the color of the blood in the capillaries seen through the nonpigmented areas. Mucous membrane color may be evaluated by looking at the gums, conjunctiva, and mucosal surface of the vulva or prepuce.

Pale mucous membranes may indicate a state of poor tissue perfusion or anemia (Figure 5-8). Preanesthetic diagnostic blood tests, such as complete blood count (CBC) and measurements of hematocrit and hemoglobin, will identify the anemic patient. Preferably, the severely anemic patient will not go to surgery before receiving appropriate blood component therapy. Pale mucous membrane color can also be an indicator of shock. Efforts must be made before the anesthetic episode to identify and begin correction of the poor color.

Dark-red mucous membranes may be seen if an animal is septic, meaning that the patient has a severe blood infection. Bacteria may be cultured from the blood. The immune system is reacting to the infection by releasing vasoactive chemicals that cause postcapillary venous dilation and increased permeability in the vessel walls. This can lead to congestion in the capillary beds and thus the brick-red color of the mucous membranes.

A bluish color to the mucous membranes (cyanosis) suggests that the red blood cells are not carrying adequate oxygen. The red cells may not have exchanged oxygen in the lungs, suggesting a respiratory problem such as obstruction of oxygen flow to the lungs or lack of breathing. The ET tube should be evaluated immediately for a kink or obstruction. A bluish color in the buccal mucosa may also result if a tie on the ET tube is too tight around the cheeks, causing stagnant blood flow. The buccal

mucosa should be compared with the conjunctival mucosa to determine whether a tight tie could be the cause of the bluish color and needs to be loosened.

Capillary Refill Time

The capillary refill time (CRT) normally should be less than 2 seconds. The same areas used to assess the color of mucous membranes may be used to assess CRT. When CRT is longer than 2 seconds, perfusion in these tissues is poor. This condition may be caused by low arterial blood pressure or peripheral vasoconstriction. Release of epinephrine can cause peripheral vasoconstriction, and slow CRT is often seen in nervous and frightened animals. α_2-adrenergic agonist drugs such as medetomidine cause significant peripheral vasoconstriction, thus slowing the CRT. A normal CRT can be detected shortly after some animals are deceased, reinforcing the importance of constant monitoring of several vital signs, not just one.

Pulse and Blood Pressure

Pulse strength can be defined as the ease or difficulty of palpating the blood flowing through the artery. Pulse strength is a general indicator of the blood pressure. If the patient's pulse becomes more difficult to palpate, the blood pressure has fallen. If the patient's pulse becomes more easily palpable or bounding, the blood pressure has increased. Pulses can be monitored at the following arteries: lingual, femoral, carotid, dorsal metatarsal, and digital (see Figures 5-1 to 5-3). Additionally the heart may be palpated directly through the chest wall. In cats the examiner's thumb and fingers are placed on either side of the chest, and light pressure is applied to feel the beating heart (see Figure 5-4). Obese patients and larger patients, such as medium-sized to large dogs, are more difficult to palpate.

An ultrasonic Doppler or oscillometric device is needed to assess arterial blood pressure accurately (see Chapter 1). Normal mean arterial pressure (MAP) ranges in awake animals are from 85 to 120 mm Hg. MAP should be maintained above 70 mm Hg while the patient is under anesthesia and never allowed to drop below 60 mm Hg.

Hypotension

Hypotension (low blood pressure) in an anesthetized patient may be caused by the following factors:

Hypovolemia: Excessive blood loss or dehydration reduces the volume of the vascular space. With little blood to pump through the vessels, the blood pressure will be low.

Cardiac insufficiency: Patients with preexisting heart disease may have a weak myocardium or leaking heart valves, which can lead to inefficient pumping action.

Excessive vasodilation: Many preanesthetic and anesthetic drugs cause vasodilation to varying degrees. The effects can be additive and significant. When the blood vessels dilate, the blood pools, venous return to the heart is decreased, and blood pressure drops.

Anesthetic depth: In general, as the patient goes deeper under anesthesia, the blood pressure drops. The correlation between blood pressure and anesthetic depth is quite accurate.

Respiratory Rate and Rhythm

One inhalation and one exhalation are considered one breath. Counting only the inhalations or only the exhalations is necessary to determine the correct *respiratory rate* (RR). The number of breaths counted in 15 seconds is multiplied by 4 to calculate the breaths per minute, or the respiratory rate. A dog or cat in the surgical plane of anesthesia has a rate of 8 to 20 breaths/min. A respiratory rate of less than 8 breaths/min is cause for concern and most likely indicates an excessive anesthetic depth. As anesthetic depth becomes dangerously deep, respiration ceases before the heart stops beating.

The respiratory rate can be determined by watching the patient's chest movement. The reservoir bag on the anesthesia machine can also be observed. The reservoir bag collapses and fills synchronously with the patient's breathing. The anesthetist can listen for breath sounds through the stethoscope and should note their character and intensity. An increase in intensity, crackles, or wheezing indicates pulmonary airway narrowing through constriction or the presence of fluid. Devices such as the capnograph display the respiratory rate on a digital display.

The depth and rhythm of the respirations should also be assessed. The inspiratory phase is about half as long as the expiratory phase. A short pause occurs before the next inspiration. If the animal feels pain during the surgery, the respiratory rate will increase. Dissociative anesthetic agents will cause the animal to inhale, hold its breath, then exhale. This irregular breathing pattern is characteristic of dissociative anesthetics. As anesthetic depth increases, respiratory rate usually decreases. Gasping or labored breathing is of particular concern. An obstruction of the trachea or ET tube or a lack of fresh gas flow can cause exaggerated respiratory effort. Check the patency of the ET tube, check for the appropriate oxygen flow rate on the anesthesia machine, and confirm that the pressure in the reservoir bag is not too high. If the ET tube is not patent, it may need to be suctioned, or the patient may need to be re-intubated. If the desired setting on the oxygen flowmeter is not being maintained, the oxygen tank supplying the anesthesia machine may need to be changed. If the reservoir bag is overinflated and has a high pressure, assuming the pop-off valve is open, the anesthetist can try decreasing the oxygen flow rate on the anesthesia machine.

The animal that spasmodically contracts its diaphragm may be exhibiting *agonal ("death agony") breathing.* Agonal breathing, or agonal gasping, is not "real" breathing; that is, no physiologic exchange of gases is occurring in the lungs. Agonal gasps can be mistaken for deep breaths if the respiratory rate has not been sufficiently monitored. Agonal gasps typically occur after a long period of apnea and are often detected as rapid movement in the patient's diaphragm, jaw, or larynx. Agonal gasps occur after cardiac arrest, and the veterinarian must be alerted immediately of their presence.

The practice of manually ventilating the patient every 5 to 10 minutes during the anesthetic period is recommended. Assisted ventilation ("bagging") opens up collapsed alveoli, preventing atelectasis. Anesthetized patients tend to breathe more shallowly; combined with the weight of other internal organs on the lungs, the shallow breathing contributes to atelectasis (Box 5-1).

While administering a ventilating breath, the anesthetist should listen at the animal's mouth for any sound of air rushing past the ET tube. Some anesthetic agents, such as isoflurane, have a pungent odor, which indicates leakage if detected. If a sound is heard or the odor of gas detected, the cuff seal is incomplete. The cuff on the ET tube should be further inflated or the patient re-intubated with a larger ET tube.

Body Temperature

Body temperature is monitored before and during the anesthetic period. Monitoring every 15 minutes is common practice, although unless an esophageal thermometer probe or a rectal probe is used, this schedule may prove challenging.

In rare instances, hyperthermia may develop when inhalation anesthetics are used. Dangerously high body temperatures spontaneously manifest in patients that develop malignant hyperthermia. If the high temperature goes unnoticed, life-threatening cerebral edema can develop. Genetic predisposition may play a role in the phenomenon of malignant hyperthermia, which has been documented in humans, pigs, and dogs. If an abnormally high body temperature is detected, or if a temperature significantly higher than the preanesthetic body temperature is recorded, the anesthetic procedure should be terminated as soon as possible.

The development of hypothermia is common and a constant concern in patients undergoing general anesthesia. The following factors contribute to the decrease in body temperature:

- Anesthetic drugs relax muscles, significantly diminish the shivering response, and decrease the overall metabolic rate. Production of body heat decreases.

BOX 5-1 | Technique for Administration of a Ventilating Breath

1. The pressure relief valve is closed.
2. The reservoir bag is squeezed while the technician ensures that the manometer does not exceed 20 cm H_2O or that the chest does not exceed a normal excursion.
3. The pressure relief valve is opened.

- The surgical site is shaved, washed with soap and water, then rinsed with alcohol. Evaporation from the skin surface has a cooling effect on the body.
- Room-temperature fluids are administered.
- Cold gases are inspired.
- A body cavity may be opened, and internal organs are exposed to ambient temperatures.

Measures to prevent body heat loss should be taken, as discussed earlier.

Neurologic Parameters

Reflexes

As anesthetic depth increases, reflex activity diminishes and eventually disappears. A *reflex* is an automatic reaction to a stimulus made by the animal without conscious awareness of the reaction. These reflex actions protect the animal from harm. For example, the swallowing reflex is triggered by the presence of saliva or other matter in the pharynx. The animal swallows the material into the gastrointestinal system rather than aspirating it into the respiratory system. Most reflexes monitored during anesthesia are located around the face, eyes, and throat. The return of the reflex or increasing strength of the reflex response indicates that the level of anesthesia is becoming lighter. The technician anesthetist may monitor the following reflexes:

- Auricular (ear flick) reflex: The fully conscious animal flicks its ear when the pinna is lightly touched or tickled. The intensity of the reaction varies among individuals. If the reflex is tested in rapid succession, the reaction to the stimulus may diminish quickly. Although this reflex can persist well into a moderate level of anesthesia, its variable nature renders it somewhat unreliable. It is best to monitor all available reflexes.
- Pedal (withdrawal) reflex: When pressure is applied to a toe, the limb is withdrawn. The pressure applied should be significant. The withdrawal reflex is useful when the animal is being masked. The mask interferes with the ability to monitor other reflexes around the face. Once the pedal reflex disappears, the animal may be sufficiently anesthetized to attempt intubation.
- Palpebral (blink) reflex: The blink reflex protects the globe from injury by the eyelids quickly closing. The reflex can be elicited by lightly touching the medial canthus of the eye. The reflex disappears or is significantly diminished as the animal enters the surgical plane of anesthesia. The palpebral reflex usually returns just before the laryngeal reflex as the animal is recovering.
- Corneal reflex: The animal blinks or retracts the globe when the cornea is touched. This reflex persists well into the deep levels of anesthesia. The corneal reflex is seldom used in monitoring anesthesia; it is used more often to help assess the point of death during euthanasia.

- Laryngeal (swallow) reflex: When saliva, food, or water is in the pharynx, the epiglottis and arytenoid cartilage close the entrance to the trachea, and the animal swallows. The laryngeal reflex can also be initiated by rubbing the ventral throat. The swallow reflex must be lost in order for intubation to proceed easily.

Cats tend to retain the laryngeal reflex longer than dogs, so they need to be more deeply under anesthesia before intubation can be accomplished. If intubation is attempted too soon, the larynx may go into a spasm and remain closed. Cats also are more likely to develop laryngeal spasm than dogs during the intubation process. See Chapter 2 for a list of methods to avoid or reduce the likelihood of these spasms.

Muscle Tone

Muscles usually relax as the animal goes deeper under anesthesia. Dissociative anesthetics cause muscle rigidity; however, some muscle relaxants, such as benzodiazepines (e.g., diazepam, zolazepam), are usually added when these anesthetics are used. The most important muscles to relax are those that control the opening of the mouth. Once the mouth can be easily opened, intubation can be performed more easily.

It is important to monitor the intensity of the jaw tone during anesthesia. When jaw tone increases, the animal's depth of anesthesia is becoming lighter. The anesthetist can test the resistance to opening the mouth by carefully prying apart the upper and lower teeth with just two fingers (Figure 5-9).

Depending on the procedure being performed, jaw tone may not be available for monitoring by the anesthetist. If the animal is undergoing a dental procedure or oral surgery, a mouth speculum may be placed in the mouth to keep it open. In such cases the anal opening may be inspected because it can indicate the degree of muscle relaxation the patient is experiencing. In the conscious animal, the anal opening is closed. In general, as the animal goes deeper under anesthesia, the anal tone becomes more relaxed and the anus opens more.

FIGURE 5-9 Method for testing jaw tone involves prying the mouth open with just two of the examiner's fingers barely inserted into the mouth.

FIGURE 5-10 The eyes have rotated ventrally. This dog is in stage III (plane 2) of anesthesia.

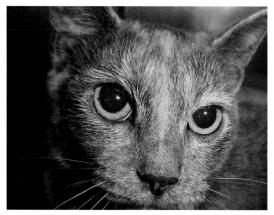

FIGURE 5-11 Glycopyrrolate and Terazol (tiletamine/zolazepam) were administered intramuscularly to this cat 15 minutes ago. Eye ointment should be applied as soon as possible to protect the eyes from drying out. Tear production and the blink reflex are diminished. Note the widely dilated pupils.

Eyes

The position of the eye in the socket, the pupil size, and the eye's responsiveness to light can be used to assess anesthesia depth. Although the responses may vary with the individual animal and the drugs given, the following general observations can be useful in assessing anesthetic depth:

- The eye rotates ventrally when the animal is in a moderate or surgical level of anesthesia (Figure 5-10).
- At light and deep levels of anesthesia, the eye is in a central position.
- When dissociative anesthetics are given, the eye position may never change (Figure 5-11).
- As the anesthetic depth increases, the pupil constricts more slowly in response to a light shined at it (pupillary light response [PLR]).
- Deeper stages of anesthesia and anticholinergic drugs cause pupillary dilation (mydriasis). The use of these drugs in the preanesthetic protocol interferes with the reliability of this reflex.

It should be noted here as well that when a patient undergoes cardiac and respiratory arrest and expires, the pupils are fully dilated.

Special Surgical Case Considerations

Although parameters to monitor for surgical patients are fairly similar for all cases, certain anesthetic complications, reactions, and considerations must be given in special situations. Young, healthy animals that are undergoing an elective procedure are still at risk for anesthetic complications, although the risk is significantly lower. Patients experiencing a trauma or a disease process pose more of a challenge. An animal that is experiencing dystocia and now requires a cesarean section is compromised differently from a patient that has been hit by a car and now requires surgery to repair a fractured tibia.

Cranial Procedures

In most surgical procedures, the eyes are available for palpebral reflex evaluation, the jaw is available for muscle tone assessment, and the eye position is evaluated throughout the procedure. Mucous membrane color and capillary refill time are monitored by means of the gingiva for appropriate monitoring. Procedures that require the surgeon to be working on or near the head present unique monitoring challenges. When surgical procedures necessitate the removal of these options, technicians must redefine the options for monitoring. Ophthalmic, aural, or mouth procedures require the anesthetist to "rethink" the approach to anesthesia monitoring—using the vulva or prepuce to monitor mucous membrane color, for example. Attaching a reflectance probe to the underside of the base of the tail instead of on the tongue is another option. Using the femoral artery for pulse assessment instead of the lingual artery is also another method to continue to effectively monitor the patient, despite obstacles to the traditional methods used.

Respiratory Compromise

Patients that are experiencing dyspnea, for whatever reason, create a challenge for the technician anesthetist. For the patient in which thoracic trauma is the source of dyspnea, the use of a ventilator extremely may be beneficial. Once the chest cavity is opened, ventilatory support needs to be provided anyway, so employing it earlier will do no harm. Patients in which abdominal issues are the cause of the respiratory compromise also benefit from ventilatory support. Pressure on the aorta, for whatever reason (gastric dilatation, gravid uterus, hemoabdomen, etc.), compromises return of venous supply as well as respiratory issues.

Patient Positioning Factors

Depending on the surgery being performed, certain necessary patient positions can create challenges for the anesthetist. Neurologic procedures that require the patient to be in ventral recumbency risk the development of respiratory problems. Animals lying on their abdomen and chest are not able to breathe as easily and effectively as if they were positioned in a different way. A patient in dorsal recumbency, with the neck in full extension or hyperextension (e.g., for thyroidectomy, ventral slot), will have respiratory issues due to the decreased ability to expand their chest. Animals undergoing perineal surgery (perineal urethrostomy, anal sac ectomy, etc.) also present a respiratory challenge. With their hind legs draped over the end of the surgery table, much pressure is on their abdominal organs and diaphragm, inhibiting normal respiratory function.

Anesthesia Monitoring Devices

The monitoring of a patient that is under the effects of anesthetic drugs is a highly involved and critically important responsibility of the veterinary technician. The veterinary technician must be willing and prepared to anticipate and troubleshoot potential problems to provide the safest anesthetic episode for the patient. Although there is no ideal monitoring device, multiple devices used together can provide useful information on the patient's status.

A well-trained, educated, sensitive, alert technician is probably the best "device." The senses of the technician are constantly relied on to monitor a patient. The technician's sense of sight can watch for changes in mucous membrane color or patient movement or changes in respirations; the sense of sound is applied to listen to heart rate and rhythm; the sense of smell can detect the presence of anesthetic gas; and the sense of touch can feel for changes in peripheral pulses indicating changes in blood pressure.

Even the best technician has limitations, however, so the use of auxiliary monitoring devices is extremely helpful. Many types of monitors are available with varying capabilities and limitations. Some monitoring devices combine multiple capabilities into one unit for convenience and optimal anesthetic evaluation.

Table 5-2 lists normal values for anesthetic monitoring of dogs and cats.

Pulse Oximeter

Pulse oximetry is based on the ability to evaluate the level of oxygen saturation in the blood to help assess tissue perfusion. Pulse oximeters also monitor pulse rates. Oxygen in the blood is carried by the hemoglobin in the red blood cells. The pulse oximeter measures how much (or the percentage) of the available hemoglobin is saturated with oxygen. This measurement is achieved using two different wavelengths of light transmitted through tissue with a pulsatile blood flow. The sensors (or probes) emit wavelengths of both red light and infrared light. The infrared light determines oxygen saturation, and the red light determines the pulse rate. The light is transmitted

TABLE 5-2 Anesthetic Monitoring: Normal Parameters for Cats and Dogs

Sao_2 (arterial oxygen saturation)	95%-99%
$ETco_2$ (end-tidal carbon dioxide level)	35-45 mm Hg
Blood pressure:	
Systolic	90-160 mm Hg
Diastolic	50-90 mm Hg
MAP (mean arterial pressure):	
Awake	85-120 mm Hg
Under anesthesia	70-99 mm Hg

through the tissue, and the photodetector (located opposite the transmitter) senses the light. The software within the unit compares the absorption ratio of the two different wavelengths. Oxygen-rich blood (arterial) absorbs less light, so more of the light wavelength is sensed by the detector; therefore a higher arterial oxygen saturation (Sao_2) reading is displayed.

Models
Some pulse oximeters are single-function units that measure only Sao_2 and pulse. Units can be small handheld versions, whereas other versions are larger and more cumbersome (Figure 5-12). Most models allow the user to set alarms for high and low limits of acceptable readings. These alarms emit an audio tone when the high or low limits of Sao_2 or pulse are reached, and they can alert the person monitoring the patient to potential problems. Other models are capable of monitoring multiple parameters, including Sao_2, heart rate, respiratory rate, and end-tidal CO_2 ($ETco_2$).

Sensors
The choice of sensor depends on the placement site and species of animal being monitored (Figure 5-13). One of the most common sensors is the lingual sensor, which resembles a clothespin in design and is available in large and small versions. Other common sensors are the reflectance probe and universal C clamp. The lingual sensor, as the name implies, is most frequently used on the tongue but can be used on the ear pinna, toe webbing, external genitalia (vulva or prepuce), or any body region with no hair. Using this probe on sites other than the tongue does cause increased pressure on the probe spring and can result in premature degradation of the probe. The reflectance probe can be used with a protective sleeve and placed in the rectum or used alone on the underside of the tail, at the base of the tail. The universal C clamp sensor can be used on feet, hocks, and other areas. Regardless of what sensor is used, certain factors can affect the efficacy of the unit and the reliability of the information. Some factors are related to patient wellness, some to

FIGURE 5-12 Basic pulse oximeters: **A and C,** handheld styles; **B,** tabletop style.

FIGURE 5-13 Pulse oximeter sensors. *Top to bottom:* Lingual sensor, reflectance probe, universal C clamp.

FIGURE 5-14 Multiparameter anesthesia monitor.

patient anatomy, and others to machine function. If at any time the information being displayed by the unit appears unreasonable, the factors listed here should be evaluated to ascertain the true status of the patient.

Unit Options

Some Sao_2 units provide only basic information, that is, a pulse rate and an Sao_2 readout. Even these basic units, however, also have a pulse bar graph to indicate the strength of the peripheral pulse being evaluated. Other models include additional information, such as noninvasive blood pressure (NIBP) monitoring, $ETco_2$ readings (capnography), and electrocardiograph (ECG) readouts (Figure 5-14). The more parameters measured by the device, the more information acquired by the anesthetist, but there is also greater potential for machine malfunction.

Troubleshooting

Maintaining an appropriate level of oxygen in the patient's blood is paramount. With a patient attached to the anesthesia machine with 100% O_2 running, the Sao_2 reading should be 95% or greater. If the reported data fall below this level, the veterinary technician needs to evaluate the situation to determine whether the machine is malfunctioning or whether in fact the patient's Sao₂ levels are dropping. Assessing the patient and the equipment quickly is important to correct the problem appropriately. Sometimes the sensor has slipped from its original position, and simply repositioning it may correct the problem. Sometimes with the lingual probe, wetting the tongue with tap water can aid in obtaining a more accurate reading. Also, it has been found that when the lingual probe is used with felines, folding the tongue can be beneficial. Folding the tongue lengthwise provides a thicker tissue mass and generally a more accurate reading. If the animal is not exchanging gases well even though a normal respiration rate is present, ventilation of the animal may need to be provided manually. Artificial ventilation helps expand the lungs more completely, thereby allowing better gas exchange.

Capnometer or Capnograph

Capnometry is the measurement and evaluation of the level of CO_2 in the patient's exhaled breath, or the $ETco_2$. This component of anesthesia is important because it can help the anesthetist evaluate the patient's respiratory rate and the quality of the respirations, therefore allowing better interpretation of the patient's depth of anesthesia. An arterial blood gas sample evaluation is the best method to determine blood CO_2 levels, but this is not usually performed in most practices. The alternative, $ETco_2$ monitoring, is an option that accurately reflects the arterial CO_2 levels.

Measurement

The capnometer can measure $ETco_2$ by one of two methods (Figure 5-15). The sensors used are either a mainstream or a sidestream device. A mainstream device evaluates the patient's CO_2 levels as the breath passes through the airway. This sensor requires the patient to be intubated and correlates to the patient's breathing pattern. A sidestream device uses a vacuum to draw a portion of the exhaled breath down a tiny tube to the main unit for evaluation. The delay in the collection of the sample translates into a displayed pattern that is "out of sync" with the patient's breathing pattern.

Display Wave

The display on the capnometer is a digital readout of the $ETco_2$. The display of a capnograph is in the form of a wave. The incline of the wave indicates the exhaled portion of a breath. The plateau at the peak height of the wave indicates the $ETco_2$ value. As the patient begins to inhale, the wave begins the decline because inspired CO_2 levels should be close to zero (Figure 5-16). Some monitoring devices are capnometers, whereas others are capnographs. Either can combine the measurement of $ETco_2$ with other monitoring parameters to provide the anesthetist with the

FIGURE 5-15 Capnograph.

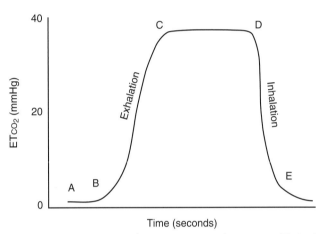

FIGURE 5-16 Capnograph tracing. *(A)* start of expiration; *(B)* dead space gas replaced by alveolar gas; *(C-D)* pure alveolar gas; *(E)* Dilution of alveolar gas by inspired fresh gas. (From Wright B, Hellyer P: Respiratory monitoring during anesthesia: pulse oximetry and capnography. Compendium 18:1083, 1996.)

most complete picture of the patient and the anesthetic episode.

Normal Values

Normal levels of expired CO_2 are 35 to 45 mm Hg for both dogs and cats. Levels that depart from the accepted range require quick, efficient evaluation by the anesthetist to determine the appropriate course of action. Values below 35 mm Hg, or *hypocarbia*, can be attributed to overzealous artificial ventilation, increased respiratory rate, too light a plane of anesthesia, pain, or hypoxia. Administering analgesics, easing up on ventilation, increasing anesthesia depth, or treating an underlying hypoxia may help resolve the hypocarbia. Values above 45 mm Hg are caused by hypoventilation, which leads to higher levels of CO_2. If more CO_2 is being produced than removed, a dangerous situation can quickly develop. *Hypercarbia* can be the result of a decreased respiratory rate, decreased respiratory minute volume, exhausted soda lime, malfunction of one of the unidirectional valves

FIGURE 5-17 Doppler unit in carrying case.

FIGURE 5-18 Concave side (the side placed next to animal) of Doppler crystal.

FIGURE 5-19 Oscillometric blood pressure monitor with a cuff placed on the metacarpus. The following measurements are indicated: systolic BP, 99 mm Hg; diastolic BP, 59 mm Hg; mean arterial blood pressure (MAP), 76 mm Hg; pulse, 57 bpm. *Inset,* Selecting an appropriately sized blood pressure cuff, the width of which should be 30% to 50% of the circumference of the extremity.

on the anesthesia machine, or a kinked endotracheal tube. Elevated CO_2 levels generally imply that some or all of the gas that was just exhaled has been rebreathed. Corrections to lower the CO_2 include checking the machine and increasing ventilation to remove the excess CO_2.

Blood Pressure Monitor

Blood pressure monitors are used to assess the blood pressure of a patient that is either awake or under anesthesia. It is important to monitor all aspects of physiology while an animal is anesthetized. Using only one monitoring device may provide information on only one parameter. Blood pressure monitors should be used in conjunction with other devices to enable the anesthetist to provide the best anesthetic care possible.

Indirect Monitoring

In private small animal hospitals, blood pressure is most often monitored by indirect methods (Figure 5-17). Doppler crystals are placed on the skin over arteries to produce an auditory assessment of pulse quality and blood pressure trends (Figure 5-18). Common arteries that are used with the Doppler crystal include the coccygeal, dorsal pedal, and digital. Theoretically any artery can be used, but these are usually the most accessible. A sphygmomanometer and a cuff can be added to the ensemble to allow estimated numeric assessment of diastolic and systolic pressures (Figure 5-19).

Noninvasive blood pressure machines, (Figure 5-20), which eliminate the need for a manual sphygmomanometer, are available. The units have cuffs that are placed on

FIGURE 5-20 A, Combination unit with blood pressure monitor and pulse oximeter. B, Blood pressure monitoring unit.

Direct Monitoring

Direct blood pressure monitoring is performed by placing a catheter in an artery and then attaching a transducer to the catheter. The transducer is connected to an oscilloscope that can display the information being received through the transducer. Usually, numeric values for diastolic pressure, systolic pressure, and mean arterial pressure (MAP) and a waveform for the pulses are displayed. This procedure is more technically challenging than indirect monitoring and requires more expensive equipment. The advantage of direct monitoring is that a "true" evaluation of the pressure can be made. With indirect monitoring, only trends can be observed because accurate numbers are not available.

Electrocardiograph

Continuous ECG monitoring of anesthetized patients provides valuable information. In addition to providing a heart rate and wave formation tracing, many ECG machines are capable of monitoring other parameters, including pulse oximetry readings, temperature, and respiratory rate. "High-end" electrocardiographs can also provide direct blood pressure monitoring options and tracing printouts. Regardless of the additional functions provided with an ECG unit, the basic ECG tracing (electrocardiogram) is a valuable source of information for the anesthetist. Continuous, or even intermittent, monitoring of the heart rate and rhythm with an ECG can alert the anesthetist to current or impending problems that may be avoided. For example, the appearance of a premature ventricular contraction (PVC) alone may be an isolated incident, but repeated multiple PVCs can be a sign of impending, severe cardiac distress. Other situations, such as atrial dysfunction (evident as changes in the P wave), myocardial hypoxia, and electrolyte disturbances (evident as changes in the T wave), can be observed with continuous ECG monitoring.

the patient, and the cuff inflation line is attached to the machine. The machine inflates the cuff at either preset intervals or manually determined intervals, the cuff is deflated, and a blood pressure measurement is acquired. The reliability of the numeric value displayed depends on the use of an appropriately sized cuff. Cuffs that are either too large or too small give inaccurate results. To ensure that the proper-sized cuff is being used, the following guidelines should be used: (1) the cuff width should be 40% of the circumference of the limb on which it is to be used and (2) the length should be appropriate so as to fall into the securing range indicated on the cuff.

KEY POINTS

1. "Light and lively" is better than "deep and dead." It is safer to keep the patient in a light to moderate plane of anesthesia.
2. Hands-on monitoring can be more reliable than mechanical device monitoring. Mechanical devices can register incorrect readings. Do not rely exclusively on mechanical monitoring devices.
3. For a full evaluation of the patient's condition and stage of anesthesia, the anesthetist should assess multiple parameters, including reflexes.
4. There is a direct correlation between progression of hypotension and progression of anesthetic depth.
5. To determine a decreasing or increasing trend in body temperature, pulse, and respiratory rate (TPR), the technician must be sure to measure these preanesthetic values of the patient. Preanesthetic TPR is invaluable information.
6. Patients undergoing long surgical procedures may need intraoperative doses of analgesia. "Turning up the gas" is often not sufficient.
7. Pulse oximeters measure the level of oxygen saturation of the blood.
8. Capnometry is the measurement of the level of exhaled CO_2; a normal reading is 35 to 45 mm Hg.
9. Blood pressure can be monitored by direct or indirect methods.

REVIEW QUESTIONS

1. How frequently should physiologic parameters be recorded in the anesthesia log during a surgery?
   a. Every minute.
   b. Every 5 minutes.
   c. Every 10 minutes.
   d. Whenever the technician has the time.

2. Which of the following contributes to hypothermia in the anesthetized patient?
   a. Anesthetic-induced muscle relaxation.
   b. The surgical prep using water and alcohol.
   c. Administering room-temperature IV fluids.
   d. All of the above.

3. Hypotension can be caused by:
   a. Increased heart rate.
   b. Vasoconstrictive drugs.
   c. Cardiac insufficiency.
   d. Patient obesity.

4. Which reflex significantly diminishes or is absent when the patient enters the surgical plane of anesthesia?
   a. Palpebral.
   b. Laryngeal.
   c. Pedal.
   d. Corneal.

5. Which class of drugs causes muscle rigidity?
   a. Local anesthetics.
   b. Anticholinergics.
   c. Dissociative anesthetics.
   d. Antibiotics.

6. Which of the following surgical procedures may create challenges for monitoring the patient owing to patient positioning?
   a. Total hip replacement.
   b. Perineal urethrostomy.
   c. Prostate biopsy.
   d. Lateral ear ablation.

7. Which monitoring device measures exhaled CO_2 levels?
   a. Pulse oximeter.
   b. Electrocardiograph.
   c. Sphygmomanometer.
   d. Capnometer.

8. A change in which wave of an electrocardiogram is likely when myocardial hypoxia is occurring?
   a. P.
   b. Q.
   c. S.
   d. T.

9. To ensure the most accurate blood pressure reading, the cuff should be what percentage of the width of the limb?
   a. 25%.
   b. 40%.
   c. 60%.
   d. 75%.

ANSWERS

1. b	4. a	7. d	9. b
2. d	5. c	8. d	
3. c	6. b		

BIBLIOGRAPHY

Edwards NJ: ECG manual for veterinary technicians, Philadelphia, 1993, Saunders.

Muir WW III, Hubbell JAE, Bednarski RM: Handbook of veterinary anesthesia, ed 4, St Louis, 2007, Mosby.

Simpson K: Let's talk about capnography. Surgivet, August 2003. Available at http://www.surgivet.com.

Thomas JA, Lerche P: Anesthesia and analgesia for veterinary technicians, ed 4, St Louis, 2011, Mosby.

Surgical Assisting—Duties during Surgery

6

Teri Raffel

LEARNING OBJECTIVES

After completion of this chapter, the reader will be able to:
- Describe the procedure for performing an instrument count.
- Describe the procedure for performing a sponge count.
- Discuss the correct method of loading and passing a scalpel blade and handle.
- Describe the techniques used to pass various types of surgical instruments safely to the surgeon.
- Discuss the role of the sterile surgical assistant as related to care of the surgical field.
- Discuss the desired method of handling tissue to avoid trauma.
- Describe the various methods of maintaining hemostasis on the operative field.
- Describe the correct procedure for draping a surgical patient.
- Discuss the various options for administering/introducing drugs onto the operative field and surgical site.
- Recognize common suture patterns.
- Describe the proper procedure for removing sutures.

Instrument Handling and Passing

Accepting sterile packs and equipment from a circulating nurse is a critical responsibility of the assistant. For a double-wrapped pack, the outer wrap should be properly unfolded by the circulating nurse and then offered to the assistant. Care must be taken so that the assistant does not contaminate himself/herself when taking the pack. When taking a peel packed item from the circulating nurse, it is equally important that the assistant be aware of the nonsterile portions of the packaging and avoid touching those areas. It bears saying that the assistant needs to be attentive to the situation when taking any sterile item from the circulating nurse. Miscommunication, a quick movement, or not securely grabbing the item can result in disaster. Either dropping the equipment or contaminating the equipment/supply would mandate a flash sterilization procedure. Worse yet, dropping the equipment/supply and having it break or be damaged as it hits the floor are a catastrophe in the operating room. The surgical assistant is responsible for properly passing the instruments to the surgeon, maintaining the instrument (or back) table, and ensuring the working order of the instrumentation throughout the procedure. Setting up and managing the instrument table allows the technician to assist the surgeon more efficiently. An organized table makes it easier for the technician to find the requested instrument quickly. Instruments should be laid out so that the ring handles (or shafts) of the instruments are closest to the assistant. Where the technician stands in relation to the table and patient dictates which direction the instruments should face.

Some technicians scrub into a procedure with the sole responsibility of managing the instrument table (e.g., for cardiovascular procedures, total hip replacements). Procedures involving extensive instrumentation and equipment greatly benefit from having a technician "run the table." At other times the technician may be required to scrub in to assist the surgeon with the procedure.

Properly passing the instruments to the surgeon is a skill that must be mastered not only for efficiency in movement but for safety as well. The shape and purpose of the instrument determines the method used to pass it safely and properly to the surgeon.

Scalpel Blades and Handles

Scalpel blades should be handled with the greatest respect. Needle holders are the only instrument that should be used to place the blade onto and to remove the blade from the scalpel handle. The use of any other instrument or device (e.g., hemostat, finger) is inappropriate and can be dangerous. Needle holders are designed to hold metal and therefore can withstand the stress of clamping a metal blade and then placing it on the handle. Hemostat tips are designed to grasp tissue or vessels and will be damaged if used to place a blade on a scalpel handle.

To load a handle with a scalpel blade, the needle holder should firmly grasp the blade on the noncutting edge and slip it onto the handle (Figure 6-1). Once loaded, the handle and blade should be passed to the surgeon in a specific manner. The technician should hold the scalpel handle with the blade facing away from the hand, with the point toward the technician (Figure 6-2). The thumb and index finger should be holding the handle with the hand in a supinated position. Pronation of the technician's hand follows as the handle is passed into the waiting hand of the surgeon (Figure 6-3). As the surgeon grasps the handle, the technician should maintain the forward momentum of the hand so as not to contact the cutting edge of the blade. This method of passing the instrument allows the cutting edge of the blade to face away from the assistant as well as the surgeon for optimal safety and handling.

Threading Eyed Needles

The needle holder should be placed at about two-thirds into the needle's curve for secure and controlled handling. The suture to be passed through the eye of the needle should pass from the inside of the needle's curve to the outside. This orientation in the eye allows the short end

FIGURE 6-2   Step 1 in properly passing loaded scalpel handle. The scalpel blade is pointed toward the assistant, with cutting edge of the blade away from the assistant's hand.

FIGURE 6-1   Loading the scalpel blade onto the scalpel handle.

FIGURE 6-3   Step 2 in properly passing loaded scalpel handle. The assistant pronates the hand and places the handle firmly in the waiting hand of the surgeon.

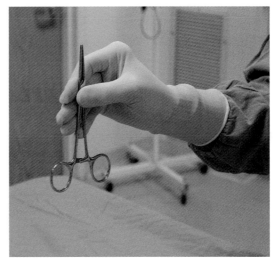

FIGURE 6-5 Proper technique for passing a straight-tip instrument.

FIGURE 6-4 Proper hand position for passing a loaded needle holder. The needle is loaded for a right-handed surgeon.

FIGURE 6-6 Proper technique for passing a curved-tip instrument.

of the suture to fall away from the outside curve of the needle, reducing the chance that the suture will pull out of the needle. When loading a needle holder with a needle and suture, whether threaded or swaged, the assistant must remember which hand is the surgeon's dominant hand. The needle and suture should be placed in the needle holder so that the surgeon can use it immediately without having to adjust the needle's position. For a right-handed surgeon, the point of the needle should face to the left, whereas for a left-handed surgeon, the needle point should face to the right (Figure 6-4). Suture used with eyed needles is most often cut from a reel or cassette. Careful technique must be used in order to avoid any contamination of the sterile field. To begin the process, the circulating nurse removes the cap from the cassette. He/she then grabs the exposed suture and pulls it straight up, exposing approximately 6 inches of suture. Care must be taken to avoid contaminating the suture by touching the inside of the cassette stopper lip. The sterile assistant or surgeon then grasps the suture *below* the level that was initially exposed. The sterile person, using a sterile operating scissors, then cuts the suture close to the hand, between his/her hand and the circulating nurse's hand. This act then allows the circulating nurse to remove the originally exposed/contaminated suture from the area. The sterile person, using a hand-over-hand motion, then pulls up as much suture as is needed. The sterile person then cuts the suture close to the cassette without contaminating the scissors.

Passing Ring-Handled and Other Instruments

When passing an instrument to the surgeon, it is important to remember to place the instrument firmly in the palm of the waiting hand to decrease the chance that the instrument will be dropped. The surgeon must know that the instrument is in hand without having to look up from the field.

The first ratchet of a ring-handled instrument should be closed before the instrument is passed. The ring handles should be facing the floor, and the tip of the instrument facing the ceiling. The box lock should be held between the assistant's thumb and index finger, with the shaft of the instrument stabilized by the remaining fingers of the delivering hand (Figure 6-5).

The technician should hold an instrument with a curved tip with the curve facing the thumb holding the instrument (Figure 6-6). When held in this fashion, after being passed to the surgeon, the instrument is positioned for immediate placement on the tissue.

When passing an instrument without ring handles, such as a thumb tissue forceps, the technician should hold it with the tips facing the floor. The other end of the instrument should be held firmly with the thumb and index finger while the remaining fingers stabilize the

FIGURE 6-7 Proper technique for passing an instrument without a ring handle.

instrument (Figure 6-7). When held in this manner, once placed in the hand of the surgeon, the instrument is ready to be used.

Tissue Handling

The careful handling of tissue in the surgical field is an extremely important responsibility of the surgical assistant. Healthy tissue needs to be handled appropriately so as not to cause trauma. Unhealthy tissue requires extreme care in handling so as not to compromise its viability further. The surgical assistant must be aware of the status of the tissue in the field and must be familiar with appropriate methods of tissue retraction. Healthy tissue may withstand the pressure of a handheld retractor, but too much pressure may cause vascular tissue damage. If too little retraction is provided, however, the surgeon will not be able to see clearly, and the procedure may be compromised. "Finding a happy medium" is the job of the surgical assistant.

When a self-retaining retractor (e.g., Balfour retractor for abdomen, Finochietto retractor for chest) is used, a moist lap pad is generally placed between the blades of the retractor and the tissue. The lap pad acts as a cushion to alleviate excessive pressure on the tissue and helps keep the tissues moist. For some situations the surgeon may choose to place stay sutures in an organ to facilitate retraction or manipulation of the organ. Assistants holding stay sutures must be careful not to hold them too firmly because of the risk of ripping the suture from the tissue.

Another situation that requires careful tissue handling is during an enterotomy or anastomosis. Often the surgeon has the assistant use his/her fingers as "clamps." After milking as much intestinal content away from the proposed intestinal incision site, the assistant will use the index and middle fingers to clamp the tissue. Care must be taken to provide adequate stabilization of the tissue without putting excessive pressure on the delicate structure.

Keeping Tissues Moist

Another important duty of the surgical assistant is to keep the exposed tissues moist. Systemic hydration should be achieved and maintained through the infusion of intravenous (IV) fluids, but the tissue must be kept moist topically as well. Generally, an isotonic solution such as lactated Ringer's solution or 0.9% normal saline is used as a lavage fluid. Depending on the surgical procedure, an antibiotic may be added to the solution for topical application.

One of the most important guidelines in surgical assisting states that "moist tissue is happy tissue." If the tissues are kept moist, rather than allowed to dry out, the circulation is less compromised and tissue function remains intact. The heat from lights and exposure to room air makes tissue vulnerable to adverse conditions.

A bowl on the sterile field can be filled with warm isotonic solution. A single gauze square can be soaked in this lavage solution, and then squeezed while suspended above the exposed tissues to drip the lavage solution onto the tissues. It is important to avoid wiping or rubbing the gauze sponge on the tissue directly. The friction created even with gentle wiping or rubbing irritates the tissue and promotes the formation of adhesions between the irritated surface of the affected tissue and other abdominal organs or body tissues. Adhesions may become problematic for the patient, requiring more surgery later to correct. The bowl containing the warm lavage solution should be kept at the back of the instrument table, preferably on a separate tray, so that if spillage does occur, there is no contamination of the sterile field. Any spilled solution remains on the tray and does not soak the covering on the table.

Maintaining Hemostasis

Maintaining hemostasis on the surgical field is also an important duty of the scrubbed-in surgical assistant. If vessels are cut, the assistant should be ready to pass the necessary hemostat. Blotting the hemorrhaging site before the surgeon places the hemostat helps the surgeon place the clamp on the vessel without including excessive tissue in the hemostat. It is important to remember that bleeding tissue should be blotted, not wiped, when trying to achieve hemostasis. Wiping with a sponge may cause coagulation already initiated to be wiped away. Firm, but not excessive, pressure blotting is more effective. The blood-soaked sponge count can serve as an estimate of blood loss. A 3 × 3–inch sponge holds approximately 6 mL of blood. A 4 × 4–inch sponge holds approximately 10 mL of blood. Ideally, only radiopaque sponges should be included in surgical packs. Less expensive, nonradiopaque sponges can be used for routine external use.

Other items available for controlling hemostasis are products such as absorbable gelatin or cellulose sponge (Gelfoam, Pfizer, New York; Surgicel, Johnson & Johnson Ethicon, Somerville, NJ) and bone wax (Figure 6-8).

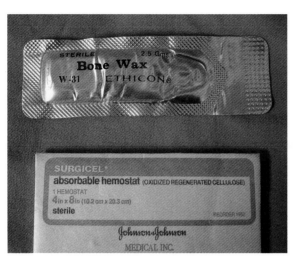

FIGURE 6-8 Bone wax and Surgicel.

FIGURE 6-9 A radiopaque sponge.

Gelfoam is gelatin sponge material that is absorbent and, when placed in a tissue defect (e.g., a punch biopsy site on the liver), encourages hemostasis by swelling to fill the defect. Surgicel is a cellulose product that, when laid on a tissue surface, promotes hemostasis by enhancing clot formation. Although Surgicel is absorbable, some sources suggest its removal after achievement of hemostasis because the product may inhibit callus formation and encourage infection. Bone wax, as the name implies, is a hemostatic agent made of beeswax and a softening agent that is used on a cut bone surface to assist with hemorrhage control. It is a poorly absorbed product and thus should be used sparingly.

Hemostasis can also be achieved by the use of electrocautery. The assistant, at the direction of the surgeon, may cauterize tissue or a vessel or may elevate the hemostat that is on the vessel so that the surgeon can activate the cautery.

FIGURE 6-10 A laparotomy pad.

Equipment Count

Instrument Count

The first duty that the surgical assistant should perform is an instrument count. An instrument count documents how many instruments are present at the outset of the procedure. Before the surgical site is closed, a second count of the instruments should be done. Most anesthesia logs have a space to record the initial surgical instrument count and the instrument and "sharps" count at closure. The circulating nurse helps the surgical assistant keep track of how many instruments (if any) were removed from the sterile field and how many sharps were used.

Sponge Count

Next, the assistant should perform a sponge count. Only radiopaque sponges should be used in surgical situations (Figure 6-9). These gauze sponges have a radiopaque string woven into the fiber that is visible on a radiograph if a sponge is inadvertently left in a patient.

The initial quantity of sponges in the pack is counted before any sponges are used. As the sponges are used, they should be discarded in a dedicated sponge bowl or kick bucket. The sponge bowl should be a basin located off the sterile field or a back table. As the sponges are discarded, the circulating nurse can unfold and count each sponge. It is important to unfold the sponges in case two or more sponges are stuck together. All sponges, whether gauze squares or laparotomy ("lap") pads (Figure 6-10), subsequently added to the sterile field must be accounted for as well.

Before the surgical site is closed, the sponges on the sterile field must be counted (by the surgical assistant) and the number of discarded sponges counted (by the circulating nurse), then totaled. The sum of these two groups of sponges must equal the number of sponges documented as entering the sterile field. If the numbers do not agree, the hunt for the missing sponge(s) begins. First, other trash receptacles in the room should be checked to see whether a sponge was discarded in an inappropriate place. If the missing sponge is not found there, the sterile team should evaluate the surgical field. Sponges may accidentally become tucked between the folds of the drapes. If the missing sponge is still not recovered, an intraoperative radiograph should be taken. If radiology is not an option, the wound should be closed and a radiograph taken in the immediate postoperative period. Using only radiopaque sponges intraoperatively aids in identifying sponges left in the patient. The incident must be thoroughly documented in the medical record in the event the sponge(s) is not recovered.

Draping—Basic Principles

Assistants are often involved with draping the patient, if not entirely responsible for this task. Draping materials can be quite varied. Some practices use cloth hand towels as the ground drape, or first layer, when draping a patient. Other larger top sheets can also be made of cloth or paper. Fenestrated drapes can be of the cloth variety or paper, but the paper option requires the surgeon to make the fenestration once the drape is opened on the sterile field. The use of ground drapes (towels) and then four top sheets is highly preferable to the use of a fenestrated drape. Linen drapes are advantageous because they can assist with patient thermal regulation better than the lightweight paper drapes. Linen drapes require laundering and refolding, a service that can be provided by an outside company or completed by the veterinary technician assistants in the practice. Paper drapes are available on bulk rolls and can be cut to custom fit the patient. Commercially prepared paper or paper/plastic combination drapes are also available. Regardless of the manufacturer, paper drapes are intended to be used as disposable, one-time-use items and should not be cleaned/laundered and reused. The type of procedure to be performed as well as the surgeon's preference influences the choice of cloth or paper. Surgical procedures expected to be very messy (cesarean section, enterotomy, etc.) may be better served by the use of disposable paper drapes.

Foundational principles regarding draping can be applied to most surgical procedures. The edges where hands are holding ground drapes should be turned over to protect sterile gloves from being contaminated by the patient's skin or hair. Sterile personnel placing drapes must also be careful to not contaminate gown sleeves or the front of the gown on the surgical table or anesthesia equipment/cables that may be near the patient. Ground towels, if used, should be placed on the patient in a specific order. The first drape is placed on the side of the patient that is closest (nearest) to the person draping. The drape for the opposite side of the patient should be placed second. A sterile person must never reach across a nonsterile field; therefore, the second drape can be placed after the sterile person walks to the other side of the table. After the two lateral drapes are placed, the cranial drape is placed. Placement of the drapes in relationship to the

FIGURE 6-11 Securing of the ground drapes.

FIGURE 6-12 Proper holding of the towel clamp.

proposed incision site depends on the veterinarian's preference and the procedure being performed. A general rule of thumb is to place the edge of the drape $\frac{1}{2}$ to $\frac{3}{4}$ inch from the incision line.

Once the cranial drape is in place, penetrating towel clamps must be used to secure the towels (Figure 6-11). Proper use and handling of the surgical instrument is imperative. The assistant's ring finger and thumb should be placed in the ring handle of the instrument. This position allows the index finger to be extended to stabilize the box lock, thereby easing the task of placing the towel clamp properly (Figure 6-12). Penetrating towel clamps are designed to pierce the skin and secure the drapes to the patient (Figure 6-13). Care must be taken to ensure that the towel clamp points have penetrated through the drape material and into the patient's skin. Towel clamps should be placed close to the intersecting corner of the two towels in order to avoid "bunching" of the drape. The fourth and final ground drape, the caudal drape, can be placed once the other three towels are secured. When placing cranial and caudal towels, in most cases, the person performing the draping must stand on the long side of the surgical table and rotate the waist and shoulder

FIGURE 6-13 Placement of the penetrating towel clamp.

FIGURE 6-15 Finished draped surgical site.

FIGURE 6-14 Placement of the nonpenetrating towel clamp.

to place the towel. The habit of draping from the short end of the table should be avoided because often access to that end is blocked by equipment (e.g., anesthesia machine) or the instrument table.

After the ground drapes have been secured, the top drape(s) should be placed. There are two options at this point for continuing the draping process. If a single fenestrated paper drape is to be used, the fenestration must be created before the drape is laid on the patient. Once the drape touches the patient, the underside is considered nonsterile and should not be manipulated. It is impossible to cut the fenestration after the drape is on the patient without contaminating the sterile field. To avoid this scenario, the fenestration should be cut, based on the basis of size of the opening created by the ground towels, before the drape is opened and placed on the patient. Once the drape (paper or linen) is on the patient, nonpenetrating towel clamps are used to secure the paper/top drape to the towels underneath. Nonpenetrating towel clamps should clamp around the neck of the penetrating towel clamp located under the paper drape (Figure 6-14). The second option for top drapes is to use four paper or linen large drapes and place them on the patient in exactly the same order the ground towels were placed. As with the fenestrated drape, these top sheets are secured to the towels underneath with the nonpenetrating towel clamps (Figure 6-15). The margins for draping a patient depend on the procedure being performed, the surgeon's preference, and the potential for extended incisions or alternate surgical sites. Communication between the assistant and the surgeon is imperative to guarantee a properly draped patient.

Drug Administration

Administration of systemic drugs is not usually a task that is handled by the surgical assistant. A nonsterile member of the team, such as the circulating nurse or the anesthetist, is usually responsible for this task. Addition analgesics, antibiotics, and cardiac medications are all examples of types of drugs that could be administered intraoperatively. A surgical assistant may be involved with drug administration if it is a medication that needs to be administered via the surgical site. Infusion of a local anesthetic and addition of an antibiotic to lavage fluid are examples of intraoperative drug administration. If a medication is to be administered by syringe and needle in the sterile field, the circulating technician must aseptically open the desired size of syringe and needle onto the sterile field. The circulating nurse then holds the bottle of medication upside down. A sterile member of the team then takes the assembled sterile syringe and needle and inserts it into the bottle. After the sterile member withdraws the desired amount of medication, it is a good idea to recap the needle, have the circulating nurse take that needle off the syringe, and open another sterile needle to be used.

Suture-Related Responsibilities

In addition to loading the needle holder, as described earlier, there are other suture-related responsibilities for the surgical assistant. One responsibility is cutting the sutures once the veterinarian has completed the suture placement. Depending on the type of sutures used (absorbable versus nonabsorbable), the length to cut the sutures varies. Absorbable sutures are generally cut quite short, leaving only ⅛ to ¼ inch of suture beyond the knot. Minimal amounts of absorbable suture are left in the patient to reduce the possibility of complications. Nonabsorbable suture is generally cut so that the suture ends extend about ½ inch beyond the knot. Suitable length is necessary to facilitate suture removal in 10 to 14 days.

Another suture-related responsibility is "running" the suture when the surgeon is placing a continuous pattern. The technician's responsibility is to keep the suture out of the incision and out of the way of the surgeon. If the path is clear, all the surgeon needs to do is place the stitches. Running the suture significantly reduces anesthesia time because the surgeon can suture much faster.

The third responsibility involving suture is recognizing suture patterns. Although closing wounds and placing sutures is not typically a skill that veterinary technicians need to master, some state Practice Acts do allow technicians to perform suturing. It is, however, essential that veterinary technicians are qualified to recognize suture patterns for various reasons. The technician must not only know what a suture line should look like but also be able to identify whether or not a suture line has been compromised (loosened sutures, missing sutures, etc.). It is also important to know the different suture patterns to appropriately remove the suture once the wound has healed.

Common Suture Patterns

Suture patterns are categorized by either the way they appose tissue edges (appositional, everting, inverting) or by the tissue layer where they are placed (subcutaneous, subcuticular, skin). Suture patterns are also named by the method of placement (interrupted or continuous).

Subcuticular versus Subcutaneous

A *subcutaneous suture pattern* is placed in the subcutaneous tissue layer. This pattern brings the skin edges into apposition but generally does not appropriately close the skin. This pattern is often used to decrease dead space in a wound, with skin sutures still being needed.

A *subcuticular suture pattern* is placed in the subcuticular space just under the skin. Often subcuticular patterns are placed to eliminate the need for skin sutures. The skin edges are close enough in apposition that further external sutures are unnecessary. This pattern may be used with canine castration incisions or cesarean section incisions or for animals that may chew at skin sutures. Most often these two patterns are placed in a continuous manner, but sometimes an interrupted pattern is indicated.

Continuous Patterns

The most frequently used continuous pattern is a *simple continuous*. Figure 6-16 shows an example of a simple continuous pattern. There is a knot at either end of the suture line and continuous suture in between. Simple

FIGURE 6-16 Simple continuous suture pattern.

FIGURE 6-17 Ford interlocking suture pattern.

continuous patterns can be employed in subcutaneous space, subcuticularly, as a skin suture on muscle layers on the linea alba or any other area where a relatively air-tight/fluid-tight apposition is needed.

The *Ford interlocking* pattern (Figure 6-17) is another continuous pattern. Though not used as frequently in small animal surgery as it is in large animal surgery, it creates a very strong suture line.

Other types of continuous patterns are Lembert, Connell, Cushing, and horizontal mattress. A Lembert pattern is an inverting pattern generally used to close a hollow organ (stomach, urinary bladder, intestine, etc.). A Connell or Cushing pattern historically was used to close hollow organs but is not used very frequently anymore. These patterns can be placed to appose tissue edges but if pulled more tightly create an inverting pattern. The differentiating factor between the two patterns is how the stitches are placed and whether or not they enter the lumen of the organ. A continuous horizontal mattress pattern can be placed in a continuous pattern but is more frequently used in an interrupted fashion.

FIGURE 6-18 Simple interrupted suture pattern.

FIGURE 6-20 Cruciate suture pattern.

FIGURE 6-19 Horizontal mattress suture pattern.

FIGURE 6-21 Vertical mattress suture pattern.

Interrupted Patterns

The *simple interrupted pattern* is probably the most frequently used suture pattern in veterinary surgery (Figure 6-18). It is an easy, quick, and versatile pattern to place. It is frequently used to close the skin, linea alba, muscle layers, subcutaneous space, and so on. It is also the pattern used to secure implants such as Penrose drains. The simple interrupted pattern results in appositional tissue edges unless excessive tension is used, in which case it results in an inverting pattern. Wound healing is poor with an inverting pattern, so care must be taken to ensure that the edges remain in apposition. The disadvantage to using the simple interrupted pattern is that it is time consuming to place as well as results in having more foreign material (suture) in the wound.

Another interrupted pattern in the *horizontal mattress*, seen in Figure 6-19. The horizontal mattress pattern is time consuming to place but is ideal in areas of tension. If pulled too tightly it will result in an everting pattern, so care must be used to keep the tissue edges appositional if that is the intention. A *cruciate pattern* (Figure 6-20) is a modification of the horizontal mattress. Once placed it results in an "X" over the wound edges.

A *vertical mattress* pattern (also called "far-far, near-near" because of how the needle is passed through the tissue) is a stronger suture pattern in areas of tension but is also time consuming to place. Its advantage over the horizontal mattress is that there are fewer incidences of unintentional everting of wound edges (Figure 6-21).

Suture Removal

When removing suture from a wound, the following instruments should be employed: a suture (stitch) removal scissors and a thumb tissue forceps. Some people like using a hemostat instead of a thumb tissue forceps, but because hemostats are intended for holding vessels, it is an inappropriate use of the instrument to have it grab suture. However, if the hemostat is not used in a surgical situation and is labeled as such ("exam room only"), then its use is permitted for suture removal. Sutures are generally removed 10 to 14 days postoperatively. If any medication has been administered that may delay healing, the suture removal date will need to be delayed. Before removal of any sutures, the incision must be inspected to ensure that healing has occurred. There should be no gaps in the incision, nor any drainage, redness or swelling.

When removing the suture from an interrupted pattern, use the thumb tissue forceps to grab one of the suture ends (tags) and gently apply tension away from the wound. Then place the hooked blade of the suture removal scissors beside the knot. With one quick motion, cut the suture and pull it out of the skin. This same method is employed until all sutures have been removed. If there is some scabbing on the wound, there will be increased discomfort for the patient. Also, if sutures have been allowed to remain in place longer than the recommended 10 to 14 days, the skin can begin to grow over the suture and bury the stitch. Removal of these sutures can be very uncomfortable for the patient and, depending on the amount of over growth, may require sedation of the patient.

For a continuous pattern, the removal process begins in the same fashion. Using a thumb tissue forceps, grab the free end of the suture at one end of the suture line and, using the hook blade of the suture removal scissors, cut the suture just next to the knot. It is unwise to pull the entire suture line through the wound because it may introduce bacteria to the entire wound. Therefore, every third or fourth stitch of the continuous pattern should be snipped, and then the shorter piece of suture pulled out. This method is also less uncomfortable for the patient. When the entire line of suture has been removed, the final stitch of the continuous pattern needs to be removed like an interrupted stitch.

KEY POINTS

1. It is the usually the surgical assistant's responsibility to perform both an instrument count and a sponge count before the procedure begins and again before the incision is closed.
2. Proper technique, for safety and efficiency reasons, must be used when passing various types of surgical instruments to the surgeon.
3. Tissue handling is a delicate process and must be properly performed by the surgical assistant.
4. Keeping exposed tissues moist intraoperatively is an essential task of the surgical assistant.
5. Effectively assisting the surgeon includes providing hemostasis on the surgical field.
6. The use of ground drapes and then four top sheets is highly preferable to the use of a fenestrated drape.
7. The edges of ground drapes where the hands are holding them should be turned over to protect the sterile gloves from being contaminated by the patient's skin or hair.
8. A sterile person must never reach across a nonsterile field; therefore, the second drape can be placed after the sterile person walks to the other side of the table.
9. Proper use and handling of the surgical instrument are imperative.
10. Communication between the assistant and the surgeon is imperative to guarantee a properly draped patient.
11. If a medication is to be administered by syringe and needle in the sterile field, the circulating nurse must aseptically open the desired size of syringe and needle onto the sterile field.
12. The technician's responsibility is to keep the suture out of the incision and out of the way of the surgeon.
13. Suture patterns are categorized by either the way they appose tissue edges or by the tissue layer where they are placed.
14. Sutures are generally removed 10 to 14 days postoperatively.

REVIEW QUESTIONS

1. Why is it important to perform an instrument count and a sponge count at the beginning and end of the procedure?

2. Which of the following methods should be used to place a scalpel blade on a scalpel handle?
   a. Thumb and index finger of the assistant's non-dominant hand.
   b. Any hemostat with secure ratchets.
   c. Needle holder.
   d. Allis tissue forceps.

3. *True* or *False:* When passing ring-handled instruments to the surgeon, the assistant should firmly place the rings into the surgeon's palm.

4. *True or False:* Rubbing or wiping a "bleeder" with a gauze square is the best means of maintaining hemostasis.

5. Why is it important to know the approximate volume of blood a sponge can absorb?

6. *True or False:* The *best* drape material is 200–thread count linen.

7. The first ground drape placed for four corner draping is on which side of the patient?
   a. The cranial side.
   b. The side closest to the person draping.
   c. The side closest to the assistant.
   d. The caudal side.

8. *True or False:* Penetrating towel clamps are used to secure drapes to the patients.

9. What does it mean when a drape is fenestrated?

10. All of the following are interrupted suture patterns except:
    a. Cruciate.
    b. Lembert.
    c. Horizontal mattress.
    d. Vertical mattress.

ANSWERS

1. If the numbers at the end of the procedure do not match the number of instruments and sponges at the beginning, it is possible that an instrument or sponge was accidentally left in the patient's body cavity and needs to be removed before closure is completed.
2. c
3. True
4. False
5. To estimate the amount of blood volume the patient lost intraoperatively.
6. False. There is no best drape material.
7. b
8. True
9. That there is a hole or an opening in the drape that will be place over the proposed incision site.
10. b

BIBLIOGRAPHY

Bassert JM, McCurnin DM, editors: McCurnin's Clinical textbook for veterinary technicians, ed 7, St Louis, 2010, Saunders.

Fossum TW, Hedlund CS, Hulse DA, et al: Small animal surgery, ed 3, St Louis, 2007, Mosby.

7

Surgical Procedures

Marianne Tear

LEARNING OBJECTIVES

After completion of this chapter, the reader will be able to:
- Understand and give a description of each surgical procedure discussed.
- Properly position patients for specific surgical procedures.
- Drape the patient for specific surgical procedures.
- Discuss the advantages and disadvantages of specific surgical procedures.
- Identify surgical instruments and supplies that may be used for specialized surgical procedures.
- Discuss surgical options for various ophthalmic conditions.
- Discuss surgical options for aural hematomas.
- Identify and prevent common complications that may arise during surgical procedures.
- Properly identify the bones and joints of the dog and cat.
- Identify different types of fractures.
- Identify the different types of fixation devices related to fracture repair.
- Discuss the different repair options for cruciate ligament rupture.
- Identify specific biopsy instruments and understand tissue preservation techniques for biopsy samples.
- Discuss minimally invasive options to general surgery, such as endoscopy, laser surgery, and laparoscopy.

KEY TERMS

Abdominocentesis
Ablation
Aerophagia
Anastomosis
Anuria
Blepharospasm
Celiotomy
Coaptation
Conjunctivitis
Cryptorchid
Crystalluria
Cystectomy
Cystostomy
Cystotomy
Cystourethrogram
Dehiscence
Disarticulation
Dysuria
Endotoxemia
Enophthalmos
Enterotomy
Entropion
Evisceration
Gastrectomy
Gastritis
Gastropexy
Gastrotomy
Hematuria
Herniation
Iatrogenic
Ileus
Insufflation
Intussusception
Ischemia
Keratitis
Lacrimation
Laparotomy
Lavage
Ligate
Malunion
Neoplasia
Non-union
Nosocomial infection
Orchiectomy
Onychectomy

Responsibilities of the Surgical Technician

During a surgical procedure the veterinarian's complete attention needs to be directed to the procedure being performed. Even the simplest of procedures can take a turn for the worse if the veterinarian is made to shift focus. The job of the veterinary technician is to ensure the vet does not become distracted or have to shift focus. To do this job, the technician must perform careful preplanning, as outlined in previous chapters. The technician should also strive to make sure that everything that could be required is ready in surgery prior to moving the animal into the surgery room.

Intraoperative duties usually involve assisting the surgeon during surgery as a "scrub nurse" (scrubbed-in, gowned, and gloved) or a circulating nurse. As a scrub nurse, the technician may give assistance for retraction of tissues, bone reduction, wound sponging, suction, and hemostasis. As a circulating nurse, the technician may give nonsterile circulating assistance. In many practices the technician may also be responsible for monitoring the anesthetized patient while acting as a scrub nurse or surgical assistant.

Being a competent surgical technician, or scrub nurse, requires (1) proficient knowledge of the surgical procedure, the surgical instruments, and aseptic and sterile techniques and (2) anticipation of the surgeon's needs.

There are too many surgical procedures to list them all in the confines of this text. The goal of this chapter is to discuss some common procedures. At the end of the chapter, laparoscopic, endoscopic, and laser procedures are covered in more depth.

Abdominal Procedures
Abdominal Exploratory Surgery

Definition

Abdominal exploratory surgery refers to surgical exploration of the abdominal cavity. Related terms include the following:

Celiotomy: Surgical incision into the abdominal cavity.
Laparotomy: Flank incision into the abdominal cavity.

Indications

Exploratory surgery may be indicated for a variety of reasons. Most often an exploratory procedure is indicated for diagnostic or curative purposes. Diagnostic purposes include obtaining surgical biopsy specimens of abdominal organs for analysis because of a chronic disease process. Curative surgery may be required because of an *acute abdomen*, a sudden onset of clinical signs associated with the abdomen. Some causes of acute abdomen can be life threatening and may require an emergency exploratory laparotomy. Common indications for abdominal exploratory surgery are abdominal masses and traumatic injury to the abdomen.

Special Instruments

A routine surgical instrument pack should be sufficient for this procedure. A Balfour abdominal retractor—a self-retaining abdominal retractor—should be available (Figure 7-1). The Balfour retractor holds the abdomen open and allows for full exposure of abdominal contents.

Balfour retractors are available in different sizes, and selection of the appropriate size is based on the size of the patient. Other special instruments may be needed, depending on the results of the abdominal exploratory surgery.

Sterile laparotomy sponges (Figure 7-2) should be available. Heated lavage fluid and suction may also be indicated.

Patient Positioning and Preparation

For abdominal exploratory surgery the patient should be positioned in dorsal recumbency for a ventral midline approach. The ventral abdomen should be clipped from just above the xiphoid process to the pubis. Adequate hair clipping is important because the incision may have to be extended either cranially or caudally for better exposure. Unless otherwise indicated, the bladder should be expressed before the animal is moved into the surgery room.

FIGURE 7-1 Balfour retractor.

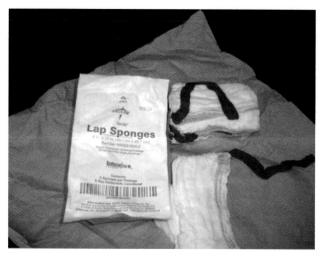

FIGURE 7-2 Sterile laparotomy (lap) sponges.

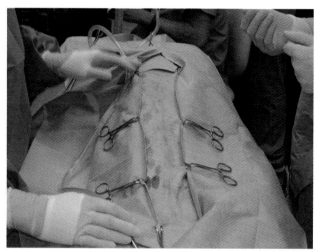

FIGURE 7-3 Four-quarter draping technique.

Patient Draping

Forany abdominal procedure, a four-quarter draping method should be considered (Figure 7-3).

Abdominal Exploratory Procedure

A blade is used to incise the subcutaneous tissues, and the abdominal wall should be tented to make a sharp incision into the linea alba. The sterile surgical assistant can moisten laparotomy sponges and place them on either side of the incision. Exposure to the air and surgical lights cause the abdominal organs to become dry. Care should be taken to ensure exposed organs remain moist and covered with sterile laparotomy sponges. The sterile surgical assistant should also take care when handling the exposed viscera; gloves or sponges used should be moistened to reduce tissue damage.

The Balfour retractor may be placed to allow full exposure of the abdominal cavity. When placing a Balfour retractor, the assistant should visualize the insertion on the side of the surgeon, and the surgeon should visualize

---

BOX 7-1   Systematic Exploration of the Abdominal Cavity

1: Explore the Cranial Quadrant

- Examine the diaphragm (including the esophageal hiatus) and the entire liver (palpate the liver).
- Inspect the gallbladder and biliary tree; express the gallbladder to determine its patency.
- Examine the stomach, pylorus, proximal duodenum, and spleen.
- Examine both pancreatic limbs (palpate gently), the portal vein, hepatic arteries, and caudal vena cava.

2: Explore the Caudal Quadrant

- Inspect the descending colon, urinary bladder, urethra, and prostate or uterine horns.
- Inspect the inguinal rings.

3: Explore the Intestinal Tract

- Palpate the intestinal tract from the duodenum to the descending colon, and observe the mesenteric vasculature and nodes.

4: Explore the "Gutters"

- Use the mesoduodenum to retract the intestine to the left, and examine the right "gutter." Palpate the kidney, and examine the adrenal glands, ureter, and ovary.
- Use the descending colon to retract the abdominal contents to the right. Examine the left kidney, adrenal gland, ureter, and ovary.

From Fossum TW, Hedlund CS, Hulse DA, et al: Small animal surgery, ed 3, St Louis, 2007, Mosby.

---

the insertion on the side of the assistant. This visualization is done to avoid entrapping any organs within the Balfour retractor.

The surgeon then performs a systematic exploration of the entire abdomen and its contents. Most surgeons have a system for exploring the abdomen and conduct the exploration the same way each time they perform the procedure. Such an approach ensures that all organs and structures are observed and a possible disease process is not overlooked. The technician should note any abnormalities seen within the abdominal cavity and record the findings in the pathology section of the surgery report (Box 7-1). A postoperative sponge count should take place prior to closure of the abdominal incision.

Abdominal Wall Closure

Surgical closure, including material is the veterinarian's preference, but the technician should have the material prepared. There are typically three layers of closure:

1. Linea alba, for strength.
2. Subcutaneous layer, to reduce dead space.
3. Skin.

Skin can be closed with a simple interrupted or continuous suture pattern or skin staples (see Chapters 1

FIGURE 7-4 These photographs were taken four hours after surgery. **A,** A celiotomy incision following routine ovariohysterectomy. **B,** A celiotomy incision following severe traction on the skin during surgery for exposure. Note the minimal redness, swelling, and drainage from incision in **A** compared with that in **B.** (From Bassert JM, McCurnin DM, editors: McCurnin's clinical textbook for veterinary technicians, ed 7, St Louis, 2010, Elsevier.)

and 6). The information on suture type, pattern, and closure layers should be included in the surgery report.

Postoperative Considerations and Instructions

The incision should be checked at least once a day for redness, swelling, or discharge; twice-daily checks would be optimal (Figures 7-4 and 7-5). This careful examination should continue until the sutures are removed—typically 10 to 14 days postoperatively. Complications from a laparotomy procedure include dehiscence, evisceration, and sepsis. *Dehiscence,* separation of all layers of an incision or wound, may occur because of suture removal by the animal or as a result of suture breakage, knot slipping or untying. The sooner the problem is detected, the less likely more severe problems will occur. Dehiscence of all layers of the incision can lead to *evisceration,* exposure of the abdominal organs (Figure 7-6). Evisceration can result in sepsis and blood loss as a result of self-mutilation of the exposed intestine. If dehiscence with or without evisceration occurs, the situation must be attended to immediately.

Animals may also begin vomiting or become inappetent. Manipulation of the viscera can lead to ileus and or pancreatitis. If vomiting or anorexia is persistent 24 to 48 hours postoperatively, intravenous fluid therapy and additional diagnostic work may be necessary.

Surgery Report

A surgery report should be completed for each surgical procedure performed at the hospital. This is valuable information for any future procedures that may be performed on the animal as well as any legal issues that could arise. The surgery report provides patient information as well as protection for the hospital. The surgery report should consist of the hospital's name; the owner's name, address, and phone number; and the patient's name, date of birth (DOB), species, breed, and hospital identification number, if applicable. A complete record of the procedure

FIGURE 7-5 Note the swelling beneath the incision on the cranial thigh of this dog. The swelling was nonpainful, and the dog's vital signs were normal. The swelling was diagnosed as a seroma. (From Bassert JM, McCurnin DM, editors: McCurnin's clinical textbook for veterinary technicians, ed 7, St Louis, Elsevier, 2010.)

FIGURE 7-6 Complete dehiscence of an abdominal incision. Note the intra-abdominal contents protruding through the incision. (From Bassert JM, McCurnin DM, editors: McCurnin's clinical textbook for veterinary technicians, ed 7, St Louis, 2010, Elsevier.)

BOX 7-2   Surgery Report: Celiotomy

Animal Hospital Name
Owner: John Doe
Address: 555 Sterling Lane
   Jupiter, NY 55555
Phone number: 555-5555
Animal Name: Sasha
Animal #: 65656501
Species: Canine
Breed: Labrador
DOB: 05/05/10
Date of Surgery: 01/03/2011
Primary Surgeon: Dr. Vet
Assistant: Nurse Scrub
Diagnosis or Preoperative Signs: Persistent vomiting and lethargy.
Surgical Procedure: Exploratory celiotomy.

Description of Surgical Procedure
Surgical Approach: A ventral midline skin incision was made extending from approximately 2 cm below the xiphoid process to approximately 6 cm cranial to the pubis. Subcutaneous tissue was bluntly dissected to expose the linea alba. The linea alba was incised to expose the abdominal cavity and viscera.
Surgical Pathology: No perforations or necrosis of the stomach were noted. All other organs were grossly unremarkable.
Surgical Procedure: The abdominal cavity was thoroughly explored for any gross abnormalities or perforations in the gastrointestinal tract. The abdominal cavity was lavaged with 3 liters of warm saline and closed routinely.
Closure:
Gastric mucosa and submucosa: 3-0 PDS in simple continuous suture pattern.
Gastric seromuscular layer: 3-0 PDS in Cushing pattern.
Linea alba: 2-0 PDS in simple continuous suture pattern.
Subcutaneous tissue: 3-0 PDS in simple continuous suture pattern.
Subcuticular layer: 3-0 Monocryl in simple continuous suture pattern.
Skin: skin staples.

performed should be recorded on this form and placed in the animal's record. Box 7-2 shows an example of a surgery report for an abdominal exploratory procedure.

Gastric Foreign Bodies and Gastrotomy
Definition
A gastric foreign body is any ingested foreign object that becomes lodged in the stomach and is unable to be digested; it may also be referred to as a "gastric obstruction." A distinction is made between *gastric foreign bodies*, which are found in the stomach, and intestinal foreign bodies, which are found anywhere in the intestines (duodenum, jejunum, ileum, or large intestine). *Linear foreign bodies* are objects that usually consist of string or thread and are seen most often in felines. With linear foreign bodies, a part of the foreign object may become lodged under the tongue or in the stomach, while the rest of the object continues through the intestines. Linear foreign bodies may cause *plication* (pleating or folding) of the intestines (Figures 7-7 and 7-8).

Indications
A primary reason to perform a *gastrotomy* (incision into the stomach) is to remove a foreign body. In dogs, foreign bodies include rocks, plastic, toys, bones, coins, corncobs,

FIGURE 7-7 Contrast radiograph detailing a linear foreign body. (From Thrall DE: Textbook of veterinary diagnostic radiology, ed 5, St Louis, 2007, Saunders.)

FIGURE 7-8 Plication of the intestines of a cat with a linear foreign body. (Courtesy Dr. J. Hauptman, Michigan State University. From Fossum TW, Hedlund CS, Hulse DA, et al: Small animal surgery, ed 3, St Louis, 2007, Mosby.)

and cassette tapes. Dogs tend to be indiscriminate eaters and eat or swallow an assortment of objects. Another indication to perform a gastrotomy is for the retrieval of full-thickness gastric biopsy specimens or removal of neoplasia. Common gastric neoplasias in dogs and cats include adenocarcinoma, lymphosarcoma, leiomyosarcoma, and leiomyoma.

Common foreign bodies in cats are trichobezoars (hairballs), string, yarn, and thread. In cats, linear foreign bodies are frequently affixed under the tongue or at the pyloric sphincter and may cause intestinal plication. If a linear foreign body is suspected, the base and underside of the tongue should be inspected for the presence of a foreign object. Younger animals are presented most often with foreign bodies because of their behavior, but an animal of any age can have a gastric or intestinal foreign body. Animals at higher risk for foreign bodies are those that have a history of foreign body ingestion or have conditions that predispose them to *pica* (craving for unnatural articles of food).

The most common clinical sign associated with a foreign body is vomiting. Vomiting may be intermittent, and some animals may otherwise act normal. Vomiting may be absent if the object is in the fundus of the stomach rather than obstructing the pyloric sphincter. Other clinical signs are lethargy, abdominal pain, anorexia, and depression. Clinical signs can be much worse if the foreign body has perforated the stomach and caused *peritonitis* (inflammation of the peritoneum).

Diagnostic testing for gastric foreign bodies should include radiographs of the abdomen. Radiopaque foreign bodies may be apparent on survey films. Many foreign bodies are radiolucent and therefore may require contrast medium to identify. One common contrast study is the barium study. The patient is administered barium orally, then a series of films is taken at predetermined intervals. Either the foreign body becomes highlighted by the surrounding barium or the barium stops moving through the gastrointestinal (GI) tract. The time required for the barium to move through the stomach and into the intestines is compared to normal gastric emptying time. If a delay in gastric emptying is noted, a foreign body may be suspected.

Radiographs should be taken immediately prior to surgery to verify the location of the object. Even if only a short time has elapsed since the initial radiographs were taken, the object may have exited the stomach and entered the intestines or even traveled as far as the colon. In that case, unless the object has sharp edges, it is usually allowed to exit without intervention. If the object has moved to the colon and needs intervention to be removed, endoscopy is the preferred technique.

Special Instruments

A general soft tissue surgical pack should be sufficient for this procedure if only a gastrotomy is required. A Balfour abdominal retractor and sterile laparotomy sponges should be available. Heated lavage fluid and suction may also be indicated.

The technician should ensure that all instruments used within the stomach are kept away from the rest of the surgical instruments. The technician and surgeon must avoid contaminating the sterile abdomen with bacteria from the stomach. A good way to approach this situation is to have a sterile towel on which all gastric instruments can be placed during the gastrotomy. Once the gastrotomy is complete, the scrubbed-in personal (scrub team) should change gloves, and those instruments should be removed from the instrument table and replaced with new, sterile instruments.

Patient Positioning

The patient should be positioned in dorsal recumbency for a ventral midline incision. The patient should be clipped and prepared for an abdominal procedure.

Patient Draping

A four-quarter draping method should be considered.

Gastrotomy Procedure

Once the patient has been positioned and prepared for surgery, a ventral midline incision through the skin, subcutaneous tissue, and linea alba is made from the xiphoid process caudal to the umbilicus. This incision may have to be extended caudally for more exposure. The surgeon should inspect the abdominal contents before proceeding with the foreign body removal. The stomach should be identified and isolated. The surgical assistant can isolate the stomach by packing it off from the rest of the abdominal contents. The surgeon then locates the area of the stomach to incise (Figure 7-9). Stay sutures are placed on either side of the proposed incision site (Figure 7-10). Stay sutures allow for manipulation of the stomach and prevent leakage of gastric fluid into the abdomen. A stab

FIGURE 7-9 Placement of stay sutures in the gas-distended stomach of a dog with a gastric foreign body.

FIGURE 7-11 Removal of gastric foreign body (peach pit).

FIGURE 7-10 Gastrotomy incision is made between the stay sutures. Note that stay sutures are gently lifted upward to avoid leakage of gastric fluid.

incision is made with a new scalpel blade (not the same one used to make the initial skin incision) between the stay sutures, in a hypovascular region of the ventral stomach. The surgical assistant should have the suction ready to place into the stab incision and drain the gastric fluid. The surgeon then extends the incision with Metzenbaum scissors. An Allis tissue forceps can generally be used to grasp the foreign body and remove it from the stomach (Figure 7-11).

Stomach and Abdominal Wall Closure

The stomach can be closed in two layers. The first layer is a simple continuous pattern of a 2-0 or 3-0 absorbable suture. This suture pattern provides apposition. The second layer is a continuous inverting pattern of 3-0 absorbable suture. It may be beneficial to perform a local lavage of the gastric incision site to help dilute any pollutants. The gloves of the scrub team should be changed, and all instruments that were used within the stomach should be removed from the table. Any instruments used to close the abdomen should be instruments that were kept out of the stomach during surgery. A warm lavage

of the entire abdomen should be performed, and the abdomen is closed routinely.

Postoperative Considerations and Instructions

One postoperative goal for gastrotomy patients is to correct any prior fluid loss or electrolyte imbalance. If the patient continues to vomit after surgery, food and water should be withheld and intravenous fluids should be continued. A centrally acting antiemetic can be administered to help control the vomiting. In the absence of vomitus, a bland diet can be introduced 12 to 24 hours postoperatively. Prognosis for the gastrotomy patient should be considered good if there were no perforations in the stomach from the foreign body. If perforations were evident, and peritonitis was present, the prognosis may be considered guarded. Box 7-3 shows an example of a surgery report for a gastrotomy.

Intestinal Foreign Bodies and Enterotomy

Definition

Foreign bodies of the intestines are any intraluminal obstruction of intestinal contents caused by an ingested object or objects; these bodies may also be referred to as "intestinal obstructions."

Indications

A primary indication to perform an *enterotomy* (incision into the intestines) is to remove a foreign body. Some foreign bodies have the ability to pass through the esophagus and stomach but are too large to pass through the intestines. The objects found in dogs and cats as gastric foreign bodies can also be found in the intestines (e.g., corncobs, balls, bones, peach pits, linear objects such as string). Intestinal foreign bodies may cause a partial or complete obstruction of the intestinal bowel. Some foreign bodies may slowly make their way through the intestinal tract, causing damage or perforations along the way. Others may become lodged in a segment of intestine where they cause a complete obstruction. A complete obstruction prevents intestinal chyme

BOX 7-3 Surgery Report: Gastrotomy

Animal Hospital Name
Owner: John Doe
Address: 555 Sterling Lane
  Jupiter, NY 55555
Phone number: 555-5555
Animal Name: Sasha
Animal #: 65656501
Species: Canine
Breed: Labrador
DOB: 05/05/10
Date of Surgery: 01/03/2011
Primary Surgeon: Dr. Vet
Assistant: Nurse Scrub
Diagnosis or Preoperative Signs: Gastric foreign body.
Surgical Procedure: Gastrotomy.

Description of Surgical Procedure
Surgical Approach: A ventral midline skin incision was made extending from approximately 2 cm below the xiphoid process to approximately 6 cm cranial to the pubis. Subcutaneous tissue was bluntly dissected to expose the linea alba. The linea alba was incised to expose the abdominal cavity and viscera.
Surgical Pathology: Foreign bodies (tennis ball remnants) were present in the stomach. No perforations or necrosis of the stomach was noted. All other organs were grossly unremarkable.
Surgical Procedure: The abdominal cavity was thoroughly explored for any gross abnormalities or perforations in the gastrointestinal tract. Stay sutures were placed in the stomach using 3-0 PDS. The stomach was gently retracted from the abdominal cavity, where an incision approximately 5 cm long was made over a relatively avascular area of the gastric body between the greater and lesser curvatures of the stomach. All foreign material was removed from the stomach. The abdominal cavity was lavaged with 3 liters of warm saline and closed routinely.
Closure:
Gastric mucosa and submucosa: 3-0 PDS in simple continuous suture pattern.
Gastric seromuscular layer: 3-0 PDS in Cushing suture pattern.
Linea alba: 2-0 PDS in simple continuous suture pattern.
Subcutaneous tissue: 3-0 PDS in simple continuous suture pattern.
Subcuticular layer: 3-0 Monocryl in simple continuous suture pattern.
Skin: Skin staples.

(intestinal contents) to proceed beyond the obstruction. A partial obstruction may allow some intestinal contents to move beyond the point of the foreign object.

The most common clinical signs associated with an intestinal foreign body include abdominal pain, vomiting, diarrhea, depression, anorexia, and weight loss. The location (proximal vs. distal), type (partial vs. complete), and duration of the obstruction can be related to the clinical signs. Complete obstructions cause more acute and serious signs. More proximal obstructions may cause persistent vomiting and dehydration. Clinical signs of distal (e.g., ileum) and partial obstructions may include lethargy, intermittent anorexia, and intermittent vomiting.

Linear foreign bodies can manifest any or all of these clinical signs. A portion of the linear foreign body may become embedded at the base of the tongue or pylorus, while the rest of the object moves down the intestinal tract due to peristaltic movement. Continuous peristalsis and resultant *plication* of the intestines (folding or bunching up of the intestines on themselves along the length of the linear foreign body) can cause the linear foreign body to be pulled tightly. This tightly pulled string now acts as a knife along the compromised intestinal tissue and cuts into the mucosa of the intestines, causing perforations along the way. The damage to the mucosa and the perforations can result in peritonitis. The intestinal plication and peritonitis cause great abdominal pain. When the abdomen is palpated on a patient with plicated intestines and peritonitis, the abdominal muscles frequently tighten, indicating abdominal pain.

Another indication to perform an enterotomy is collection of a biopsy specimen from an intestinal segment. Malignant intestinal tumors are common and can cause partial or complete obstruction. The different types of intestinal neoplasias are mentioned in the following section on intestinal resection and anastomosis.

Special Instruments
A general use soft tissue surgery pack in conjunction with Doyen intestinal clamps will be needed for an enterotomy.

FIGURE 7-12 Doyen clamps. These intestinal clamps are considered nontraumatic to the intestines.

FIGURE 7-13 Midjejunal intestinal foreign body in a dog.

The Doyen clamps allow the surgeon to clamp the intestines on either side of the incision site (Figure 7-12). Doyen clamps are considered nontraumatic and prevent intestinal contents from leaking into the abdomen while the procedure is performed. If Doyen clamps are unavailable, the fingers of the assistant can serve the same purpose. If they do, it is important to make sure that the assistant's gloves are moist to prevent tissue trauma. Sterile laparotomy sponges should be available. Heated lavage fluid and suction may also be indicated.

The surgical assistant must ensure that all instruments used within the intestines are kept away from the rest of the surgical instruments. This practice aids in avoiding contamination of the abdomen with intestinal bacteria. All instruments used in the intestines should be placed on a sterile towel during the enterotomy and then removed from the instrument table once the intestines are closed. The other option is to have an instrument set solely used for the GI tract, then replaced with a clean set after the intestinal closure. Once the enterotomy is complete, all scrubbed personnel should change gloves, and a new set of instruments can be introduced for closure of the abdomen. A Balfour retractor should also be available for better exposure of the abdomen.

Patient Positioning
The patient should be positioned in dorsal recumbency to perform a ventral midline incision. The patient should be clipped and prepared for an abdominal procedure.

Patient Draping
A four-quarter draping method should be considered for an enterotomy.

Enterotomy Procedure
The skin, subcutaneous tissue, and linea alba can be incised from the xiphoid process to just cranial to the pubis. Once the abdominal cavity is opened, moistened

FIGURE 7-14 The normal intestine is pink with visible vessels and motility. Note the difference in color between the normal intestine (**A**) and the devitalized segment of bowel (**B**). (From Bassert JM, McCurnin DM, editors: McCurnin's clinical textbook for veterinary technicians, ed 7, St Louis, 2010, Elsevier.)

lap sponges can be placed on either side of the body wall, and a Balfour may be inserted for maximum exposure. A full exploratory procedure should be performed before an enterotomy is begun. The GI tract should be examined completely. Once the intestinal foreign body is located (Figure 7-13), the affected intestine can be isolated from the abdomen by being packed off with lap sponges.

The surgeon needs to decide, from an analysis of the intestine, whether an enterotomy or a resection and anastomosis should be performed. If necrosis or perforations of the intestinal segment are absent, an enterotomy may be sufficient (Figure 7-14). The intestinal contents should be milked away from the foreign body site. Doyen clamps or the fingers of an assistant can be placed a few

FIGURE 7-15 Enterotomy incision performed at the antimesenteric border of the jejunum. The incision is made over the distal aspect of the foreign body.

FIGURE 7-16 Removal of an intestinal foreign body (cloth) in jejunum of a dog.

FIGURE 7-17 Partial-thickness closure of a jejunal enterotomy site in a dog.

FIGURE 7-18 Complete closure of the jejunal enterotomy site using absorbable suture material in a simple interrupted suture pattern.

centimeters away on either side of the proposed enterotomy. The enterotomy incision should be made just distal to the foreign body on the *antimesenteric border* (the side of the intestine without the attached mesentery) of the intestine (Figure 7-15). This region is selected because the viability of the intestines proximal to the foreign body may be in question, and it is preferable to suture healthy intestine. The incision may need to be extended with Metzenbaum scissors to allow the removal of the foreign body (Figure 7-16). Forceps or gloved fingers may be useful in grasping and slowly removing the object.

Intestine and Abdominal Wall Closure

Once the foreign body is removed, the enterotomy incision can be closed (Figures 7-17 and 7-18). An absorbable monofilament taper point suture in a simple interrupted suture pattern may be used to close the incision. Multifilament suture should never be used in the GI tract; the braid of the suture can act as a wick for bacteria. A local

lavage of the enterotomy site is warranted as is a warm abdominal lavage of the entire abdomen. All scrubbed personnel should change gloves, and the instruments used to perform the enterotomy should be placed aside. Clean instruments (those not used in the intestines) should be used to close the layers of the abdominal cavity. The abdominal cavity can be closed routinely.

Postoperative Considerations and Instructions

One postoperative goal for enterotomy patients is to correct any previous fluid loss or electrolyte imbalances. The owner should be informed of possible complications that could arise postoperatively. Complications include necrosis and perforations of the bowel, as well as leakage and dehiscence of the intestines. All these complications can lead to peritonitis. The prognosis for a patient with peritonitis may be considered "guarded." If a simple enterotomy was performed and the bowel appeared healthy intraoperatively, a good prognosis can be given. Early identification of an intestinal foreign body is important for a positive outcome. Box 7-4 shows an example of a surgery report for an enterotomy.

BOX 7-4   Surgery Report: Enterotomy

Animal Hospital Name
Owner: John Doe
Address: 555 Sterling Lane
    Jupiter, NY 55555
Phone number: 555-5555
Animal Name: Sasha
Animal #: 65656501
Species: Canine
Breed: Labrador
DOB: 05/05/10
Date of Surgery: 01/03/2011
Primary Surgeon: Dr. Vet
Assistant: Nurse Scrub
Diagnosis or Preoperative Signs: Intestinal foreign body.
Surgical Procedure: Enterotomy.

Description of Surgical Procedure
Surgical Approach: A 15-cm ventral midline incision was made from the umbilicus to the pubis through the skin, subcutaneous tissues, and linea alba.
Surgical Pathology: All abdominal organs were examined. A foreign body was palpable at the proximal jejunum region. All other organs were unremarkable.
Surgical Procedure: A 4-cm incision was made through the antimesenteric border of the proximal jejunum at the distal end of the foreign body. The area was packed off with lap sponges to protect the abdomen from any intestinal spillage. A stocking material (approx. 12 cm long) was removed through the enterotomy incision. The incision was closed with 3-0 PDS in a simple interrupted appositional suture pattern. The abdomen was lavaged with warm sterile saline. The enterotomy site was surrounded with omentum and replaced into the abdomen.
Closure:
Linea alba: 2-0 PDS in simple interrupted suture pattern.
Subcutaneous: 3-0 Monocryl in simple continuous suture pattern.
Skin: 3-0 nylon in simple interrupted suture pattern.

BOX 7-5   Characteristics of Intestinal Devitalization

- Lack of motility
- Discoloration: black, green, gray
- Severe thinning of the visceral wall
- Lack of bleeding on cut section
- Lack of fluorescein dye uptake
- Lack of Doppler blood flow

Modified from Bassert JM, McCurnin DM, editors: McCurnin's clinical textbook for veterinary technicians, ed 7, St Louis, 2010, Elsevier.)

Intestinal Resection and Anastomosis

Definition

Intestinal resection and anastomosis (R and A) is the excision of a segment of bowel followed by the reestablishment of the two remaining segments.

Indications

A primary indication for performing an intestinal resection and anastomosis is to remove a section of dead or diseased bowel. Box 7-5 lists the characteristics of devitalized intestinal tissue. Causes of devitalized bowel include foreign bodies, neoplasia, intussusception, necrosis, and ischemia. Ischemia or necrosis of the intestines can lead to peritonitis and a poor prognosis. Peritonitis is an inflammatory process that involves the serous membrane of the abdominal cavity. Leakage of GI contents is a main source of peritonitis.

As previously mentioned, common clinical signs associated with foreign bodies of the intestinal tract include vomiting, lethargy, abdominal pain, anorexia, and depression. Common clinical signs of neoplasia of the intestinal tract include vomiting, weight loss, flatulence, and melena. If an intestinal leakage has occurred and peritonitis is present, some common signs are abdominal pain, vomiting, shock, fever, and tachycardia.

Diagnostic tests should include radiographs and ultrasound (if available) of the abdomen as well as a complete blood analysis. If peritonitis is suspected and an abdominal effusion is identified in the abdomen, an *abdominocentesis* (puncture of abdominal cavity to obtain fluid) should be performed to determine the type of fluid present. Presence of bacteria in the abdominal fluid indicates a possible GI leak.

Special Instruments

A general use soft tissue surgical pack will be needed for the R and A procedure. A Balfour retractor will aid in abdominal exposure. Doyen clamps should be available for holding off intestinal contents. If Doyen clamps are unavailable, the fingers of an assistant can be used. Sterile laparotomy sponges should be available. Heated lavage fluid and suction may also be indicated.

As with enterotomy, the scrub team wants to avoid contaminating the abdominal cavity with intestinal contents, so sufficient laparotomy sponges should be available to pack off the intestinal segment. The scrub team will need to change their gloves as well as the instrument pack before closure of the abdomen.

Patient Positioning

The patient should be positioned in dorsal recumbency to perform a ventral midline incision. The patient should be clipped and prepared for an abdominal procedure.

Patient Draping

A four-quarter draping method should be considered for the R and A procedure.

Intestinal Resection and Anastomosis Procedure

A ventral midline abdominal incision from the xiphoid process to the pubis should be made so that a full exploratory laparotomy can be performed. Moistened lap sponges can be applied to either side of the incision, and a Balfour retractor may be placed for better abdominal exposure. A full examination of the GI tract should be performed. The segment of diseased bowel should be identified, exteriorized, and packed off with lap sponges (Figure 7-19).

The surgeon needs to assess the viability of the intestinal segment in question. The presence of peristalsis, vascular pulses, and intestinal color may aid in determining intestinal viability. If the intestinal segment is questionable, it may be the surgeon's preference to resect that region. Neoplasia and necrosis of the intestines are conditions that would require resection. The blood vessels from the mesentery to the intestinal segment need to be ligated and transected. The intestinal contents (chyme) should be milked away from the area to be resected. The diseased region can be clamped with a crushing forceps (e.g., Carmalt). The area of the intestines to remain can be clamped with Doyen clamps, which are considered nontraumatic and should be gentle on the intestinal tissues. If Doyen clamps are unavailable, the moistened fingers of an assistant will provide the same function.

The surgeon then transects the intestines with a scalpel blade along the outside of the Carmalt forceps, and the intestinal segment along with the forceps is removed. A few millimeters of healthy tissue should be removed with the diseased segment to ensure that the anastomosis site is closed with healthy intestine (Figure 7-20).

Intestine and Abdominal Wall Closure

The technician holds the two segments of intestine close to each other so that they are aligned correctly. A single-layer, simple interrupted suture pattern is frequently used for an end-to-end anastomosis because it produces minimal stenosis or leakage and heals rapidly. A 3-0 or 4-0 monofilament absorbable suture should be used for the anastomosis site.

After the anastomosis has been completed, sterile saline can be injected into the surgical site to check for any leakage from the suture site (Figure 7-21). The intestines should be moderately distended with fluid while maintaining intestinal occlusion. Additional sutures can be placed in the event that leakage occurs. The mesenteric defect should then be closed in a simple continuous or interrupted suture pattern (Figure 7-22). If peritonitis was present, a closed suction drain may need to be placed to allow drainage of the abdominal cavity. A local lavage of the anastomosis site as well as a full abdominal lavage with warm saline should be performed in the event that leakage of the intestinal contents has occurred. If peritonitis was present, specimens for bacterial culture of the abdomen should be obtained before closure. The anastomosis site should be wrapped with omentum before closure. The scrub team needs to change gloves and the instrument pack to close the abdomen. The abdomen should be closed routinely.

Postoperative Considerations and Instructions

Animals found to have peritonitis during the procedure are usually more critical cases and will need more supportive postoperative care. If the patient is debilitated, IV nutrition may be warranted. IV antibiotics and fluids should be continued. Peritonitis has a high rate of morbidity, and this should be explained to the owner. The patient's clinical signs should be closely monitored postoperatively. Any signs of depression, vomiting, fever, abdominal pain or tenderness, or discharge from the incision site could be the result of a dehiscence of the intestinal suture and the presence of peritonitis. Other complications associated with intestinal surgery are leakage of the surgical site, stenosis of the intestinal lumen, perforation, and death. A large intestinal resection can lead to short-bowel syndrome. The clinical signs of short-bowel syndrome include malnutrition, weight loss, and diarrhea. Treatment of short-bowel syndrome is based on the clinical signs but includes correction of fluid loss and electrolyte imbalances.

Nutritional support must be provided until the intestines adapt. Prognosis for the patient receiving an intestinal resection and anastomosis can be considered good if peritonitis was absent and removal of large amounts of intestine was averted. The healing process of the intestines is generally rapid but can be interrupted by associated factors, such as debilitation of the patient. Prognosis of the patient with peritonitis should be considered

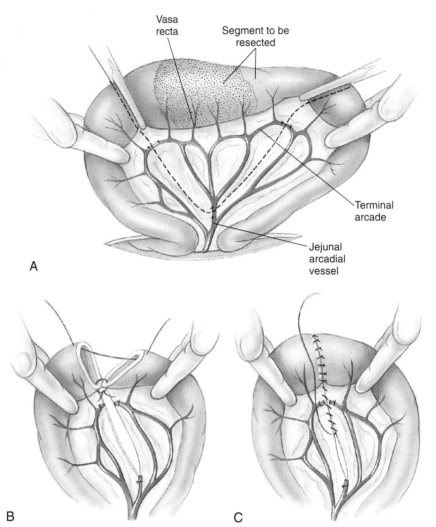

FIGURE 7-19 Jejunal resection and anastomosis. **A,** Carmalt forceps are placed on the region to be resected to avoid leakage of intestinal chyme. Fingers are used as Doyen clamps to help prevent leakage as well. Mesenteric vessels (jejunal arcadial and terminal arcade vessels) are ligated. **B,** After ligation, the mesenteric vessels are transected. Diseased portion of bowel is removed, and interrupted sutures are placed, starting at mesenteric border first. **C,** Additional interrupted sutures are placed at the antimesenteric border and continued around the bowel segment until the anastomosis is complete. (From Fossum TW, Hedlund CS, Hulse DA, et al: Small animal surgery, ed 3, St Louis, 2007, Mosby.)

FIGURE 7-20 The two segments of bowel are held appositional to each other to begin the anastomosis.

"guarded." Box 7-6 shows an example of a surgery report for an intestinal resection and anastomosis.

Gastric Dilatation and Volvulus

Definition

Gastric dilatation and volvulus (GDV) refers to the swelling (specifically gaseous distension) and rotation of the stomach on its mesenteric axis. *Dilatation* is the stretching of an organ beyond its normal dimensions. *Volvulus* refers to the rotation of an organ. A small animal patient can have gastric dilatation without the volvulus, commonly referred to as a "simple gastric dilatation." The generic term "bloat" does not distinguish between a simple gastric dilatation and gastric dilatation with a volvulus.

BOX 7-6   Surgery Report: Intestinal Resection and Anastomosis

Animal Hospital Name
Owner: John Doe
Address: 555 Sterling Lane
    Jupiter, NY 55555
Phone number: 555-5555
Animal Name: Sasha
Animal #: 65656501
Species: Canine
Breed: Labrador
DOB: 05/05/10
Date of Surgery: 01/03/2011
Primary Surgeon: Dr. Vet
Assistant: Nurse Scrub
Diagnosis or Preoperative Signs: Intestinal foreign body.
Surgical Procedure: Intestinal resection and anastomosis, exploratory laparotomy.

Description of Surgical Procedure
Surgical Approach: A 20-cm ventral midline incision was made through the skin from the xiphoid process to the pubis. The incision was carried through the underlying subcutaneous tissues and linea alba.
Surgical Pathology: A purulent and serosanguineous discharge oozed out of the tissues when the incision was made. Approximately 200 mL of serosanguineous fluid was removed from the abdominal cavity. The mesentery and omentum were grossly inflamed. A foreign body was located mid-jejunum. The region of intestines where the foreign body was located was inflamed and thickened. Perforations were evident at the mesenteric border of the jejunum. The rest of the bowel and the abdomen were unremarkable.
Surgical Procedure: The abdomen was explored and the entire length of bowel examined. The affected portion of the jejunum was exteriorized and the abdominal cavity packed off with lap sponges. Approximately 5 cm of grossly normal jejunum was resected proximal and distal to the abnormal segment. First, the appropriate jejunal mesenteric vessels were double-ligated with 3-0 PDS and divided between the ligations. Intestinal contents were milked away from the surgical site. Crushing forceps was placed across the small intestines about 2 cm from the proposed site of transection of the intestine. The intestine was transected between each set of crushing and Doyen forceps with a scalpel. The mesentery attached to the resected portion of the bowel was incised, and the abnormal jejunum was completely removed from the surgical site. The bowel edges were apposed with 4-0 PDS in a simple interrupted suture pattern, beginning first at the mesenteric border and taking bites through the submucosal layer. The mesentery was apposed with 4-0 PDS in a simple continuous suture pattern. The abdomen was thoroughly lavaged with sterile saline. Aerobic and anaerobic cultures were collected of the abdomen. A closed suction drain was placed through the skin and into the cranial abdomen. The external portion was attached to the skin with 3-0 nylon. The abdomen was closed routinely.
Closure:
Linea alba: 0 PDS in simple interrupted suture pattern.
Subcutaneous tissues: 2-0 PDS in simple continuous suture pattern.
Subcuticular layer: 3-0 Monocryl in simple continuous pattern.
Skin: 3-0 nylon in simple interrupted suture pattern.

FIGURE 7-21 **A,** To check for leaks after intestinal anastomosis, the intestine is occluded on either side of the incision, and the occluded segment of intestine is filled with sterile saline. **B,** The incision is checked for leakage while the segment is filled with saline. (From Bassert JM, McCurnin DM, editors: McCurnin's clinical textbook for veterinary technicians, ed 7, St Louis, 2010, Elsevier.)

FIGURE 7-22 Completed anastomosis of the jejunum.

FIGURE 7-23 Nine-year-old German Shorthair Pointer with gastric dilatation and volvulus (GDV). Note the severely distended abdomen that protrudes past the rib cage.

BOX 7-7	**General Treatment of Gastric Dilatation and Volvulus**

1. Decompression of the stomach.
2. Correction of fluid and electrolyte imbalances, correction of arrhythmias, and treatment for shock in most cases.
3. Correction of the malpositioned stomach and partial gastrectomy of devitalized tissue if warranted.
4. Gastropexy procedure, which involves surgically attaching the stomach to the body wall to prevent future gastric dilatation and volvulus (does not prevent future bloat).

Indications

GDV is considered a true surgical emergency. Box 7-7 summarizes the common treatment for GDV.

GDV usually occurs in deep-chested, large-breed animals but is sometimes seen in smaller breeds and rarely in cats. A GDV may occur at any age but is generally noted in middle-aged to older dogs. The precise etiology of GDV is unknown, but many cases occur after ingestion of a large meal followed by strenuous exercise. Diet, amount of food ingested, frequency of feeding, feeding behavior, and exercise after a meal may all be contributing factors to the development of GDV. Other contributing factors include anatomic predisposition, ileus, trauma, primary gastric motility disorders, vomiting, and stress. The classic clinical sign of GDV is severe abdominal distension past the rib cage (Figure 7-23). Other signs include restlessness, hypersalivation, abdominal pain, nonproductive attempts to vomit (retching, "dry heaving"), and signs of shock.

The first step in the correction of GDV is to stabilize the patient and reverse shock. Compression of vessels by the distended abdomen decreases venous return to the heart (effectively reducing vascular volume) and cardiac output, thus initiating shock; if left untreated, these animals will die from cardiac collapse. Two large-bore IV catheters should be placed in either the cephalic or jugular veins. Venous return is compromised in the caudal half of the animal so catheters placed there will not be useful. IV fluids should be administered if shock is present. Oxygen

FIGURE 7-24 Before a stomach tube is passed, the length of tube to be passed is marked by measuring from the nose to the last rib. (From Bassert JM, McCurnin DM, editors: McCurnin's clinical textbook for veterinary technicians, ed 7, St Louis, 2010, Elsevier.)

should be available and should be administered if respiratory distress is evident.

The second step in the correction of GDV is to decompress the stomach to allow gas to escape. The gas is most likely associated with one of the following: aerophagia (habitual swallowing of air), bacterial fermentation (with associated carbon dioxide production), or metabolic reactions. The gastric gas is unable to escape through normal physiologic means, such as vomiting or eructation, because the esophageal and pyloric sphincters are often twisted or rotated closed. The technician needs to choose an appropriately sized orogastric tube in correlation with the animal's size. The tube should be measured from the point of the nose to the xiphoid process (Figure 7-24). Tape can be applied to the tube to mark the appropriate length. A roll of tape placed between the upper and lower canine teeth can be used as a mouth gag to hold the

FIGURE 7-25 A roll of tape (pictured) or a mouth gag can be used to hold the mouth open while a stomach tube is passed. The assistant should hold the mouth gag in place by holding the mouth shut around the gag. (From Bassert JM, McCurnin DM, editors: McCurnin's clinical textbook for veterinary technicians, ed 7, St Louis, 2010, Elsevier.)

FIGURE 7-26 Placement of orogastric tube in a German Shorthair Pointer with GDV. Note the roll of tape between the upper and lower jaws for easier placement of the tube.

patient's mouth open for placement of the stomach tube (Figure 7-25). Lubricant can be applied to the end of the tube for easier passage. The tube can be placed through the hole of the tape roll and down the esophagus (Figure 7-26). Sedation may be required to help keep the animal relaxed and manageable. Damage to the esophagus can occur if the tube is aggressively forced down the esophagus.

Once air has been removed from the stomach, the stomach should be lavaged with warm water to help remove any gastric contents. If attempts to pass the stomach tube are unsuccessful, percutaneous decompression with a trocar can be attempted. A 14-, 16-, or 18-gauge needle or catheter can be inserted through a quickly clipped and prepared body wall and into the stomach. This allows the evacuation of gas and relieves pressure on the vessels. It is imperative to pinch the gastric tube before removing it; failure to do so can result in aspiration of stomach contents.

The patient should be taken to surgery to correct the position of the stomach as soon as stabilization has been accomplished. The volvulus of the stomach hinders gastric blood flow and can cause necrosis of the stomach tissue. Timely treatment of GDV can produce survival rates approaching 85%.

Special Instruments

A general use soft tissue surgical pack should be sufficient for GDV surgery. A Balfour abdominal retractor, Army-Navy retractors, and extra towel clamps should be available. An appropriately sized orogastric tube is needed for intraoperative decompression of the stomach. Sterile laparotomy sponges should be available. Heated lavage fluid and suction may also be indicated.

Patient Positioning

The patient should be positioned in dorsal recumbency to allow a ventral midline incision to be made. The abdomen should be clipped from mid-thorax to the pubis. Adequate cranial clipping is important so that the surgeon can extend the incision as needed. Rotation of the stomach back to its normal position can be difficult if the proper exposure is not achieved. The entire abdomen should be clipped to allow a full abdominal exploratory surgery. The lateral aspects of the abdomen should be clipped as well, in the event that placement of a gastric feeding tube is warranted.

Patient Draping

A four-quarter draping method should be considered for the GDV procedure.

Procedure for Treatment of Gastric Dilatation and Volvulus

The surgeon makes a ventral midline incision from the xiphoid process to just caudal to the umbilicus. This incision can be extended for the exploratory procedure if necessary. Moistened laparotomy sponges should be placed on either side of the incision site, and a Balfour retractor may be positioned for better abdominal exposure. Upon entry into the abdominal cavity, the first structure noted is the greater omentum, which usually covers the dilated stomach during a GDV. Blood may be evident in the abdomen, usually from rupture of the short gastric vessels. An orogastric tube should again be passed through

FIGURE 7-27 The stomach of a dog with GDV generally rotates in a clockwise direction. (From Fossum TW, Hedlund CS, Hulse DA, et al: Small animal surgery, ed 3, St Louis, 2007, Mosby.)

the mouth, down the esophagus, and into the stomach to allow decompression of gas and the release of gastric contents. A warm gastric lavage should be performed until the contents from the stomach are emptied and the lavage water collected is clear.

The surgeon then attempts to rotate the stomach back to its original position. Most stomachs twist or rotate in a clockwise direction and can rotate 90 to 360 degrees (Figure 7-27). Correction of the malpositioned stomach usually involves rotation in a counterclockwise direction. The surgeon grasps the stomach at the pylorus region with the right hand and the greater curvature of the stomach with the left hand. The greater curvature is pushed downward toward the floor while the pylorus is lifted up on. This procedure should return the stomach to its original placement. The stomach should then be explored for necrosis. If necrosis is evident, a partial gastrectomy may need to be performed. A full exploratory laparotomy should be conducted to be sure no damage has occurred to other abdominal organs. Often the spleen follows the path of the stomach, and a splenic torsion may be apparent. The spleen should be observed for damage, and a splenectomy performed, if warranted. A gastropexy procedure must be done to prevent future GDV.

Permanent Gastropexy Procedures

A *gastropexy* ("pexy") procedure permanently affixes the stomach to the body wall and prevents further occurrence of GDV. Many educated owners of large-breed dogs may decide to have an elective gastropexy performed on their pets. This procedure can be done, for example, when a large-breed pet is admitted for an ovariohysterectomy (OHE). If available, a less invasive gastropexy procedure can be done laparoscopically. A variety of pexy procedures can be performed, although they vary on rates of dependability as well as frequency of surgical complications. The goal of all these procedures is to create a permanent adhesion between the gastric serosa and the peritoneal surface of the abdominal wall. For a permanent adhesion to form, the gastric muscle must be in contact with the body wall muscle. Gastropexy procedures include the following types:

- Tube gastropexy
- Circumcostal gastropexy
- Muscular flap gastropexy
- Belt-loop gastropexy
- Incisional gastropexy

Incisional gastropexy is a general term and is not necessarily specific to a particular technique. For example, some surgery textbooks refer to a muscular flap gastropexy as an "incisional gastropexy." There is also an incisional gastropexy technique that involves tacking the stomach to the ventral midline abdominal incision by incorporating the sutures of the gastropexy into the sutures used to close the abdomen. This particular incisional gastropexy has the major disadvantage of potential problems if the abdomen needs to be opened again later. Also, the surgeon may be more likely to incise through the stomach inadvertently while making the midline incision. A third type of incisional gastropexy is probably the most common procedure for tacking the stomach to the abdominal wall. An internal incision is made into the right ventrolateral body wall, exposing the abdominal muscles. A second incision is made into the seromuscular layer of the stomach antrum. The edges of the gastric incision are sutured to the internal abdominal wall incision. This connection will form a permanent adhesion. This particular type of incisional gastropexy is considered simple and effective and has less potential for complications than other methods of gastropexy (Figure 7-28).

Abdominal Wall Closure

After the gastropexy, the abdomen should be reevaluated. If all or a portion of the spleen appears nonviable, it should be removed. The abdomen should be flushed and then closed routinely.

Postoperative Considerations and Instructions

Dogs can have many complications after GDV repair. Cardiac arrhythmias are common and can continue for 2-3 days postoperatively. The arrhythmias are usually ventricular in origin. Treatment of the arrhythmias involves correction of electrolyte imbalances and maintenance of normal hydration state. If the arrhythmias are more severe and interfere with cardiac output or the animal has premature beats or a sustained cardiac rate above 160 beats per minute, IV drug intervention may be necessary.

FIGURE 7-28 Incisional gastropexy. **A,** An incision is made into the seromuscular layer of the stomach antrum and is lined up with an incision in the ventrolateral abdominal muscle wall. **B,** Completed gastropexy showing the incision in the stomach sutured to the incision in the abdominal muscle wall. (Courtesy Dr. David Holt.)

Lidocaine may be administered by constant rate infusion. The animal should be monitored for muscle tremors, vomiting, and/or seizures, which are signs of lidocaine toxicity. If they are noted, another antiarrhythmic, such as procainamide or sotalol, should be used.

Gastritis may occur secondary to mucosal ischemia. Vomiting should be monitored and can be treated with antiemetics. If no vomiting is reported, water can be offered 1 day after surgery, and food can be introduced in small quantities 24 to 48 hours after surgery. Fluid therapy should be maintained until oral intake is adequate.

Devitalized stomach tissue must be resected to avoid possible septic peritonitis. Gastric viability at surgery is subjective, and postoperative necrosis and perforation can occur postoperatively despite careful assessment. Timely correction of GDV is imperative for a good prognosis. The prognosis may be considered "guarded" if gastric necrosis was evident. Box 7-8 shows an example of a surgery report for GDV repair.

Reproductive Procedures
Ovariohysterectomy

Definition
Ovariohysterectomy (OHE), also called spay or neuter, refers to the surgical excision of the ovaries and uterus.

Indications
The primary indication for OHE is to sterilize the animal so that it can no longer reproduce. Other indications are as follows:
- Neoplasia of reproductive tract.
- Treatment of neoplasia elsewhere in the body influenced by reproductive hormones (e.g., mammary tumors).
- Trauma or injury to reproductive tract.
- Dystocia (difficult birth).
- Uterine torsion.
- Abolition of heat cycle.
- Stabilization of other systemic diseases (e.g., diabetes).
- Congenital abnormalities.

FIGURE 7-29 Spay hooks.

The OHE is one of the most common surgical procedures performed in small animal practice. Clients may inquire about ovariohysterectomies more than any other surgical procedure. The veterinary technician should be able to communicate to clients the advantages and disadvantages of having their pets spayed or neutered. Clients may have preconceived notions about spaying their pets, and the technician may be responsible for explaining to the client the importance of OHE and correcting any misconceptions.

Special Instruments
Surgeons may or may not use a spay hook (Snook hook) for OHE. The hook is used to exteriorize the uterine horn, allowing the surgeon to make a smaller abdominal incision if desired. Spay hooks come in an assortment of sizes; the technician should pick the size appropriate for the animal (Figure 7-29).

Patient Positioning
Most patients are positioned in dorsal recumbency for OHE. This positioning is best suited for a ventral midline incision. Some surgeons may prefer a lateral (flank) approach to the abdomen for an OHE, which requires positioning the patient in lateral recumbency. The ventral abdomen should be clipped and aseptically prepared from the xiphoid process to the pubis.

BOX 7-8   Surgery Report: Gastric Dilatation and Volvulus

Animal Hospital Name
Owner: John Doe
Address: 555 Sterling Lane
    Jupiter, NY 55555
Phone number: 555-5555
Animal Name: Sasha
Animal #: 65656501
Species: Canine
Breed: Labrador
DOB: 01/05/08
Date of Surgery: 12/03/2011
Primary Surgeon: Dr. Vet
Assistant: Nurse Scrub
Diagnosis or Preoperative Signs: One-day history of retching, abdominal distension; gastric dilatation and volvulus.
Surgical Procedure: Gastric dilatation and volvulus (GDV) correction and incisional gastropexy.

Description of Surgical Procedure
Surgical Approach: The patient was placed in dorsal recumbency. A skin incision approximately 25 cm long was made from
    the xiphoid process to the pubis. The incision was continued through the fascia and linea alba, and the abdomen was
    entered. A large amount of falciform fat was resected.
Surgical Pathology: The stomach was rotated 270 degrees, grossly distended, and hypermotile. The pylorus was located
    ventrally and to the left of the fundus. There was no evidence of devitalized tissues. There was minimal hemorrhage in
    the abdomen.
Surgical Procedure: Moist laparotomy sponges were placed along the incision, and a Balfour retractor was placed. On enter-
    ing the abdomen, the omentum was seen covering a gas-distended stomach that was rotated 270 degrees clockwise. The
    stomach was decompressed with an 18-gauge needle and suction. The stomach was then repositioned by pulling up on
    the pylorus to rotate the stomach counterclockwise back to its correct anatomic position. A stomach tube was passed
    and revealed a moderate amount of brown, malodorous fluid. The stomach was lavaged with warm water until the fluid
    leaving the stomach was clear. The entire surface of the stomach was inspected and appeared healthy. The abdomen was
    explored routinely. Next, an incisional gastropexy was performed; an incision was made into the seromuscular layer of
    the stomach in the region of the pyloric antrum. A second incision was made into the right ventrolateral abdominal wall,
    exposing the abdominal muscles. The edges of the gastric incision were sutured to the abdominal wall incision using two
    suture lines and a simple continuous pattern. The abdomen was lavaged with 2 liters of sterile saline, and the body wall
    was closed routinely.
Closure:
Incisional gastropexy: 2-0 PDS in two lines of simple continuous patterns.
Linea alba: 0 PDS in simple continuous pattern.
Subcutaneous tissue: 2-0 PDS in simple continuous pattern.
Subcuticular tissue: 2-0 Monocryl in continuous suture pattern.
Skin: skin staples.

Patient Draping

The type of drape used for OHE is the surgeon's prefer-ence. Because this is an abdominal procedure, a four-quarter draping method should be considered.

Canine and Feline Ovariohysterectomy Procedures

In dogs the start of the incision can be made 3 to 6 cm caudal to the umbilicus. In cats the incision should be started 3 to 4 cm caudally. An incision should be made through the skin (Figure 7-30) and the subcutaneous tissue and linea alba (Figure 7-31). The length of the inci-sion is the surgeon's preference.

    The left abdominal wall is raised and the spay hook is slid down against the abdominal wall to grasp the horn of the uterus. The hook should be turned to trap the uterine horn, which can then be elevated from the abdomen. In dogs the suspensory ligament should be torn without tearing the ovarian vessels; this maneuver allows exteriorization of the ovary. Tearing the suspensory liga-ment is generally not necessary to exteriorize a cat's ovary. Plucking of the ligament is the most painful portion of the procedure. The animal's heart rate and respiratory rate generally increases at this time. Once the pedicle has been ligated the heart rate and respiratory rate should return to normal anesthetized levels. The method of liga-tion and transection of the pedicle is the surgeon's prefer-ence. Surgeons may decide to use clips, the two-clamp method, or the three-clamp method (Figure 7-32). Carmalt, Kelly, or Crile forceps (see Chapter 1) may be

FIGURE 7-30 Abdominal skin incision. Electrocautery is used for hemostasis of small vessels.

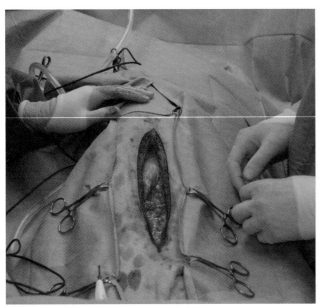

FIGURE 7-31 Abdominal incision through the subcutaneous tissue and linea alba.

FIGURE 7-32 Three-clamp technique of uterine horn. Note ovary caudal to hemostats.

FIGURE 7-33 Double ligation of the uterine body, cranial to cervix.

used for clamping the pedicles. The forceps used depends on the size of the pedicle. Two clamps should be placed across the ovarian pedicle, proximal (deep) to the ovary, and one clamp across the ovarian ligament.

The technician should be knowledgeable about what type of suture the surgeon will be using and have it loaded and ready for use on the instrument table before it is needed. An absorbable suture material is usually used for pedicle ligation. The size of the suture is the surgeon's preference and depends on the size of the pedicle. If clips are being used, the technician should have the clip applicator loaded and accessible for the surgeon.

The surgeon then places a ligature proximal to the ovarian pedicle clamp and securely ties the ligature. One clamp may be removed or "flashed" (unclamped and then reclamped) while the surgeon tightens the ligature. Flashing is done to compress the pedicle and secure the ligature so that it is less likely to slide off once the pedicle is transected. If the ligature is not secure and slides off the pedicle, the pedicle will bleed, and the patient could lose a significant amount of blood and die. If the ligature slides off, the pedicle must be isolated (this may require extending the incision more cranially) and the ligature replaced. A second ligature is placed proximal to the first (therefore flashing is not necessary to secure the second ligature) to provide additional security in preventing hemorrhage. The pedicle can then be transected at the level of the third clamp, between the clamp and the ovary. The same procedure can be done for the other uterine horn.

The body of the uterus should then be exteriorized, and a two-clamp or three-clamp method can be used. The clamps are placed onto the uterine body, cranial to the cervix. A ligature is placed closer to the cervix (Figure 7-33). A clamp should be placed distal to the ligatures. The surgeon then transects the uterine body between the clamp and the ligatures. The uterine stump should be checked for hemorrhage.

Excessive bleeding can occur if the ovarian pedicle and/or the uterine stumps are not properly ligated. The abdominal cavity should be carefully inspected for hemorrhage prior to closure.

Abdominal Wall Closure

The abdomen should be flushed and then closed routinely.

Postoperative Considerations and Instructions

Intra-abdominal hemorrhage can occur postoperatively; if not treated it can be fatal. If ligation of a bleeding stump is attempted without proper visualization, renal dysfunction may occur secondary to ureteral ligation.

Cesarean Section

Definition

Cesarean section, also referred to as "cesarotomy" or "hysterotomy," is delivery of a fetus or fetuses by incision through the abdominal wall and uterus. The word "cesarean" has no relation to the birth of Julius Caesar, as some believe; it takes its name from the Latin word *caedere*, to cut.

Indications

The primary indication for a cesarean section is *dystocia* (difficult birth). Dystocia can develop from the following situations:

- Maldeveloped fetuses.
- Oversized fetuses.
- Malpositioned fetuses.
- Small pelvic canal size of dam.
- Previous pelvic trauma of dam.
- Insufficient dilation.
- Uterine inertia (lack of contractility of uterus; can result from overstretching of uterus, toxemia, obesity, or exhaustion).

The objective of a cesarean section is to remove all the fetuses from the uterus as swiftly as possible. Although it may be performed as an intervention in an emergency, cesarean section is frequently planned for brachycephalic breeds (e.g., boxers, bulldogs, Pekingese, pugs) or animals with a history of dystocia.

Special Instruments

A general use soft tissue surgery pack should provide the surgeon with the necessary instruments needed for cesarean section. Extra hemostats should be available. Extra hands will also be needed to help warm and resuscitate the puppies or kittens.

Patient Positioning

For cesarean section the patient should be positioned in dorsal recumbency. For all three procedures, the ventral abdomen should be clipped, preliminary abdominal preparation performed, and urinary bladder emptied before the patient is taken to the surgery room. The animal should be rapidly anesthetized in the surgery room, and a final surgical prep should be performed while the surgeon and scrub assistant are preparing for surgery.

Patient Draping

A four-quarter draping technique should be used for cesarean section.

Cesarean Section Procedure

See Box 7-9 for an overview of three different methods of performing a Cesarean section:

After the animal is draped, a ventral midline incision should be made into the skin and subcutaneous tissue, from just cranial to the umbilicus and continuing caudally to the pubis. The external rectus sheath should be elevated with forceps before the stab incision is made into the abdomen, to avoid lacerating the uterus.

Cesarean without ovariohysterectomy. The uterine horns should be gently exteriorized from the abdomen (Figure 7-34). It is extremely important that this process be done carefully to avoid tearing the uterine vessels. The uterus should be isolated with moistened laparotomy sponges to help prevent contamination of the abdomen. The scrub nurse should have the sponges moistened in

---

BOX 7-9   Cesarean Section Procedures

Cesarean Without an Ovariohysterectomy

The owner may elect not to spay the animal. The veterinarian should inform the owner of the possibility of future dystocia in this pet. In addition, the client should be made aware that the surgeon may open the abdomen, inspect the uterus, and discover that it has deteriorated to such an extent that leaving it in the abdomen is no longer an option.

Cesarean Followed by an Ovariohysterectomy

An indication to perform this procedure may be to prevent the animal from having dystocia in the future.

En Bloc Resection (radical resection of the uterus; neonates removed after resection of uterus)

En bloc removal of the uterus may be optional or essential because of possible fetal compromise or uterine viability.

FIGURE 7-34 Gentle exteriorization of a gravid uterus.

FIGURE 7-35 The fetus is being "milked," or gently squeezed, toward the hysterotomy incision.

FIGURE 7-36 Removal of the fetus from the uterus. Note the abundance of laparotomy sponges isolating the uterus from the abdomen.

warm saline and ready to place under and around the uterus.

The surgeon then incises the uterine body. The uterine body should be tented on incision to avoid damage to the fetuses. The incision is made on the ventral aspect of the uterus and can be extended using Metzenbaum scissors (not a blade). Each horn should be emptied by squeezing each fetus cranially toward the incision (Figure 7-35). The fetus can then be gently lifted out of the uterus (Figure 7-36), and its amniotic sac manually ruptured. The scrub nurse should have hemostats available for clamping off the umbilical cord of each neonate. Once the cord is clamped, the surgeon severs it.

Care should be taken at this point to make every attempt to avoid contamination of the abdomen and surgical field with amniotic fluid. An abundance of lap sponges will aid in this endeavor. If the placenta easily separates from the uterus, it is removed with the neonate. Each neonate should be passed to a nonsterile assistant. When the fetuses are being passed to the nonsterile assistant, breaks in sterility can occur and should be monitored closely by a nonsterile technician.

The scrub nurse should always be focused on the surgical procedure and the patient in front of him or her. After removal of all obvious fetuses, a meticulous examination of the uterus should be performed from the ovaries to the cervix to make certain that no fetuses remain. A local lavage of the external uterus should be performed after closure of the uterine incision. The specific technique used for closure of the abdomen and the suture used to close the incision are the choice of the surgeon. An absorbable suture should be used for closure of the uterus. After closure of the uterine body, the abdominal cavity should be lavaged with warm saline in case the abdomen was contaminated with uterine contents (amniotic fluid). The adage "The solution to pollution is dilution" holds true for any surgical procedure in which bacteria may have entered the sterile abdomen (e.g., GI tract).

Cesarean followed by ovariohysterectomy. An OHE may be performed after the cesarean section, as previously described.

En bloc resection. The first step in an en bloc resection is to isolate the ovarian pedicles. Separation of the broad ligament from the uterus is done at the point of the cervix. Any fetuses within the vagina have to be directed back into the uterine body. The uterine body should be clamped at the cranial aspect of the cervix. Once the ovarian pedicles and the uterine body are clamped, the surgeon transects between the clamps, and the ovaries and uterus are removed. The uterus is handed off to nonsterile personnel. Again, breaks in sterility can easily occur at this time and should be monitored. The nonsterile personnel need to remove the fetuses from the uterus (see following discussion). Once the uterus is removed en bloc ("as a whole"), the surgeon ligates the ovarian and uterine pedicles with two ligatures. The pedicles should be examined for bleeding before closure. A warm lavage of the abdomen helps with any contamination of the abdomen from uterine spillage and also helps warm the dam.

Abdominal Wall Closure
Closure of the abdomen is done according to the surgeon's preference. Some surgeons may finish with a subcuticular layer or intradermal layer rather than placing skin sutures (closing in three layers). This is done to avoid irritation of the neonates from the skin suture ends during the nursing process.

Neonatal Care
The care of the neonates generally is the responsibility of the nurse or technician. This job can be extremely rewarding, especially if the neonates are resuscitated successfully and can leave the hospital with their mother. If the neonates are transferred still in the uterus, the technician needs to incise the uterus, by tenting the uterus and using Metzenbaum scissors. Extreme caution must be used when incising the uterus so as not to injure the neonates. The amniotic sac on each neonate needs to be broken as well.

FIGURE 7-37 Initiation of tactile stimulation for a neonate.

FIGURE 7-39 Various neonatal endotracheal tubes and pediatric laryngoscope.

FIGURE 7-38 Aspiration of fluid from the oropharynx using an infant suction bulb.

The technician should have a warm, dry area prepared for the neonates before surgery. The area should include some or all of the following: plenty of clean, warm towels; a radiant lamp; a hair dryer; and circulating warm-water heating pads. Drugs that should be available include naloxone (opioid antagonist), doxapram (respiratory stimulant), and epinephrine (cardiovascular stimulant). Suture and scissors should also be available to ligate the umbilical cords. The neonates should be dried off immediately with warm towels (Figure 7-37). A heating unit should be used to aid in the warming process. The neonates should be briskly rubbed to initiate spontaneous respiration.

The nurse or technician also must ensure that the clamp on the umbilicus is secure and there is no unnecessary pulling on the umbilicus. Strain on the umbilical cord can cause abdominal herniation from the umbilical site. An infant suction bulb can be used to help aspirate fluid from the oropharynx and nares (Figure 7-38). If opioids were used as a premedication for the dam, a drop of naloxone can be placed under the tongue of each neonate to reverse the effects of the opioids on the neonates. If respiratory efforts of the neonate are slow to commence, a drop of doxapram placed under the tongue can be used to aid in respiratory stimulation. If the

newborn has an appropriate heart rate (120-150 beats/min) but is still having respiratory-related issues, tactile stimulation and administration of oxygen by mask may be successful in instituting respiration. If respiratory efforts do not commence within about 30 seconds, or if bradycardia occurs, the nurse may need to administer positive-pressure ventilation by mask. The newborn may need to be intubated and ventilated until he/she starts to take breaths on his/her own (Figure 7-39).

Once respiration has been achieved, cardiovascular stability must be addressed, especially if the patient is bradycardic or has a weak heartbeat. If no heartbeat can be identified, chest compressions should be administered by fingers across the lateral chest wall. If chest compressions appear unsuccessful, epinephrine can be administered under the tongue.

Some neonates never achieve respiration or a heartbeat once retrieved from the uterus, but every attempt should be made to revive them. A newborn's survival can depend on each individual situation. How long the fetus was wedged in the canal or how long the dam was in labor can determine the outcome. Whimpering and crying sounds from the newborns are always a good sign.

Once the newborn has been stabilized with an adequate respiratory rate and an adequate heart rate, the umbilical cord can be ligated and transected approximately 1 to 2 cm from the body (Figure 7-40). The newborns should be kept in a warm environment (about 90° F) until the mother's surgery is complete, and oxygen supplementation may be a necessary part of a successful resuscitation (Figure 7-41).

The mammary glands of the dam should be cleaned after surgery to remove any surgical prep solutions as well as any blood. The newborns should be reunited with their mother, and nursing should commence as soon as possible. The mother's behavior toward the newborns should be observed during the first few hours. Care should be taken not to return the newborns to their mother too

FIGURE 7-42 Lateral abdominal radiograph of a dog with pyometra. Note the enlarged uterus *(arrows)* in the caudoventral abdomen displacing the viscera cranially and dorsally. (From Fossum TW, Hedlund CS, Hulse DA, et al: Small animal surgery, ed 3, St Louis, 2007, Mosby.)

complications. The adage "Never let the sun set on a pyometra" has its merits. A pyometra can rupture at any point, releasing all the purulent material into the abdominal cavity and leading to septicemia and/or endotoxemia. In addition, the rate of recurrence of pyometra after medical therapy is as high as 77%.

Most animals affected are 6 years or older intact females. It is possible for a condition known as *stump pyometra* to develop in a previously spayed female if ovarian tissue was left behind during the original procedure. The remnants of the uterus left near the cervix can become infected. Clinical signs are seen within 4 to 8 weeks after the last heat cycle and can include decreased appetite, lethargy, increased thirst and urination, and in some, but not all cases, foul-smelling vaginal discharge. A fluid-filled uterus may be detected on abdominal radiographs (Figure 7-42).

Special Instruments
A routine surgical instrument pack should be sufficient for this procedure. Sterile laparotomy sponges should be available. Heated lavage fluid and suction may also be indicated.

Patient Positioning
Patients are positioned in dorsal recumbency. The ventral abdomen should be clipped and aseptically prepared from the xiphoid process to the pubis.

Patient Draping
The type of drape used for a pyometra is the surgeon's preference. Because this is an abdominal procedure, a four-quarter draping method should be considered.

Pyometra Surgery
A routine ovariohysterectomy is performed (see previous discussion). Care must be taken because the uterus is typically engorged and friable (Figure 7-43). The surgeon

FIGURE 7-40 Ligation of the umbilical cord 1 to 2 cm from the body wall.

FIGURE 7-41 Successful resuscitation of five puppies.

soon. She could inadvertently injure them if she is not fully recovered. Some mothers may reject or kill their young, so careful observation is important.

To reduce stress and exposure to pathogens and nosocomial infections, the bitch and the newborns should be released from the hospital as soon as possible.

Box 7-10 shows an example of a surgery report for a cesarean section.

Pyometra
Definition
Pyometra describes a pus-filled uterus. The condition is more prevalent in dogs than cats but can be seen in both species. The condition can be referred to as either open or closed, depending on the cervix. In an open pyometra, the cervix is open, allowing the purulent discharge to drain. Both types are considered serious; as the purulent material accumulates, uterine rupture can occur.

Indication
An OHE is the recommended treatment for pyometra. Owners may wish to elect medical management of the condition if the animal is a valuable breeder. This should be discouraged because it is associated with severe

BOX 7-10   Surgery Report: Cesarean Section

Animal Hospital Name
Owner: John Doe
Address: 555 Sterling Lane
    Jupiter, NY 55555
Phone number: 555-5555
Animal Name: Sasha
Animal #: 65656501
Species: Canine
Breed: Labrador
DOB: 05/05/09
Date of Surgery: 1/05/2011
Primary Surgeon: Dr. Vet
Assistant: Nurse Scrub
Diagnosis or Preoperative Signs: Dystocia.
Surgical Procedure: Cesarean section.

Description of Surgical Procedure
Surgical Approach: A ventral midline skin incision was made cranial to the umbilicus and extended caudally 10 cm.
Surgical Pathology: Three neonates were removed from the uterus.
Surgical Procedure: An incision was made through the subcutaneous tissue and linea alba into the peritoneal cavity. The fetus-distended uterus was identified, exteriorized, and packed off with moistened lap sponges. A 5-cm longitudinal incision was made into the ventral aspect of the uterine body, and three puppies were milked out one by one. A hemostat was placed on the umbilical cords, and the umbilical cords were transected. The puppies were handed to the assistants. The remaining placenta was grasped with forceps and removed from the uterine body. The uterus was closed, and the abdomen was lavaged with sterile saline before closure of the peritoneal cavity. Hemostasis was maintained throughout the surgery with the aid of monopolar cautery.
Closure:
Uterine body: 3-0 PDS in two continuous layers.
Linea alba: 2-0 PDS using simple interrupted suture pattern.
Subcutaneous tissue and subcuticular layer: Each closed with 2-0 PDS using simple continuous suture pattern.
Skin: Tissue adhesive was applied to the skin.

FIGURE 7-43 The uterus must be carefully handled in cases of pyometra because it is often large, friable, and heavy. Compare the pyometra uterus in **A** with the normal uterus in **B**. (From Bassert JM, McCurnin DM, editors: McCurnin's clinical textbook for veterinary technicians, ed 7, St Louis, 2010, Elsevier.)

may require an assistant to scrub in to help lift and remove the uterus.

Postoperative Considerations and Instructions

The animal should be monitored postoperatively as it would be for an OHE. IV antibiotics are typically given until the animal is considered stable. Oral antibiotics should continue for 7 to 10 days postoperatively at the veterinarian's discretion.

Canine and Feline Castration

Castration may also be referred to as a "*neuter*," "*alter*," or orchiectomy.

Routine Canine Castration

Definition. *Canine castration* refers to the surgical removal of the testicles in the dog.

Indications. The primary indication for performing a canine castration is for sterilization of the dog. Other indications include the following:

- Prevention of roaming.
- Prevention of aggressive behavior or fighting.
- Prevention of urine marking.
- Correction of congenital abnormalities.
- Treatment of scrotal or testicular neoplasia.
- Treatment of scrotal abscess, infection, or trauma.
- Treatment of disease elsewhere in the body related to hormones (e.g., prostatic disease, perineal hernias, perianal tumors).

Instrumentation. A general use soft tissue surgical instrument pack should be sufficient for canine castration.

Patient positioning. The canine patient should be placed in dorsal recumbency for castration. The scrotum should be examined and palpated for the presence of both testicles before anesthesia is induced. If both testicles are present, a routine castration can be performed. If only one testicle is present, the dog is considered "cryptorchid" and may require an inguinal or abdominal surgery to remove the other testicle.

For a routine castration the surgical site should be clipped from the tip of the prepuce to just above the scrotum. The clipped region should extend laterally into the inguinal section on both sides. The scrotum should not be clipped. The skin of the scrotum is delicate and sensitive and may be susceptible to clipper burns or tears. Irritation of the scrotum can cause the animal to lick or bite at the affected region postoperatively. The surgical site should be aseptically prepared.

Patient draping. A single fenestrated drape is appropriate for orchiectomy. The surgeon may elect to use a four-corner draping method. A single fenestrated drape is placed over the surgical region (the testicles and scrotum are draped out of the surgical field).

Canine castration procedure. The surgeon may decide to do an "open castration" or "closed castration." In the closed procedure, the tunics are not incised, and the entire spermatic cord encased in its parietal vaginal tunic is ligated and transected. In the open procedure, the tunics are incised, and the contents of the cord are ligated and transected separately.

Open castration. The surgeon selects the first testicle and applies pressure cranially to advance the testicle into the prescrotal region. The skin and subcutaneous tissues and spermatic fascia are incised (Figure 7-44). The surgeon then incises the parietal vaginal tunic (Figure 7-45), and the testicle is gently extruded (Figure 7-46). A hemostat should be placed across the tunic at the attachment of the epididymis. The ligament of the tail of the epididymis is separated from the tunic. Three clamps can be placed across the spermatic cord (Figure 7-47). The

FIGURE 7-44 A skin incision is made in the prescrotal region for canine castration.

FIGURE 7-45 Incision into the parietal vaginal tunic of the canine scrotum for orchiectomy.

FIGURE 7-46 Gentle extrusion of the canine testicle for orchiectomy.

vascular cord and the ductus deferens are recognized and can be individually ligated using an absorbable suture. The surgeon may decide to ligate the vascular cord and ductus deferens together. A circumferential ligature is then placed around both the ductus deferens and the vascular cord. A hemostat is placed on the cord close to the testicle. The cord is then transected between the

FIGURE 7-47 Three hemostats are used to clamp the spermatic cord in canine castration.

FIGURE 7-48 Ligation and transection of the ductus deferens and vascular cord in canine castration. The cord is checked for hemorrhage before closing.

hemostat and ligatures (Figure 7-48). The cord is examined for bleeding and returned within the tunic. The second testicle can be removed in the same manner.

Closed castration. Closed castration is performed much like open castration except for the incision of the parietal vaginal tunics. Once the skin, subcutaneous tissue, and spermatic fascia are incised, the spermatic cord is exteriorized. Ligatures are placed around the entire spermatic cord and tunics, and the cord is then transected.

Postoperative considerations and instructions. Common complications associated with canine castration include hemorrhage and scrotal hematoma. A scrotal hematoma may be the result of a hemorrhaging vessel (or vessels). Care should be taken during the surgery to provide appropriate hemostasis to avoid such complications. Cold compresses can be placed to aid in hemostasis postoperatively if hemorrhage has occurred. A complete scrotal ablation (removal of scrotum) may be necessary if

FIGURE 7-49 Fenestration is made in single drape just large enough to reveal both testicles for feline castration.

hemostasis was unsuccessful. Other complications include self-inflicted trauma to the incision and infection or dehiscence of the incision site.

Box 7-11 shows an example of a surgery report for a canine castration.

Routine Feline Castration

Definition. *Feline castration* refers to the surgical removal of the testicles in the cat.

Indications. The primary indication to perform a castration is for sterilization of the male cat. Other indications include the following:
- Prevention of roaming.
- Prevention of aggressive behavior or fighting.
- Prevention of urine spraying or marking.
- Correction of congenital abnormalities.
- Treatment of scrotal neoplasia.
- Treatment of scrotal abscess, infection, or trauma.
- Treatment of endocrine abnormalities.
- Treatment of disease elsewhere in the body related to hormones (e.g., prostatic disease, perineal hernias).

Instrumentation. No special instrumentation is required to perform a feline castration. The surgeon may prefer to use metal clips rather than the spermatic cord to tie a knot, or may prefer using suture for ligation.

Patient positioning. The feline patient may be positioned for castration in lateral or in dorsal recumbency with the legs tied cranially. The positioning of the patient is the surgeon's preference.

Patient draping. A single fenestrated drape should be sufficient for orchiectomy (Figure 7-49).

Feline castration procedure. An examination of the testicles should be conducted before anesthesia is induced, to ensure that both testicles have descended into the scrotum. The male cat should be positioned according to the surgeon's instructions (lateral or dorsal recumbency). The testicles should be prepared for surgery by gently plucking the hair from the scrotum. The scrotum should then be prepped and draped with proper aseptic technique. One testicle is held in place while the surgeon

BOX 7-11   Surgery Report: Canine Castration

Animal Hospital Name
Owner: John Doe
Address: 555 Sterling Lane
    Jupiter, NY 55555
Phone number: 555-5555
Animal Name: Sasha
Animal #: 65656501
Species: Canine
Breed: Labrador
DOB: 05/05/10
Date of Surgery: 01/03/2011
Primary Surgeon: Dr. Vet
Assistant: Nurse Scrub
Diagnosis or Preoperative Signs: Intact male.
Surgical Procedure: Open castration.

Description of Surgical Procedure
Surgical Approach: A 3-cm ventral midline incision was made in the prescrotal region while one testicle was advanced
    cranially into the incision line. The incision was extended through the subcutaneous tissues.
Surgical Procedure: The right testicle was pushed up through the incision. The vaginal tunic was then incised, and the
    testicle pushed through. The ligament of the tail of the epididymis was bluntly dissected. The ductus deferens and
    the vascular cord were individually ligated with 2-0 PDS, then both were ligated together with a circumferential ligature.
    The testicle was then transected distal to the ligatures. The same procedure was performed on the left testicle.
Closure:
Subcutaneous tissue: 2-0 PDS in simple continuous suture pattern.
Subcuticular tissue: 3-0 Monocryl in simple continuous suture pattern.
Skin: 3-0 nylon in simple interrupted suture pattern.

FIGURE 7-50 Incision is made through the skin and parietal vaginal tunic of the feline scrotum for orchiectomy.

FIGURE 7-51 The testicle is extruded from the feline scrotum with gentle force.

makes an incision over it (Figure 7-50). The parietal vaginal tunic is incised, and the testicle can then be extruded from the scrotum with gentle force (Figures 7-51 and 7-52).

The spermatic cord can be ligated and transected using different techniques. Metal clips can be used for ligation of the spermatic cord. Once the clips are in place, the testicle can be transected. Another option for ligation of the spermatic cord is using hemostats and suture. Three

hemostats are placed on the spermatic cord, and the testicle is then transected. A ligature is placed around the cord just below the forceps.

Another type of procedure uses the reproductive anatomy to tie knots. In one such procedure the ductus deferens and the spermatic vessels are separated and used to tie square knots. Another such procedure uses an overhand technique (Figures 7-53 to 7-55). This is done by placing a hemostat on top of the spermatic cord and

FIGURE 7-52 Full extrusion of the feline testicle, allowing visualization of the spermatic cord.

FIGURE 7-55 The spermatic cord is pulled through and a knot is made with the cord in the overhand technique for feline castration.

FIGURE 7-53 Overhand technique for feline castration. A hemostat is placed on top of the spermatic cord, and the cord is wrapped over and around the hemostat. The cord is grabbed with the hemostat and clamped near the testicle.

FIGURE 7-54 Feline testicle is transected in overhand technique.

wrapping the cord over and around the hemostat. The cord is then grabbed by the hemostats and clamped near the testicle. The testicle is transected and the cord pulled through to make a knot on itself.

All these procedures are acceptable methods for feline castration; the choice is left to the surgeon's discretion. The scrotum itself is left unsutured.

Postoperative considerations and instructions. Scrotal bleeding can be a common complication associated with feline castration. A cold compress can be placed on the scrotum for several minutes to aid in hemostasis. If hemorrhage continues, another surgery may be required to ligate a bleeding vessel. General discharge instructions are listed in Chapter 10. Box 7-12 shows an example of a surgery report for a feline castration.

Cystotomy

Definition

Cystotomy refers to a surgical incision into the bladder to expose the lumen or interior of the urinary bladder.

Indications

A primary indication for performing a cystotomy is to remove cystic calculi. Removal of bladder stones is probably the most common bladder surgery performed in small animal surgery. In the dog the most frequent urolith observed is the struvite (45% to 50% of all calculi). Other uroliths found in the dog include calcium oxalate, urate, silicate, and cystine crystals. Uroliths are most frequently noted in middle-aged dogs, although they can occur at any age.

Clinical signs associated with bladder stones include hematuria, stranguria, dysuria, and pollakiuria. Stones may also become wedged in the urethra of male dogs and cause obstructions of the urethra. Animals with suspected cystic calculi should have radiographs. Abdominal radiographs of animals with calculi frequently reveal radiopaque densities in the urinary system. Obstruction of

BOX 7-12 Surgery Report: Feline Castration

Animal Hospital Name
Owner: John Doe
Address: 555 Sterling Lane
    Jupiter, NY 55555
Phone number: 555-5555
Animal Name: Kitty
Animal #: 65656501
Species: Feline
Breed: Domestic shorthair
DOB: 05/05/10
Date of Surgery: 01/03/2011
Primary Surgeon: Dr. Vet
Assistant: Nurse Scrub
Diagnosis or Preoperative Signs: Intact male.
Surgical Procedure: Feline castration.

Description of Surgical Procedure
Surgical Approach: A 1-cm incision was made through the skin on the left and right caudal scrotum to exteriorize each
    testicle.
Surgical Pathology: None.
Surgical Procedure: Applying pressure cranially, the right testicle was exteriorized. An incision was made over the testicle,
    and the spermatic fascia and parietal vaginal tunic were incised. The ligament of the tail of the epididymis was separated
    from the tunic using a hemostat. The ductus deferens and the vascular cord were then tied to each other and transected
    distal to the knot. The same procedure was repeated on the left side.
Closure:
The scrotal incisions were left open to heal by second intention.

the urethra can lead to a buildup of urine in the bladder and can cause bladder distension. Bladder distension can lead to a rupture if left untreated. Rupture of the bladder can also result from trauma (e.g., being hit by a car) or from improper placement of a urinary catheter or forceful expression of the bladder. Most abdominal procedures require expression of the bladder before transport into surgery. *The bladder of a trauma patient should not be expressed before surgery.* The condition of the bladder may be in question, and attempts to express a traumatic bladder may lead to a bladder rupture. Clinical signs of bladder rupture can include shock, fever, hematuria, anuria, and abdominal pain. Urine in the abdominal cavity can cause uremia and dehydration. A bladder rupture can lead to death if identification of the rupture is delayed. Uroabdomen can be diagnosed by the performance of an abdominocentesis. Creatinine and urea measurements of the abdominal cavity fluid are compared with blood serum levels. If the levels of creatinine and urea in the abdominal fluid are greater than in the blood serum, an uroabdomen can be diagnosed. A contrast cystourethrogram can also be performed to diagnose the exact region of the bladder leakage.

Other indications to perform cystotomy include neoplasia and congenital abnormalities. The most common neoplasia associated with the bladder in dogs and cats is transitional cell carcinoma. In the dog, bladder cancer makes up less than 1% of all canine cancers. The incidence of bladder cancer in cats is much lower.

Table 7-1 lists treatment options and preventive measures for different types of canine urolithiasis. Box 7-13 lists canine predispositions for urinary calculi.

Special Instruments
A general use soft tissue surgery pack will be sufficient for cystotomy. A bladder spoon should be available (Figure 7-56). Bladder spoons can aid in the retrieval of cystic calculi, especially those located in the neck of the bladder. A Balfour abdominal retractor should also be available.

Patient Positioning
The patient should be positioned in dorsal recumbency to perform a ventral midline incision.

Patient Draping
A four-quarter draping method should be considered for cystotomy.

Cystotomy Procedure
The entire abdomen should be clipped from xiphoid process to the pubis. The patient should be prepped from the xiphoid process to the pubis in the event an

TABLE 7-1	Treatment and Prevention of Canine Urolithiasis	
Urolith Type	Treatment Options	Preventive Measures
Struvite	Surgical removal or dissolution Hill's s/d diet Control infection Urease inhibitor? Keep urine pH <6.5, blood urea nitrogen (BUN) <10 mg/dL, and urine specific gravity <1.020	Hill's c/d diet Monitor urine pH and urine sediment; eliminate infections quickly and appropriately
Calcium oxalate	Surgical removal	Hill's u/d diet or Hill's w/d diet plus potassium citrate
Urate	Surgical removal or dissolution Hill's u/d diet Allopurinol Control infection	Hill's u/d diet Allopurinol if necessary Correct congenital portosystemic shunts
Silicate	Surgical removal	Hill's u/d diet Prevent consumption of dirt
Cystine	Surgical removal or dissolution Hill's u/d diet d-Penicillamine N-(2-Mercaptopropionyl)-glycine (MPG)	Hill's u/d diet Thiol-containing drugs if necessary

From Fossum TW, Hedlund CS, Hulse DA, et al: Small animal surgery, ed 3, St Louis, 2007, Mosby.

BOX 7-13   Breed, Gender, Age, and Other Predispositions for Urinary Calculi in Dogs

Struvite Uroliths
Miniature Schnauzer, Bichon Frise, Cocker Spaniel
Female more than male dogs; middle-aged dogs
Urinary tract infection (UTI)

Calcium Oxalate Uroliths
Miniature Schnauzer, Lhasa Apso, Yorkshire Terrier
Male dogs, middle-aged to older dogs

Calcium Phosphate Uroliths
Yorkshire Terrier

Urate Uroliths
Dalmatian, English Bulldog
Dogs with portosystemic shunts

Silicate Uroliths
German Shepherd, Golden Retriever, Labrador Retriever
Male dogs, middle-aged dogs

Cystine Uroliths
Dachshund, English Bulldog (possibly Basset Hound and Rottweiler)
Male dogs, middle-aged dogs

FIGURE 7-56 Bladder spoon.

either side of the incision, and a Balfour retractor positioned for better exposure of the abdomen. The bladder should be isolated, and lap sponges positioned beneath the bladder to segregate it from the rest of the abdomen. Stay sutures should be placed at the apex of the bladder to assist in manipulation as well as to prevent spillage of urine into the abdomen (Figure 7-57). The scrub nurse should grasp the stay sutures and gently lift upward to avoid spillage of urine.

The surgeon makes a stab incision on the ventral aspect of the bladder in a hypovascular region. The technician should have suction ready to place into the stab incision to remove the urine from the bladder before leakage occurs. The stab incision can then be extended with Metzenbaum scissors. A bladder spoon can be used to aid in the removal of cystic calculi, especially at the neck region of the bladder (Figure 7-58). A red rubber catheter can be passed through the urethra, and sterile saline should be flushed through the catheter to confirm the urethral passage is clear of cystic calculi and is patent. Cystic calculi should be flushed back into the bladder if possible to avoid having to perform an *urethrotomy* (incision into the urethra).

unexpected finding requires an extended incision. This additional clipping and prepping allows the surgeon to extend the incision cranially if desired. A ventral midline incision beginning at the umbilicus and extending caudally to the pubis should be sufficient for cystotomy. The subcutaneous tissues and linea alba should be incised on the midline. Moistened lap sponges should be placed on

FIGURE 7-57 Cystotomy incision into the ventral aspect of the bladder. Note that stay sutures are used to lift gently upward on the bladder to avoid leakage of urine. A red rubber catheter is placed to flush any stones in the urethra back into the bladder. (Modified from Fossum TW, Hedlund CS, Hulse DA, et al: Small animal surgery, ed 3, St Louis, 2007, Mosby.)

FIGURE 7-58 The bladder spoon is used to remove stones from the neck of the bladder.

Cultures of the bladder should be obtained. Some surgeons may also prefer to take a sample of the bladder for biopsy or culture. The bladder should be examined for deficiencies and closed according to the surgeon's preference. Closure of the bladder can consist of a two-layer or three-layer continuous closure or a simple interrupted suture pattern (Figure 7-59). The stay sutures can be removed, and the abdomen should be lavaged with warm saline. The abdomen should be closed routinely. Bladder stones retrieved from the bladder should be submitted for analysis.

Onychectomy

Definition
Onychectomy, or declawing, is the removal of the claw and its associated third phalanx (Figure 7-60).

Indications
An onychectomy is usually an elective procedure to prevent the cat from scratching furniture of the owners.

FIGURE 7-59 The cystotomy incision is closed in a simple interrupted suture pattern using an absorbable suture.

Occasionally it is a non-elective procedure, required to remove neoplasia of the claw and or phalanx or to remove an infected nail bed. Elective declaws are usually performed between 3 and 12 months of age and are typically done on the front paws only. A declawed cat should be kept indoors, but in the event that the cat were to get outside it would still have its back claws as a means of defense. This is a painful procedure, and proper analgesia and pain management protocols need to be initiated prior to surgery.

Special Instruments
The procedure can be done in one of three methods, use of the Rescoe Nail Trimmer technique (Rescoe, Walled Lake, MI) scalpel blade, or the CO_2 laser. Each requires its own instrumentation. A tourniquet will be required to control hemorrhage.

Patient Positioning
The cat is typically placed in lateral recumbency. The feet are not clipped unless the cat is a long-haired breed, and are surgically scrubbed. If the laser method is used, alcohol should not be used as it will likely ignite when the laser beam hits the prepared area. The toe nails should not be clipped because their length will aid in nail manipulation during the procedure (Figure 7-61). A tourniquet is placed on the limb, but not tightened, prior to aseptic preparation.

Patient Draping
A fenestrated drape should be sufficient.

Declaw Procedure
Once the foot has been scrubbed, a tourniquet should be positioned distal to the elbow and tightened. Placing the tourniquet proximal to the elbow can lead to radial nerve damage (Figure 7-62). At this time a nerve block may be performed (Figure 7-63).

For the Rescoe technique, extend the claw cranially and position the blade on the dorsal surface of the digit

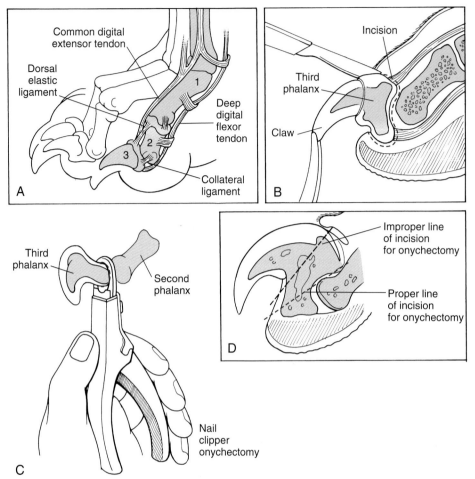

FIGURE 7-60 **A,** Distal phalangeal anatomy for onychectomy. **B,** Dissection onychectomy disarticulates the third phalanx by transecting tendons, ligaments, and other soft tissue attachments. **C,** Nail clipper onychectomy should remove the entire ungual crest but often leaves a portion of the ventral flexor process of P3. **D,** Proper and improper lines of transection. (Modified from Fossum TW, Hedlund CS, Hulse DA, et al: Small animal surgery, ed 3, St Louis, 2007, Mosby.)

FIGURE 7-61 Declaw. To aid in nail manipulation, the nail is not trimmed before surgery. (From Bassert JM, McCurnin DM, editors: McCurnin's clinical textbook for veterinary technicians, ed 7, St Louis, 2010, Elsevier.)

between the second and third phalanges. Care must be exercised to avoid cutting the footpad. As the cutting blade of the nail trimmer is advanced, the pad should be moved caudally and the nail should be rotated dorsally and caudally. This process is repeated for each digit.

With the blade technique, a No. 12 scalpel blade is used to excise the third phalanx. First the collateral ligaments are cut, and then the nail itself is cut away from the pad and underlying tissue.

For both the Rescoe and blade techniques, sutures or surgical glue can be placed to appose the skin edges after nail removal. If glue is used it should not be placed on exposed bone or dropped into the wound. The wound should be closed first, and then a drop of glue added. Paws are bandaged snugly with gauze and tape. Care must be taken not to make the bandage too tight, as vascular compromise and skin sloughing could occur. Once the bandage has been placed, the tourniquet can be removed.

FIGURE 7-62   Declaw. A tourniquet should always be placed, distal to the elbow (**A**) rather than proximal to the elbow (**B**) to help prevent permanent radial nerve damage. (From Bassert JM, McCurnin DM, editors: McCurnin's clinical textbook for veterinary technicians, ed 7, St Louis, 2010, Elsevier.)

FIGURE 7-63   Sites for nerve blocks of sensory innervation to the feline forepaw. **A,** Extend the carpus and palpate the superficial digital flexor tendon along the palmar aspect of the paw. Block the median nerve with bupivacaine just medial to the superficial digital flexor tendon. Similarly, block the palmar branches of the ulnar nerve along the lateral superficial digital flexor tendon. **B,** Block dorsal digital nerves II to V by inserting the needle from lateral to medial just distal to the carpus. Inject bupivacaine as the needle is withdrawn. Block dorsal digital nerve I at the articulation between metacarpal I and II with bupivacaine. (From Fossum TW, Hedlund CS, Hulse DA, et al: Small animal surgery, ed 3, St Louis, 2007, Mosby.)

The last technique uses a laser to disarticulate the third phalanx. A tourniquet is not necessary with this procedure because the site does not typically bleed when cut with the laser. Saline-soaked sponges are needed to cover the remainder of the cat's foot, all instruments, and the surgeon's fingers. The sponges prevent burning by absorbing the extra energy given off by the laser.

The patient preparation for a laser declaw is similar to that for the standard declaw. Care must be taken not to use flammable liquids when prepping the paw skin. The surgeon will choose the wattage, mode, and tip size used for the procedure. The technician will ensure that the surgery room and its occupants are "laser safe." A hemostat can be positioned on the claw for manipulation and extension of the nail. A 360-degree circumferential incision is made through the skin and the underlying fascia between the second and third phalanges. This incision exposes the common digital extensor tendon. The laser is then used to transect the common digital extensor tendon as well as the deeper synovial layer at its insertion on the distal phalanx. Gentle distraction of the nail at this point exposes the collateral ligaments. The collateral ligaments are then incised bilaterally, and the joint (second/third phalanges) can be disarticulated. The third phalanx is further freed up by laser transection of the deep digital flexor tendon caudal to its ungual process. Care should be taken to avoid thermal damage to the digital pad and other soft tissue attachments, which can be caused by misdirection of the laser beam. This procedure should be repeated on each remaining claw.

At the end of the laser procedure, each digit should be meticulously examined. Any char noted on the digit should be removed with sterile gauze. Bandages can be placed for significant hemorrhage, but the laser declaw procedure is usually associated with minimal or no hemorrhage.

Postoperative Considerations and Instructions

It is imperative that multimodal pain management be used for this procedure. Pain medication should be given for at least 4-5 days postoperatively. Bandages are removed within 24 hours, before the cat leaves the hospital. The owner should be advised to provide shredded paper or pelleted litter to prevent contamination of the paws with clay litter. Regular litter can be re-introduced after 10 days. The cat's activity should be restricted and excessive grooming should be discouraged until the paws have healed.

In addition to the general postoperative and discharge instructions for any declaw surgery, more specific recommendations exist for laser declaw surgery. As stated, postoperative pain tends to be decreased with a laser declaw, but not absent. As with any procedure, appropriate analgesics should be administered postoperatively. Slight epithelial swelling is normal after surgery and may aid the redundant epithelium in covering the surgical site. Closure of the laser declaw site is usually not indicated. In most cases the patient bears weight on the paws the same day or 1 day postoperatively.

Ear Procedures
Aural Hematoma Repair

Definition

Aural hematoma refers to the formation of a hematoma within the auricular cartilage on the concave surface of the ear. The hematoma forms when the cartilage in the ear pinna fractures, usually from violent head shaking or scratching at the ears secondary to otitis, foreign bodies in the ear canal, atopy, or ear mites. It is important to treat the underlying cause of the aural hematoma to prevent further injury and recurrence. Auricular hematomas occur most frequently in pendulous-eared dogs, but they also occur in cats and erect-eared dogs.

Indications

Surgical correction of an aural hematoma should be performed as soon as possible to relieve the animal's pain and to prevent a permanently thickened, cauliflower-like ear.

Instrumentation

A soft tissue surgery pack will provide the surgeon with the necessary instruments for surgical correction of an aural hematoma.

Patient Positioning

Patients are usually placed in lateral recumbency with the affected ear dorsal.

Patient Draping

A single fenestrated drape should be sufficient for the aural hematoma procedure.

Treatment Options

A variety of treatment options exist for the repair of aural hematomas. The objectives of these treatments are to eliminate the hematoma and prevent reappearance of the condition. This section describes only one common treatment option.

Incision drainage procedure. Incision drainage is probably the most widely used procedure for the treatment of aural hematomas. Its purpose is to eliminate dead space between the layers of cartilage until scar tissue can form. An incision (S-shaped or straight) is made directly over the entire hematoma. Fibrin and blood clots are removed, and the area is lavaged. Several vertical mattress sutures are placed on the concave surface of the ear around the incision (Figure 7-64) to avoid pocket formation where fluid can collect. The incision itself should remain open to allow continual drainage.

Box 7-14 shows an example of a surgery report for incision drainage.

Lateral Ear Canal Resection
Definition
Resection of the lateral ear canal involves lateralization of the horizontal ear canal.

Indications
Lateral ear canal resection is indicated for animals with chronic otitis externa or neoplasia. Lateral wall resection allows drainage of the ear canal while affording ventilation of the canal. Bacteria thrive in moist and humid environments, so allowing ventilation reduces the risk of infection. Surgery improves the chronic condition in many patients, but it is not a cure. Appropriate medical management is usually required in conjunction with surgery.

Instrumentation
A soft tissue surgery pack should be sufficient for lateral ear canal resection.

FIGURE 7-64 Sutures should be placed vertically rather than horizontally for aural hematoma repair. Sutures may be placed through the cartilage without incorporating the skin on the convex surface of the ear, or full-thickness sutures may be used. (From Fossum TW, Hedlund CS, Hulse DA, et al: Small animal surgery, ed 3, St Louis, 2007, Mosby.)

Patient Positioning
The patient should be positioned in lateral recumbency with the affected ear upward and the head slightly elevated. A sandbag can be placed under the head for elevation.

Patient Draping
A four-quarter draping method should be used for lateral ear resection. The inner and outer aspects of the pinna should be aseptically prepared and can be left in the surgical field.

Lateral Ear Resection Procedure
The entire ear, including both sides of the pinna and the adjacent skin, should be clipped and aseptically prepared. The ear canal should be lavaged and cleaned before the

FIGURE 7-65 Lateral ear resection (Zepp procedure). (From Fossum TW, Hedlund CS, Hulse DA, et al: Small animal surgery, ed 3, St Louis, 2007, Mosby.)

patient enters the surgery room. Once the animal is prepped and draped, the surgeon makes two parallel skin incisions from the tragus ventrally past the horizontal ear canal. The incision should extend past the region where the canal becomes horizontal. The skin flap is then excised at the proximal region. A vertical incision is made in the subcutaneous tissue over the vertical canal. The subcutaneous tissue is then reflected dorsally, exposing the auricular cartilage of the vertical canal. The cartilage of the vertical canal is then cut distally along the same incision line. The cartilage flap is reflected distally, and the opening of the horizontal canal observed. The proximal two thirds of the cartilage flap are excised, and the remaining third is reflected ventrally to form a "drainboard," which is then sutured to the ventral skin incision. The drainboard technique was established by Zepp to maintain horizontal canal patency (Figure 7-65).

Postoperative Considerations and Instructions
A bandage may be placed over the ear after the lateral ear canal resection. The owner should be made aware of possible mutilation of the surgical site by the pet. An Elizabethan collar should be sent home with the owner to avoid self-mutilation complications. Although complications are uncommon, insufficient drainage and sustained ear infections may be seen postoperatively. Most lateral ear resections still require medical management by the owner. Before leaving the hospital, the owner should also

---

BOX 7-14   Surgery Report: Incision Drainage Procedure

Animal Hospital Name
Owner: John Doe
Address: 555 Sterling Lane
    Jupiter, NY 55555
Phone number: 555-5555
Animal Name: Sasha
Animal #: 65656501
Species: Canine
Breed: Labrador
DOB: 05/05/10
Date of Surgery: 01/03/2011
Primary Surgeon: Dr. Vet
Assistant: Nurse Scrub
Diagnosis or Preoperative Signs: Aural hematoma right ear.
Surgical Procedure: Incisional drainage of aural hematoma.

Description of Surgical Procedure
Surgical Approach: An S-shaped incision was made directly over the aural hematoma on the concave region of the pinna of the right ear. Blood and clots were evacuated.
Surgical Pathology: Aural hematoma located on concave surface of right ear.
Surgical Procedure: An S-shaped incision was made with a scalpel over the fluctuant part of the hematoma. Blood was drained out of the cavity, and several small clots were removed with forceps and by blotting with sponges. Numerous simple mattress sutures of 3-0 nylon were placed in a vertical orientation in a staggered pattern through the skin on the concave side of the ear and the underlying cartilage. The S-shaped incision was left open to drain, and a bandage covering the entire ear was placed.
Closure:
See above.

---

be instructed on how to clean and administer medication in the horizontal canal. Because the anatomy of the ear canal has changed, the tympanic membrane is more susceptible to damage. Analgesics should be sent home with the owner. Suture removal should be performed 10 to 14 days after surgery.

Box 7-15 shows an example of a surgery report for a lateral ear resection.

Ophthalmic Procedures
Entropion Repair
Definition

Entropion refers to a "rolling in" of the eyelid. This can mean the upper lid only, lower lid only, or both lids. Different regions of the eyelid may be involved: the medial aspect, the lateral aspect, or the entire lid.

Indications

The primary indication for an entropion surgery is to alleviate ocular irritation caused by the eyelid or by the facial hairs adjacent to it, which come in contact with the conjunctiva and cornea.

Clinical Signs

Clinical signs of entropion may include lacrimation (tearing), blepharospasm (squinting, blinking), photo-

phobia (sensitivity to light), enophthalmos (pulling back of the eye and a secondary, raised third eyelid), conjunctivitis (inflammation of the conjunctiva), keratitis (inflammation of the cornea) with or without corneal ulceration, and self-trauma (pawing at the eye). Decreased vision may also result from constant eyelid closure or from corneal scarring caused by the constant irritation.

Developmental entropion, or conformational entropion, is the most common form seen in small animals, mostly dogs. It is believed to be inherited. The most common breeds presented with developmental entropion are the Chinese Shar-Pei, chow chow, Saint Bernard, Rottweiler, Great Dane, bull mastiff, Labrador retriever, and English bulldog. Dogs with conformational entropion may have both eyes affected at the same time, but occasionally only one eye is affected.

Spastic entropion occurs secondary to ocular pain, which may result from a corneal foreign body, uveitis (intraocular inflammation), corneal ulceration, or chronic conjunctivitis. The painful eye is pulled back, causing the eyelid to roll inward. In cases of spastic entropion, the primary problem must be addressed and resolved. Application of a topical anesthetic usually temporarily resolves a spastic entropion. Dogs with developmental (conformational) entropion still have rolling in of the eyelid even after application of topical anesthetic.

BOX 7-15 Surgery Report: Lateral Ear Canal Resection

Animal Hospital Name
Owner: John Doe
Address: 555 Sterling Lane
　Jupiter, NY 55555
Phone number: 555-5555
Animal Name: Sasha
Animal #: 65656501
Species: Canine
Breed: Cocker spaniel
DOB: 05/05/07
Date of Surgery: 01/03/2011
Primary Surgeon: Dr. Vet
Assistant: Nurse Scrub
Diagnosis or Preoperative Signs: Chronic otitis externa AU.
Surgical Procedure: Lateral ear canal resection.

Description of Surgical Procedure
Surgical Approach: Two parallel skin incisions were made from the tragus ventrally past the horizontal canal.
Surgical Pathology: The right and left ear canals were inflamed, with a marked amount of ceruminous discharge present.
Surgical Procedure: The skin incision was extended past the vertical canal, and the proximal skin flap was excised. A vertical incision was made in the subcutaneous tissue over the canal, and the tissue was reflected dorsally. The cartilage of the vertical canal was incised distally along the incision line. The proximal region of the cartilage flap was excised. The remaining cartilage flap was reflected ventrally and sutured to the ventral skin incision with 3-0 nylon. The same procedure was performed on the left ear.
Closure:
See above.

Patient Positioning

The patient is placed in sternal or lateral recumbency for entropion surgery; several sandbags can be used to help position the head.

Patient Draping

Often a specialized eye drape is used for the patient undergoing entropion repair. The drape is secured with towel clamps.

Patient Preparation

Cleanliness and sterility of the surgical area are important in the patient with entropion. Shaving or clipping of the surgical area and the surrounding skin is done first. Baby shampoo diluted (1:3) with water is both effective and safe in cleansing the shaved area. Gauze squares soaked in the diluted baby shampoo are used to gently wipe away stray hairs and debris. Then, a very dilute (1:50) povidone-iodine (Betadine) solution is used in the same manner. To achieve asepsis, the dilute povidone-iodine solution should be in contact with the skin for approximately 1 minute. The area is gently wiped with gauze squares soaked in sterile saline to remove the solution. If necessary, the eye is flushed with saline to remove any dirt, particles, or mucus that may be trapped under the lids or within the surrounding conjunctiva.

FIGURE 7-66　Half-curved tissue forceps. Small forceps with fine jaws; the teeth of the forceps are structured to allow for tissue pickup without trauma. (From Sonsthagen TF: *Veterinary instruments and equipment,* ed 2, St Louis, Mosby, 2011.)

Special Instruments

Because of the delicacy of eye procedures such as entropion repair, specialized instruments are often required. Appropriate care and handling of the following ophthalmic instruments are important:

Half-curved tissue forceps is a smaller forceps used for handling eyelid and conjunctival tissue (Figure 7-66). The forceps may be straight or curved with teeth structure that allows tissue to be manipulated without causing trauma.
Chalazion forceps provide tissue stabilization and hemostasis (Figure 7-67).

FIGURE 7-67 Chalazion forceps. The ends may be circular or oval, with round, smooth edges. (From Sonsthagen TF: Veterinary instruments and equipment, ed 2, St Louis, 2011, Mosby.)

FIGURE 7-68 Jaeger lid plate.

The Jaeger lid plate has flat, curved ends that are placed under the eyelid to provide a firm surface when making an incision (Figure 7-68).

Tenotomy scissors have short, blunt, narrowed tips for dividing and dissecting the muscles and tendons of the eye during recession and resection for strabismus surgery (Figure 7-69).

Needle holders are used for handling delicate suture needles needed for placing sutures in an eye and performing neurosurgery; fine needles are held by jaws attached to spring-loaded handles that catch or release with gentle pressure (Figure 7-70).

Surgical Options

Eyelid tacking. Eyelid tacking is performed in young animals to roll out the eyelid temporarily (Figure 7-71). Young puppies (usually up to 16-20 weeks) with conformational entropion are candidates for temporary placement of sutures or staples. The Chinese Shar-Pei is a breed that commonly benefits from eyelid tacking. Even though eyelid tacking is a relatively simple procedure, standard postoperative care is important. The animal should wear an Elizabethan collar until the sutures or staples are removed. In some cases, a repeat procedure may be necessary. Permanent correction is usually delayed until the animal reaches its adult conformation.

In cases of spastic entropion, temporary eyelid tacking, in addition to treatment of the underlying cause, may result in resolution of the problem.

Holtz-Celsus procedure. Several techniques are described to correct conformational entropion. The Holtz-Celsus procedure is a widely used approach that involves excision of a crescent-shaped section of skin and muscle (a "smile") from the affected portion of the eyelid (Figure 7-72). Eversion of the eyelid is accomplished by suturing the resulting skin defect.

Subcutaneous sutures are usually not necessary with the Holtz-Celsus procedure. Skin sutures are placed approximately 1 to 2 mm apart in a simple interrupted pattern. Common sutures used are silk, gut, and polyglactin 910 (Vicryl). Small sutures are preferred, usually 5-0 or 6-0, because they have a better cosmetic result.

Complications with the Holtz-Celsus procedure may result from making the initial incision too far from the eyelid margin or placing the sutures too far apart.

Postoperative Considerations

A patient is often discharged the day of entropion surgery. Tissue swelling may occur, although it should resolve within a few days. The owner may apply warm compresses to the area to help with any swelling. Sutures are left in place for about 10 to 14 days. Nonabsorbable sutures are most frequently used. Absorbable sutures can also be used, especially if removing the sutures will be difficult because of an aggressive or uncooperative animal. A topical ophthalmic antibiotic is usually sent home with the owner to be used two or three times a day for 10 to 14 days after surgery.

The animal should wear an Elizabethan collar until the sutures are removed, to prevent them from being rubbed out before healing has been completed. The awkwardness of the Elizabethan collar, especially in large dogs, often requires restriction of activity until the collar is removed.

A recheck examination is recommended 10 to 14 days after surgery, or sooner if there are any problems. Box 7-16 shows an example of a surgery report for entropion repair.

Eyelid Mass (Neoplasm) Removal

Incidence and Differential Diagnosis

Eyelid masses are found in both dogs and cats. Breeds of dogs that are more predisposed to eyelid masses include poodles, Labrador retrievers, and mixed breeds. Generally, eyelid masses are seen in older dogs.

Canine eyelid masses are usually benign and may be differentiated based on their clinical appearance, but they should always be examined histologically as well.

Feline eyelid neoplasms are usually malignant and can rarely be differentiated from one another solely on the basis of their clinical appearance.

Eyelid neoplasms may be raised, alopecic (having hair loss), and pigmented or nonpigmented, and may or may not become ulcerated. Cytologic examination, specifically by fine-needle aspiration and biopsy samples of eyelid masses, may be helpful.

FIGURE 7-69 Tenotomy scissors. (From Sonsthagen TF: Veterinary instruments and equipment, ed 2, St Louis, 2011, Mosby.)

FIGURE 7-70 Castroviejo needle holder with catch. (From Sonsthagen TF: Veterinary instruments and equipment, ed 2, St Louis, 2011, Mosby.)

FIGURE 7-71 Eyelid tacking for entropion; sutures are placed to temporarily evert the eyelid margin. A few drops of surgical glue may be placed within the created furrow to minimize the tension on the sutures and prevent removal if the patient rubs his/her eye. (From Fossum TW, Hedlund CS, Hulse DA, et al: Small animal surgery, ed 3, St Louis, 2007, Mosby.)

Canine eyelid neoplasms. A *meibomian* (sebaceous) adenoma is the most common eyelid neoplasm in dogs. It arises from the meibomian gland and is found near the meibomian orifice. Other, less common benign neoplastic masses are melanoma, papilloma, and histiocytoma. Malignant neoplastic masses, which occur less often in dogs, include mast cell tumors, adenocarcinomas, basal cell carcinomas, squamous cell carcinomas, hemangiosarcomas, and fibrosarcomas.

Feline eyelid neoplasms. Squamous cell carcinoma is the most common feline eyelid tumor and is often found in cats with white or pink eyelids. Other neoplasms are basal cell carcinoma, fibrosarcoma, and mast cell tumor.

Indications for Surgery

An eyelid mass should be removed if (1) the mass becomes too large, (2) there is concern about malignancy, (3) corneal or conjunctival irritation is present, or (4) the patient is traumatizing the mass, with or without

FIGURE 7-72 **A,** Holtz-Celsus procedure for entropion repair. **B,** Note the use of the Jaeger eyelid plate to stabilize the eyelid during skin incision. **C-E,** The surgeon then closes the defect. (From Fossum TW, Hedlund CS, Hulse DA, et al: Small animal surgery, ed 3, St Louis, 2007, Mosby.)

FIGURE 7-73 Wedge resection for ectropion correction. (From Fossum TW, Hedlund CS, Hulse DA, et al: Small animal surgery, ed 3, St Louis, 2007, Mosby.)

bleeding. In some cases the owner may request removal of the mass to achieve an improved cosmetic appearance. Generally, the smaller the mass to be removed, the easier it is to reconstruct the lid, therefore preserving normal eyelid function. When the eyelid mass becomes too large (greater than one-third of the length of the eyelid), skin flaps may be necessary for eyelid reconstruction. If the eyelid mass is not completely removed, it may recur.

Patient Positioning
The patient is placed in sternal or lateral recumbency for eyelid mass removal; several sandbags can be used to help position the head.

Patient Draping
Often a specialized eye drape is used. An eye drape has a precut hole that is placed directly over the eye. The drape is secured with towel clamps.

Patient Preparation
See previous section on patient preparation for entropion repair.

Special Instruments
See previous section on special instruments for ophthalmic procedures.

Surgical Options
Eyelid mass removal and subsequent eyelid repair involve careful apposition of the conjunctiva, eyelid margin, and the surrounding skin for cosmetic healing and optimal function of the eyelid. The alignment of the eyelid margin, both horizontally and vertically, is critical.

Wedge resection. A wedge resection of the eyelid mass and adjacent eyelid is a simple, common procedure (Figure 7-73). A chalazion forceps or a Jaeger lid plate may be used for stabilization. A full-thickness "house-shaped" incision is made with sharp dissection. The incision is closed in two layers. Subcutaneous sutures are placed in a simple interrupted pattern using 5-0 Vicryl. Skin sutures are placed using a figure-of-8 pattern for apposition of the eyelid margin, and a few simple interrupted sutures are placed for the remainder of the incision using 6-0 Vicryl.

The mass is routinely biopsied and submitted for histopathology to confirm the diagnosis. Box 7-17 shows an example of a surgery report for wedge resection of an eyelid mass.

BOX 7-16 Surgery Report: Entropion Repair

Animal Hospital Name
Owner: John Doe
Address: 555 Sterling Lane
 Jupiter, NY 55555
Phone number: 555-5555
Animal Name: Sasha
Animal #: 65656501
Species: Canine
Breed: Rottweiler
DOB: 05/05/10
Date of Surgery: 01/03/2011
Primary Surgeon: Dr. Vet
Assistant: Nurse Scrub
Diagnosis or Preoperative Signs: Entropion OU.
Surgical Procedure: Holtz-Celsus entropion repair OU.

Description of Surgical Procedure
Surgical Approach: The patient was placed in sternal recumbency and the head positioned with sandbags. Each eye was clipped, prepped, and covered with a sterile eye drape. Towel clamps were used to secure the drape in place.
Surgical Procedures: Ophthalmic scissors were used to make a "smile" incision into the skin and subcutaneous tissue of the ventral eyelid approximately 5 mm from this lid margin. The incision was wider laterally and tapered medially over a distance of approximately 1 cm. Minimal bleeding was encountered and was effectively stopped with gentle pressure from a sterile cotton-tipped applicator. A simple interrupted 6-0 silk suture was first placed in the middle of this incision to re-appose the edges, followed by subsequent simple interrupted sutures approximately 2 mm apart to appose the skin edges.
Closure:
See above.

BOX 7-17 Surgery Report: Wedge Resection of Eyelid Mass

Animal Hospital Name
Owner: John Doe
Address: 555 Sterling Lane
 Jupiter, NY 55555
Phone number: 555-5555
Animal Name: Sasha
Animal #: 65656501
Species: Canine
Breed: Labrador
DOB: 05/05/07
Date of Surgery: 01/03/11
Primary Surgeon: Dr. Vet
Assistant: Nurse Scrub
Diagnosis or Preoperative Signs: Upper eyelid mass OS (3-4 mm in length).
Surgical Procedure: Eyelid mass resection.

Description of Surgical Procedure
Surgical Approach: The patient was placed in sternal recumbency, and the head positioned with sandbags. The left eye was clipped, prepped, and covered by a sterile eye drape. Towel clamps were used to secure the drape in place.
Surgical Pathology: A 3-mm mass on the eyelid margin at the meibomian glands.
Surgical Procedures/Correction: A chalazion forceps was placed around the eyelid mass to protect the globe, stabilize the tissue, and aid in hemostasis. With a beaver blade, a wedge-shaped incision (5 mm wide × 15 mm tall) was made at the eyelid margin. The mass was incised with a blade and removed with ophthalmic scissors.
Closure:
Subcutaneous layer: Using 5-0 Vicryl, two sutures were placed in simple interrupted suture pattern.
Skin layer: A figure-of-eight suture through the skin at the lid margin was placed using 6-0 silk. Three simple interrupted sutures using 6-0 silk were also placed.
Surgical samples: The mass was resected and submitted for histopathology.

Protrusion (Prolapse) of the Gland of the Third Eyelid

Protrusion of the gland of the third eyelid is also known as glandular hypertrophy, glandular hyperplasia, "cherry eye," and prolapse of third eyelid gland.

Third Eyelid Anatomy and Function

The third eyelid, also known as the "nictitating membrane," serves as added protection for the globe. It rises up from the ventromedial aspect of the orbit (part closest to nose) and over the globe to protect it when the animal pulls its globe back into the orbit, for whatever reason. Movement of the third eyelid also aids in removal of dirt and particles from the eye. On the underside of the third eyelid is a small gland that secretes and distributes approximately 30% of the tear production. Because the gland significantly contributes to the precorneal tear film, it should not be removed. Clinical studies have confirmed extensive clinical experience that keratoconjunctivitis (KCS, "dry eye") is frequently seen in such animals, often years later, especially in breeds susceptible to prolapse of the gland.

Mechanism of Prolapse

Prolapse of the third eyelid gland is the most common primary disorder of the third eyelid. A prolapse may result from a weakness in the connective tissue attachment between the ventral aspect of the third eyelid and the periorbital tissues; therefore the gland becomes everted while remaining attached to the cartilage of the third eyelid. This weakness allows the gland, which is normally found ventrally, to flip up dorsally, where it then becomes enlarged and inflamed because of chronic exposure. Abrasions and drying of the exposed gland may result in secondary inflammation and swelling. If the gland becomes severely infected, preoperative treatment with topical antibiotics is recommended.

Occasionally, in the early stages of prolapse, the gland returns to its normal position on its own or with manipulation. Unfortunately, prolapse of the gland usually recurs. Surgical intervention is the definitive treatment.

Clinical Signs

Common clinical signs of third eyelid gland prolapse include ocular discharge, conjunctivitis, and the pink, swollen mass on the third eyelid seen by owners. Tear production may be affected in some patients and may decrease.

Incidence

Protrusion of the gland of the third eyelid is usually seen in puppies and dogs younger than 2 years. It can occur in one or both eyes. Breeds predisposed to this disorder are the Cocker Spaniel, English Bulldog, Boston Terrier, Great Dane, and Pug.

Patient Positioning

The patient is placed in sternal or lateral recumbency for third eyelid gland surgery; several sandbags can be used to help position the head.

Patient Draping

Often a specialized eye drape is used. An eye drape has a precut hole that is placed directly over the eye. The drape is secured with towel clamps.

Patient Preparation

See previous section on patient preparation for entropion repair.

Special Instruments

Because of the delicacy of eye procedures, specialized instruments are often required. Appropriate care and handling of ophthalmic instruments are important. In addition to those instruments listed in the section on entropion repair, an eyelid speculum is useful for surgical correction of third eyelid gland prolapse; it is used to retract the eyelids without putting pressure on the eye itself (Figure 7-74).

Surgical Options

For years, surgical removal of the third eyelid gland was the treatment of choice for third eyelid protrusion. As the importance of the third eyelid gland in tear production became more apparent, however, surgical repositioning of the gland became widely recommended. Therefore, removing the third eyelid gland should be avoided, because this may and probably will predispose the eye to develop KCS (dry eye).

Numerous techniques are currently available for correcting prolapse of the third eyelid gland (Figures 7-75 and 7-76), with some achieving greater success than others. The choice is usually the surgeon's preference. A simple, common procedure is discussed next.

Morgan pocket technique. The Morgan pocket technique involves creating a conjunctival pocket where the third eyelid gland is secured. The third eyelid is grasped and suspended with forceps on the nasal and temporal sides. Two 1-cm parallel incisions are made on the posterior surface of the third eyelid. The incisions are arched

FIGURE 7-74 Eye speculum. The curved ends slide under each eyelid; then a spring device or a turning knob spreads the eyelids apart. (From Sonsthagen TF: Veterinary instruments and equipment, ed 2, St Louis, 2011, Mosby.)

FIGURE 7-75 Morgan pocket technique for repair of a prolapsed gland of the third eyelid (TE). This method involves securing the TE gland into a conjunctival pocket formed on the posterior surface of the TE. When the conjunctival margins are sutured, openings are left on either end to allow drainage of secretions. Suturing begins by oversewing and burying the knot (subcuticular pattern), then runs continuously through the conjunctiva from side to side, and finally is tied on the anterior ventral surface of the TE. This method of suturing prevents corneal irritation from the suture knots. (From Maggs D: Slatter's fundamentals of veterinary ophthalmology, ed 4, St Louis, 2008, Saunders.)

toward each other, with one incision made above the third eyelid gland and the second made below it. Apposition of the two outermost incisions, with gentle downward pressure applied to the gland, results in burial of the gland being in the conjunctival pocket. Care must be taken that the suture ends do not contact the cornea and therefore cause irritation.

Postoperative Considerations

Inadequate positioning of the third eyelid gland may result in re-prolapse. Usually a second attempt and possibly a third attempt to resecure the gland are made, typically using a different approach. Box 7-18 shows an example of a surgery report for correction of a prolapsed third eyelid gland.

Orthopedic Procedures

Definition

Orthopedic surgery is a branch of surgery dealing with the preservation and restoration of the function of the skeletal system and its articulation and association with its related structures (Figure 7-77).

Technician's Responsibilities

The purpose of this section is to familiarize the surgical technician with the basic presentation of fractures, with fracture evaluation, and with the types of repair available for the stabilization of different fractures. Understanding fracture management and repair will make the technician

an asset to any veterinary practice. Being able to triage, evaluate, and either refer or prepare the patient for orthopedic surgery are all responsibilities that may fall on the technician. Box 7-19 introduces orthopedic terms and abbreviations.

Orthopedic fracture repair is a broad and highly specialized subject; readers wanting more in-depth coverage can supplement this chapter's discussion with additional reading (see Bibliography). Orthopedic surgery requires expensive specialized instruments and equipment along with an experienced orthopedic surgeon.

Orthopedic problems are usually not life-threatening situations. These cases can be considered life-threatening emergencies, however, if the skull or spine is involved or if the patient has lost large amounts of blood because of a long-bone fracture. Other cases that can be considered nonelective but are not life threatening are open fracture or open dislocation repairs. All these cases need to be fully evaluated, and the patient should be stabilized (e.g., open airway, controlled bleeding, stable vital signs, and managed pain) before further evaluation or surgery can occur. Elective orthopedic surgical cases that may be presented to the hospital include cranial cruciate or anterior cruciate ligament rupture, medial or lateral patellar luxation, hip dysplasia, or osteochondritis dissecans. These cases also need to be properly evaluated before surgery, but they are considered elective.

Patients that are presented with fractures can be assumed to be in significant pain and need strong analgesics. It is the technician's responsibility to see that the

FIGURE 7-76 **A,** Typical appearance of a prolapsed third eyelid gland. **B,** Elliptical incision. **C,** Initial anchor suture. **D,** Initial suture carried to the opposite side of the gland. **E,** Placement of a second suture. **F,** The initial suture is drawn together and tied. **G,** Inversion of prolapsed tissue. *Dotted lines* indicate that the suture and knots lie under the conjunctiva. **H,** Appearance of third eyelid immediately after surgery.

BOX 7-18 Surgery Report: Prolapsed Gland of Third Eyelid

Animal Hospital Name
Owner: John Doe
Address: 555 Sterling Lane
Jupiter, NY 55555
Phone number: 555-5555
Animal Name: Fluffy
Animal #: 65656501
Species: Canine
Breed: Pug
DOB: 05/05/07
Date of Surgery: 01/03/2011
Primary Surgeon: Dr. Vet
Assistant: Nurse Scrub
Diagnosis or Preoperative Signs: Prolapsed gland of the third eyelid, OD.
Surgical Procedure: Morgan pocket technique.

Description of Surgical Procedure
Surgical Approach: The patient was placed in left lateral recumbency to allow access to the right eye. The leading edge of the third eyelid was grasped with two small, noncrushing forceps and reflected away from its origin.
Surgical Procedures/Correction: With sharp dissection, two 1-cm incisions were made parallel to each other through the bulbar conjunctiva dorsal and ventral to the free margin of the gland. Blunt dissection was used to free up the conjunctiva for ease of suturing.
Closure (Technique and Suture): 6-0 Vicryl suture was used in a simple interrupted, buried pattern to appose the two incisions together, thus replacing the prolapsed gland within the third eyelid.
Surgical samples: None.

BOX 7-19 Orthopedic Terms and Abbreviations

ACL: Anterior cruciate ligament.
A-O: Arbeitsgemeinschaft für Osteosynthesefragen, Swiss for the Association for the Study of Internal Fixation (ASIF). These abbreviations are frequently seen together but separated by a slash: AO/ASIF. The AO is involved in research and development of medical devices used in orthopedic surgery. Their devices are available through a company called Synthes Holding AG (West Chester, PA).
ASIF: Association for the Study of Internal Fixation.
Articular: Pertaining to a joint.
Aseptic loosening: Breakdown of bone and loosening of prosthesis in the absence of microorganisms.
CCL: Cranial cruciate ligament.
Callus: Unorganized network of woven bone formed about ends of a broken bone, which is reabsorbed as healing is completed.
Closed reduction: Nonsurgical realignment of fracture or joint.
Delayed union: Prolonged renewal of continuity in a broken bone or between the edges of a wound.
Dislocation: Complete separation of the articular surfaces of a joint.
Elective: Referring to surgical cases that can wait for later scheduling.
HOD: Hypertrophic osteodystrophy; developmental disease that causes disruption of metaphyseal trabeculae in long bones of young, rapidly growing dogs.

Hip dysplasia: Abnormal development of coxofemoral joint characterized by subluxation or complete luxation of femoral head in younger patients and mild to severe degenerative joint disease in older patients.
IVDD: Intervertebral disc disease associated with disc degeneration and extrusion, causing spinal cord compression and nerve root entrapment.
Interfragmentary: Bone pieces of a fracture that may or may not be able to be reconstructed and stabilized.
Luxation: Complete separation of a bone from its articulation.
MPL: Medial patellar luxation.
Malunion: Faulty union and alignment of the fractured bone.
Non-union: Failure of the fractured bone ends to unite.
Nonelective: Referring to surgical cases that cannot wait for later scheduling.
Nonreducible: Unable to be restored to the normal place or position.
OCD: Osteochondritis dissecans; inflammation of bone and cartilage that results in the splitting of cartilage pieces into the affected joint.
Open reduction: Surgical opening and exposure to realign a fracture or joint.
Reducible: Able to be restored to the normal place or relation of parts, as a fracture.
Subluxation: Partial or incomplete separation of a joint.

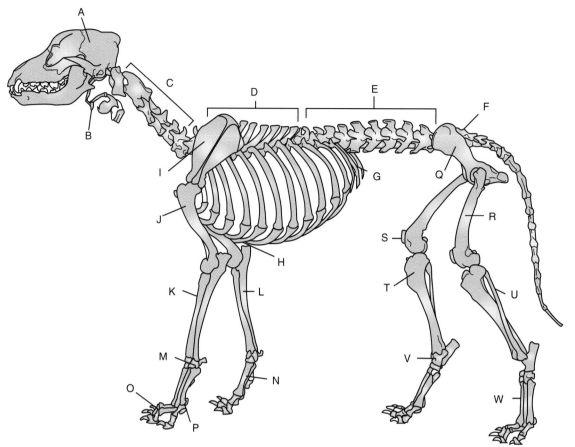

FIGURE 7-77 Skeleton of the male dog. A, Skull; B, hyoid apparatus; C, cervical spine; D, thoracic spine; E, lumbar spine; F, sacrum; G, ribs; H, sternum; I, scapula; J, humerus; K, radius; L, ulna; M, carpal bones; N, metacarpal bones; O, phalanges; P, sesamoid bone; Q, pelvis; R, femur; S, patella; T, tibia; U, fibula; V, tarsal bones; W, metatarsal bones. (From Evans H, deLahunta A: Guide to the dissection of the dog, ed 7, St Louis, 2010, Saunders.)

fracture patient receives adequate pain management as directed by the veterinarian. Any fracture noted on examination should be immobilized and bandaged accordingly. External coaptation (application of external appliance, such as a splint or cast) is important to reduce further disruption or damage to the fracture or fragments and the surrounding soft tissue and to prevent further blood loss at the fracture site. Stabilization of fractures also greatly enhances pain management and the animal's comfort level.

Types of bandages used to stabilize a fracture include the Robert Jones bandage (any long-bone fracture) (Figure 7-78) and modified Robert Jones with metal or plastic splint (carpal, metacarpal, tarsal, metatarsal, and phalangeal fractures). A fiberglass cast with adequate padding can also be used for these same types of fractures. Fiberglass applied as a cast and not as a splint can make maintenance and changes technically difficult. Other bandages used for preoperative and postoperative support are the Ehmer sling (hip luxation) (Figure 7-79), spica splint (humeral or femoral fractures) (Figure 7-80), and Velpeau sling (scapular fractures) (Figure 7-81). All these

bandages, except for the Robert Jones, can be used as external coaptation if surgery is not an option.

Owners must always be informed of bandage and fracture complications associated with splinting or slinging. A bandage should be checked three or four times a day for signs of swelling, slippage, moisture, or soiling. If any of these scenarios occurs, the bandage should be changed.

Preoperative Considerations for Fractures

The patient history can provide pertinent information to help determine whether a patient is a good candidate for surgery and what type of fixation is best suited for a positive outcome. How old is the patient? How large and active is the animal? What is the overall health status of the patient? What is the temperament of the patient?

The patient's age is significant in terms of how much more the bones need to grow and how active the animal is. Generally, the younger the patient, the faster is the healing time; however, there is also a greater risk of angular limb deformities if the growth plates are still open and have been traumatized. Also, younger patients are more active and are more difficult to confine for long

FIGURE 7-78 **A,** When applying a Robert Jones bandage, place adhesive tape stirrups on the cranial and caudal surfaces of the foot from the carpus (tarsus) to 6 inches beyond the toes. Cover any wounds with a nonadhesive pad. **B,** Then wrap 3 to 6 inches of cotton padding around the limb. **C,** After applying tape stirrups and cotton padding on the limb, wrap elastic gauze firmly over the cotton to compress it. **D,** Then apply elastic tape to the outer surface of the bandage. (From Fossum TW, Hedlund CS, Hulse DA, et al: Small animal surgery, ed 3, St Louis, 2007, Mosby.)

periods. The older the patient, the slower is the healing time. This can contribute to an increased chance of complications because of the longer recovery time. Older patients tend to be more sedentary and to have more difficulty recovering after long periods of inactivity and muscle loss.

The animal's size and weight can affect recovery times and success. Any animal that is overweight has an increased risk of failure for any type of orthopedic repair. Too much force placed on any orthopedic repair too soon can cause premature loosening of the fixation and possible failure of the repair. Some large-breed dogs and overweight dogs and cats are often too weak after orthopedic surgery to lift or support their own weight and may need assistance to rise and walk.

The importance of the orthopedic surgery patient's overall health should never be underestimated. Preoperative consideration of any preexisting conditions that would increase the patient's risk during anesthesia or for delayed healing need to be addressed. Problems with other joints or bones can contribute to poor comfort levels and increase the length of recovery.

Owner compliance is a major consideration in any orthopedic case. The animal's temperament influences how successful owners can be at following postoperative care instructions at home. Owner compliance is probably the most underestimated component of any orthopedic patient's recovery and outcome. An animal that is aggressive, difficult to handle, or difficult for the owner to treat has a lower chance for a successful recovery than the easily handled, stoic animal. If the owners are incapable of handling and treating the patient correctly postoperatively or cannot return for follow-up examinations, the consequences can be catastrophic.

Fracture Assessment

Fractures can be classified or described by the following factors:
1. Bone location (e.g., humerus, femur, tibia).
2. Open or closed fracture (open fractures have penetrated through the skin; the skin is intact in closed fractures).
3. Location of fracture on the bone (e.g., midshaft, articular).

FIGURE 7-79 Ehmer sling. **A,** After minimal padding has been applied to the tarsus, a sling of adhesive tape is passed along the medial aspect of the limb. **B,** The tape is then wrapped around the hindlimb with the stifle and hock held in maximal flexion for one or two passes. **C,** On the third pass, the tape is brought over the flank and twisted behind the hock. **D,** The tape is then passed over the front of the metatarsus. **E,** This wrapping is repeated for three or four passes. (From Bassert JM, McCurnin DM, editors: McCurnin's clinical textbook for veterinary technicians, ed 7, St Louis, 2010, Elsevier.)

4. Type of fracture (e.g., oblique, spiral, transverse).
5. Reducible or nonreducible fracture.

To assess any fracture completely, radiographs should be taken after a thorough physical examination. Some sedation is usually necessary to achieve complete relaxation and compliance of the patient for the radiographic views needed. In animals that are a sedation risk, radiographs can be taken through the bandage or splint. When radiographs are taken of any long-bone fracture, the joints above and below the fracture site should be included on the film. Articular fractures should be centered on the film using the least amount of manipulation necessary. Standard anterior-posterior (anteroposterior, AP) and ventral-dorsal (ventrodorsal, VD) views are suggested for proper fracture evaluation. Radiographs should also be taken postoperatively to confirm proper alignment and repair. X-ray films also serve as a point of reference for follow-up radiographs.

FIGURE 7-80 **A,** When placing a spoon splint on a limb, firmly apply cast padding around the limb in a spiral fashion with a 50% overlap. **B,** Wrap elastic gauze firmly over the cast padding. **C,** Place the padded limb in an appropriate-sized splint. **D,** Secure the splint to the limb with Vetrap (3M, St Paul, MN) or elastic adhesive tape. (From Fossum TW, Hedlund CS, Hulse DA, et al: Small animal surgery, ed 3, St Louis, 2007, Mosby.)

FIGURE 7-81 A 90-90 flexion sling. After minimal padding has been applied to the tarsus, a sling of adhesive tape is passed along the medial aspect of the limb (see Figure 7-78A). **A,** The tape is then wrapped around the hind limb with the stifle and hock held in 90-degree flexion. **B,** A second layer of tape is passed horizontally around the tibia to hold the previous layer in place. (From Bassert JM, McCurnin DM, editors: McCurnin's clinical textbook for veterinary technicians, ed 7, St Louis, 2010, Elsevier.)

Radiographs and a thorough physical examination should suffice in determining whether the fracture or fractures are open or closed. An *open fracture* is a fracture in which the skin and the soft tissue covering the bone were punctured, usually by the sharp ends of the fractured bone, creating a path for external contaminants to come in contact with the bone. The fracture is then considered to be "open" (no longer closed) to the external environment. If possible, open fractures should be cultured before cleaning and antibiotic therapy. Open fractures can be classified or labeled according to the mechanism of puncture and the severity of the soft tissue damage, as follows:

Grade I open fractures have a small puncture hole in the skin around the location of the fracture. The bone broke through the skin and was exposed to external factors but is no longer visible. Soft tissue damage is minimal.

Grade II open fractures have a larger puncture or tear in the skin around the location of the fracture, and more soft tissue damage associated with the external trauma is evident.

Grade III open fractures have large tears and in some cases, loss of skin at the area of impact. Soft tissue damage is extensive and usually caused by severe bone fragmentation along with the force of the external impact. Grade III open fractures can also be described as shearing injuries. The patients usually have lost so much soft tissue that the bone is exposed, and in some cases, the bone is sheared away or even missing.

Complications tend to be worse and more life threatening with open fractures than with closed fractures. Complications associated with open fractures include skin necrosis and infection leading to bone death. With both open and closed fractures, bleeding, soft tissue damage, and swelling are concerns. With any open fracture, contamination and vascular compromise are of great concern and play a large part in determining what type of repair is best suited for the condition.

A *closed fracture* is a fracture that at the time of impact did not puncture or tear the skin at or around the location of the fracture. Soft tissue damage and swelling can range from mild to severe. Figure 7-82 shows the anatomy of a long bone, and Figure 7-83 illustrates bone planes of a femur.

Types of Fractures

Five types of common fractures are shown in Figure 7-84.

Articular fractures. Articular fractures, better known as *physeal fractures*, always involve the joint. These fractures are frequently seen in young, growing animals and are referred to as Salter-Harris fractures. Any fracture involving the physis or growth plate in early stages of bone development can be detrimental to development and may cause angular limb deformities. Physeal fractures can involve the physis itself or the physis and the bone above and below it. Salter-Harris fractures are identified according to the location of the fracture line and what areas of the bone are involved (Figure 7-85).

Y fractures and T fractures are types of articular fractures that involve the distal aspect of the humerus (Figure 7-86). The fracture lines run ventrodorsally through the humeral condyle and run in transverse or oblique configurations through the medial and lateral epicondyles.

Surgical Options for Fracture Repair

Surgical options for fracture repair are initially basic but can become very detailed. In general, the purpose for any fracture fixation is to bring the opposing ends of the

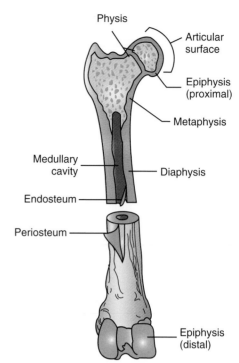

FIGURE 7-82 Anatomy of a long bone (femur). Diaphysis: long shaft or body of bone. Epiphysis (proximal/distal): ends of bone, usually wider than shaft, and either entirely cartilaginous or separated from shaft by cartilaginous disk. Metaphysis: wider end of shaft of the bone adjacent to epiphysis. Periosteum: fibrous covering around bone that is not covered by articular cartilage. This layer is important for bone growth, repair, nutrition, and attachment for ligaments and tendons. Articular surface: smooth layer of hyaline cartilage covering epiphysis where one bone forms a joint with another bone. Medullary cavity: space in diaphysis containing bone marrow. Endosteum: fibrous tissue lining medullary cavity of bone. Physis: growth plate.

fracture and joints back into alignment. After reduction of the fracture, the bone is restabilized and supported by internal or external fixation. Once the bone has been properly immobilized, the healing process and callus formation begin. *Internal fixation* is a form of rigid fixation placed under the skin and muscle directly on or in the bone surface or medullary cavity to regain stability. *External fixation* is a form of fixation applied through the exterior surface (skin and muscle) of the limb to the interior area (bone and medullary cavity) to help with stability.

Bone is the deepest tissue within the limb and therefore is afforded poor drainage in the event of infection. Bone infections (osteomyelitis) are serious and difficult to treat. Great care must be taken when preparing any patient for orthopedic surgery. A broad-spectrum antibacterial, antimicrobial, and antifungal scrub and final prep should be used before surgery, with adherence to strict sterile technique throughout the procedure to prevent contamination.

Internal Fixation

Internal fixation devices include bone plates and screws (Figures 7-87 to 7-90), interlocking nails, intramedullary pins, Kirschner wires, and cerclage wire.

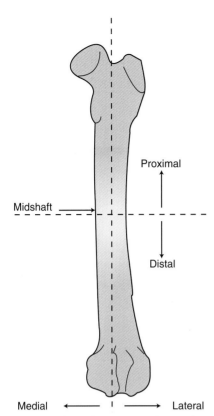

FIGURE 7-83   Bone planes (femur). Proximal: area closest to the body or point of origin. Distal: area farthest from the body or point of origin. Midshaft: center of shaft, or toward median plane. Lateral: farther from medial plane. Medial: toward median plane (inside or middle).

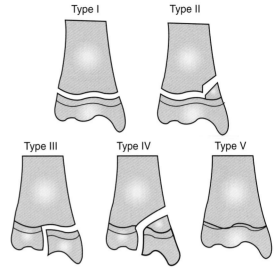

FIGURE 7-85   Salter-Harris fractures. Type I fracture runs through the physis. Type II fracture runs through the metaphysis and physis. Type III fracture runs through the physis and epiphysis. Type IV fracture runs through the metaphysis, physis, and epiphysis. Type V fracture is a crushing injury to the physis; may not always be detected initially by radiographs.

Articular fractures

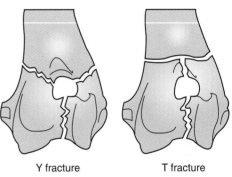

FIGURE 7-86   Y and T articular fractures.

Bone plates come in a variety of shapes, sizes, and lengths. They are designed to be used with various sizes of screw. The plates are made of titanium or stainless steel and are used with screws of the same material. Soft tissue and muscle dissection is necessary to gain adequate exposure of the fracture and to afford successful reduction of the fracture.

Interlocking nails are driven into the medullary cavity and secured in position by screws that engage the bone and the nail at its proximal and distal aspects. This type of fixation provides stabilization without extensive soft tissue dissection and muscle manipulation to expose and reconstruct the fracture (Figures 7-91 to 7-93).

Intramedullary (IM) pins are driven through the bone and into the medullary cavity with a Jacob's chuck . Their placement can be approached as an open surgical technique or a closed pinning technique (Figures 7-94 and 7-95). IM pins can be used alone (single IM pin driven into medullary canal) or stacked (multiple IM pins driven

FIGURE 7-84   Types of fractures. 1, Transverse: extending from side to side at right angle to long axis. 2, Oblique: being on an incline or slanting. 3, Spiral: curving around a center point or axis. 4, Comminuted reducible: broken or crushed into numerous fragments but able to be placed or aligned with opposite end of fracture. 5, Comminuted nonreducible: broken or crushed into numerous fragments and unable to be placed or aligned together with opposite end of fracture.

Dorsal view   Lateral view
FIGURE 7-87 Internal fixation (bone plate and screws).

FIGURE 7-89 Radiograph (lateral view) of tibial fracture repair. An internal plate and screws were used for fixation.

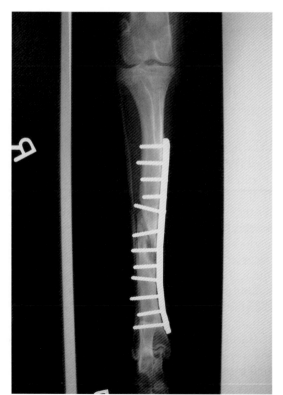

FIGURE 7-88 Radiograph (dorsal view) of a tibial fracture repair. An internal plate and screws were used for fixation.

FIGURE 7-90 Internal orthopedic plate and screw set.

FIGURE 7-93 Interlocking nail and instrument set.

A B

FIGURE 7-94 Intramedullary pins. **A,** Stacked. **B,** Single.

FIGURE 7-91 Placement of a nail within the medullary cavity using an interlocking nail jig.

Jig

FIGURE 7-92 Completed interlocking nail fracture repair. Note the two screws at proximal and distal ends of the bone used for securing the nail.

FIGURE 7-95 Jacob's chuck (used to drive pins through bone) and intramedullary pins.

FIGURE 7-96 Full-cerclage wire application for fracture stabilization.

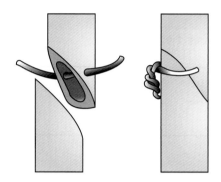

FIGURE 7-97 Hemicerclage wire application for fracture stabilization.

FIGURE 7-98 Kirschner-Ehmer (KE) bars, clamps, and wrench (for adjustment of clamps) used for external fixation.

FIGURE 7-99 SK rods, clamps, and wrench (for adjustment of clamps) used for external fixation.

into medullary canal). Intramedullary pinning is inexpensive compared with all other types of internal fixation but does not provide very rigid stability. Pins tend to migrate, and removal of the implant may become necessary.

Orthopedic wires (Kirschner or cerclage) can be used alone or combined with other fixation devices to achieve proper fixation. Cerclage wire comes in different diameters ranging from 0.4 to 1.5 mm and is used in fracture fixation for the reduction of fragments and the protection of fissures. Cerclage wires can be applied by being passed either completely around the bone (full cerclage; Figure 7-96) or wire through a predrilled hole placed through the bone (hemicerclage; Figure 7-97).

Kirschner wires, or K-wires, are small sections of precut wire that have pointed ends (trocar) for drilling through the bone. They come in multiple diameters for stiffness and can be used in combination with cerclage wire for interfragmentary reduction.

Postoperative care. Postoperative care for internal fixation is strict confinement for 6 to 8 weeks. The patient is rechecked at suture removal, usually 10 to 14 days after surgery. Follow-up radiographs are taken every 4 to 6 weeks postoperatively to monitor bone healing. Young animals may need to be followed more closely because of the rate of bone healing and increased risk of angular complications. Internal fixation is not routinely removed unless the complications involve the implant.

External Fixation

External fixation used as primary repair includes casts, rigid splints, SK fixation, Kirschner-Ehmer (KE) fixation,

and ring fixation (Figures 7-98 to 7-101). As with internal fixation, external fixation requires specialized equipment and has many more applications beyond the scope of this chapter.

External fixation devices stabilize the bones or fracture from the exterior of the limb. These devices use threaded cross-pins that are drilled into the bone, then attached to bars with clamps, nuts and bolts, or aluminum rings to make an external tension device. This will provide rigid stability until the fracture has time to heal. Once the fracture has closed, external fixation is removed. With any

FIGURE 7-100 External fixation fracture repair of tibia and fibula in a dog.

FIGURE 7-102 External ring fixator of long-bone fracture.

FIGURE 7-101 External fixation fracture repair of tibia and fibula.

FIGURE 7-103 External ring fixation set.

external fixation device, weekly to biweekly appointments are needed for fixator adjustments, cleaning of pin tracks, and bandage changes. External fixators are an affordable treatment option for long-bone fractures or temporary joint immobilization. They are not appropriate for fractures that may involve the pelvis or pelvic joints. External fixation devices can be created that best suit the fracture types and locations. The devices can be continually modified or changed throughout the healing period.

The *ring fixator*, or circular fixator, is a type of external fixator that uses different-sized rings (usually three or four) and various types of pins (Figures 7-102 and 7-103). These pins are drilled through the bone and attached to the ring using clamps. The pin is then put under tension to pull the fracture back into alignment and is secured to the ring frame. Ring fixators have many uses in orthopedic surgery (see other texts).

Postoperative care. Postoperative care for external fixators and ring fixators includes periodic visits for cleaning of pin tracts and tightening of clamps. In most cases the external bars or rings need to be padded and wrapped to prevent trauma to the patient and to reduce the risk that the fixator will be caught on objects (e.g., bedding material, crate, furniture). Radiographs should be taken postoperatively and then every 4 weeks until the fixator is removed. Activity should be restricted for the first 4 weeks, then left to the veterinarian's discretion.

Complications with Fixation

The following complications may occur with internal or external fixation:
- Non-union
- Malunion
- Delayed union
- Aseptic loosening
- Infection

Casts and Splints

Casts and splints are other external coaptation devices available for closed reduction of fractures at low cost and requiring no surgery. Anesthesia is necessary to sedate and relax the animal so that the fracture can be reduced, then splinted or cast. A radiograph is essential to ensure proper alignment before and after coaptation is applied. Splints work well on small, young, fast-healing animals. Splints are best suited for injuries that are distal to the elbow or stifle.

When fiberglass or plaster cast material is used, periodic changes can be difficult. A cast cutter or oscillating saw is needed to cut the cast, and specialized cast spreaders are needed to remove the cast easily from the limb. Most patients require sedation for cast and splint changes. They need to be still and pain free during the procedure. A sedated or anesthetized animal is less likely to react to the loud noises associated with the oscillating saw. Most casts require additional support (walking bar) to prevent normal damage to the cast from walking. Casts need to be checked at least every 1 to 2 weeks.

Splints used as primary coaptation devices are easier to manage and change than casts. As with casts, however, splints are suited only for fractures that are distal to the elbow and stifle. Any animal with a splint should have the bandage changed and the fracture rechecked once a week.

Casts and splints require similar care. They must be kept clean and dry and checked for slippage and mutilation by the animal. Any swelling in the toes or signs of malodor should also be noted. If observed, these changes need to be addressed immediately. Radiographs must be taken more often to confirm that fracture alignment and orientation have not changed. Any animal with a cast or splint must be confined to a crate or small room, with no opportunity to run, jump, play, climb stairs, or have free access to the outside until the fracture is healed.

Complications with casts and splints. The following complications may occur with casts or splints:
- Skin irritation
- Skin ulcers

- Non-union
- Malunion
- Delayed union
- Infection

Amputation

Amputation involves the complete removal of a limb from the body. Common indications for amputation include trauma resulting in severe soft tissue damage or irreparable fractures and neurologic injuries (e.g., brachial plexus avulsion). Other indications are neoplasia, ischemic necrosis, unmanageable arthritis, and severe congenital deformities. Both hindlimb and forelimb amputations are considered major surgeries and should be performed only with a thorough knowledge of the patient's physical status. Preanesthetic blood tests, including complete blood count (CBC), chemistry panel, electrolyte status, and blood type and crossmatch, should be obtained before surgery whenever possible. The patient's preoperative condition is extremely important because a large amount of fluid, electrolytes, and blood is lost when the limb is removed. Patients should be stabilized before surgery with appropriate fluid, electrolyte, and blood replacement therapy. A balanced electrolyte solution should also be administered throughout the procedure to help maintain hydration and blood pressure.

A variety of techniques exist for removal of the forelimb and hindlimb. Forelimb amputation can be achieved by disarticulation of the shoulder joint or by removal of the scapula. Scapular removal is faster, easier and allows for a more cosmetically favorable result than shoulder disarticulation. Hindlimb amputation involves either midshaft femoral amputation or disarticulation of the coxofemoral joint. Midshaft amputation is considerably easier to perform than hip disarticulation. All techniques involve severing the muscles at their origins or insertions or directly through the muscle belly (Figure 7-104). Major nerves are then isolated and directly injected with a local anesthetic (Figure 7-105) before they are transected (Figure 7-106). Local nerve blocks contribute significantly to postoperative pain control. Arteries and veins are isolated from surrounding tissues. Arteries are usually ligated first, thus allowing blood to drain through the venous system. In patients with neoplasia, however, veins are ligated first to limit the dissemination of tumor cells. Figures 7-107 and 7-108 show an amputated limb and the postoperative appearance of a disarticulated coxofemoral joint.

Pain management is critical for amputation patients. A variety of analgesic protocols is currently available and is often used in combination for effective prevention of postoperative discomfort. Epidural anesthesia should be performed preoperatively and can be achieved with various drugs; morphine is often used in forelimb amputations, and an opioid and local anesthetic are frequently used in hindlimb amputations. Epidural anesthesia with both an opioid and a local anesthetic is extremely effective

FIGURE 7-104 Dissection through the sartorius muscle belly of the medial hindlimb using electrocautery during a hindlimb amputation.

FIGURE 7-105 Injection of the femoral nerve with local anesthetic before transection.

FIGURE 7-106 Transection of the femoral nerve.

FIGURE 7-107 Disarticulated amputation of the hindlimb after surgery.

FIGURE 7-108 Postoperative surgical site of hindlimb amputation (disarticulated).

in controlling postoperative pain. As mentioned, intraoperative visualization of the nerves allows direct injection of local anesthetic before transection. Systemic injections of opioids and nonsteroidal anti-inflammatory drugs (NSAIDs) are often administered postoperatively. Transdermal fentanyl patches are also recommended as part of the postoperative pain management program. These

patches allow a slow, continuous administration of fentanyl over 72 hours. The patch is applied to a clipped area of the animal's skin immediately after surgery.

Cranial Cruciate Repair

Indications

Cranial cruciate ligament (CCL) ruptures are also referred to as anterior cruciate ligament (ACL) injury or "football player's knee" in human patients. CCL surgical repair should be performed for a partial or complete rupture of the ligament. Both the cranial and the caudal cruciate ligaments act as major stabilizing structures in the knee. The cruciate ligaments originate on either side of the femoral condyle, then course across the intercondylar fossa and attach on opposite sides of the tibia (Figure 7-109). These ligaments function as the primary check against hyperextension of the stifle joint and limit internal rotation of the tibia. Rupture of the CCL causes instability of the stifle, which leads to degenerative changes in the joint, including synovitis, degeneration of articular

Patellar ligament
Caudal cruciate ligament
Cranial cruciate ligament
Intermeniscal ligament
Medial meniscus
Lateral meniscus

Medial   **Lateral**

FIGURE 7-109 Orientation of the cruciate ligaments and menisci. (From Fossum TW, Hedlund CS, Hulse DA, et al: Small animal surgery, ed 3, St Louis, 2007, Mosby.)

cartilage, osteophyte formation, and capsular fibrosis. The medial meniscus usually is also damaged in dogs with CCL rupture. The meniscus is a fibrocartilaginous structure between the femur and tibia that functions to cushion and center the joint. CCL rupture most often causes a bucket-handle type of tear in the medial meniscus.

Rupture of the CCL is the most common cause of hindlimb lameness in the dog. Ligament failure can result from both traumatic (acute) and degenerative (chronic) causes. Currently, degenerative causes are the most common reason for CCL rupture. Osteoarthritic changes act as a precursor to CCL weakening and rupture. Reports also indicate that 37% of dogs with a unilateral CCL tear will rupture the contralateral ligament within 2 years, indicating that degenerative processes often occur in both stifle joints.

Traumatic rupture results from hyperextension of the stifle joint or excessive internal rotation of the tibia. The CCL becomes tightly twisted, and the excessive mechanical forces cause the ligament to tear. Dogs are often presented with a history of running and catching the leg in a hole, trapping the leg in a fence or gate, or jumping to catch an object (e.g., Frisbee). Traumatic injuries account for approximately 20% of CCL ruptures.

Dogs that have sustained an acute rupture present with significant hindlimb lameness. However, the degree of

lameness varies widely with the increasing chronicity of the injury. The hind leg is usually carried in flexion, and occasionally at rest the toe may touch the ground. Dogs may resist manipulation of the stifle joint because of the pain from acute inflammation. Joint effusion may also be palpable adjacent to the patellar tendon.

The major diagnostic tests for CCL injury include palpation, the tibial compression test, and the cranial drawer test (Figure 7-110). Palpation of the affected leg often reveals muscle atrophy, pain, joint effusion, and asymmetry. Flexion and extension of the stifle joint may result in an audible click associated with displacement of the medial meniscus. Examination of the affected joint reveals a positive cranial drawer sign (cranial displacement of the tibia) and increased internal rotation of the tibia with joint flexion.

Special Instruments
A variety of retractors are typically used for CCL surgery. Hohmann retractors allow inspection of the internal surfaces of the joint (Figure 7-111). Steinmann pins and a Jacob's chuck are used to drill holes in the tibia. Cruciate needles allow the passage of suture through dense tendons and tissues. SECUROS currently offers a crimping system that is used for extracapsular repairs (Figure 7-112). Both 40- and 80-lb-test nylon is available. A distractor is used to place tension on the suture loop and can be locked to check cranial drawer. Crimp tubes are then placed and crimped (with a special crimping tool) to hold the suture in place.

Patient Positioning
The patient may be placed in dorsal or lateral recumbency with the affected leg up for CCL repair. The leg should be clipped from the hip to the tarsus. An examination glove should be placed on the foot to cover the unshaven area. The leg should be suspended while it is scrubbed to ensure complete and circumferential sterility. It is important to prepare the limb in this suspended position to allow the greatest amount of manipulation during surgery (Figure 7-113).

Patient Draping
The surgeon should grasp the suspended leg in a sterile manner, and the foot and tarsus should be covered with an appropriately sized stockinette. The leg is held suspended, and a three-cornered draping technique is used at the hip.

Cranial Cruciate Ligament Repair
A variety of surgical techniques have been designed to restore stability to the stifle and limit secondary degenerative joint disease. It is recommended that the joint capsule be opened with each technique to allow visualization and removal of the damaged ligament and menisci.

Intracapsular techniques involve replacement or reconstruction of the CCL using various materials, including

FIGURE 7-110 Cranial drawer test. To examine for cruciate ligament injury, place the thumb of one hand over the lateral fabella and the index finger over the patella. Stabilize the femur with this hand. Place the thumb of the opposite hand caudal to the fibular head with the index finger on the tibial tuberosity. With the stifle flexed and then extended, attempt to move the tibia cranially and distally to the femur. (From Fossum TW, Hedlund CS, Hulse DA, et al: Small animal surgery, ed 3, St Louis, 2007, Mosby.)

FIGURE 7-111 Hohmann retractors.

FIGURE 7-113 Lateral recumbency positioning with suspended leg is usually appropriate for orthopedic surgical preparation of a limb.

FIGURE 7-112 Cruciate Repair System (SECUROS, Fiskdale, MA). *Left to right,* Crimper, crimp tubes, distractor, 80-lb fishing line, and needle.

biologic tissues (patellar tendon and fascia lata) and synthetic suture material. The joint is approached laterally (Figure 7-114), and a graft of tissue is isolated. A tunnel is then drilled through the cranial surface of the tibia. The graft is fed through the tunnel and over the top of the lateral condyle, thereby reconstructing the CCL.

Extracapsular techniques are usually faster and easier to perform than intracapsular repairs. Extracapsular repairs involve placement of sutures outside the stifle joint. The joint is approached laterally, and the appropriate suture (e.g., monofilament nylon, nylon fishing line) is loaded onto a properly sized cruciate needle. The needle

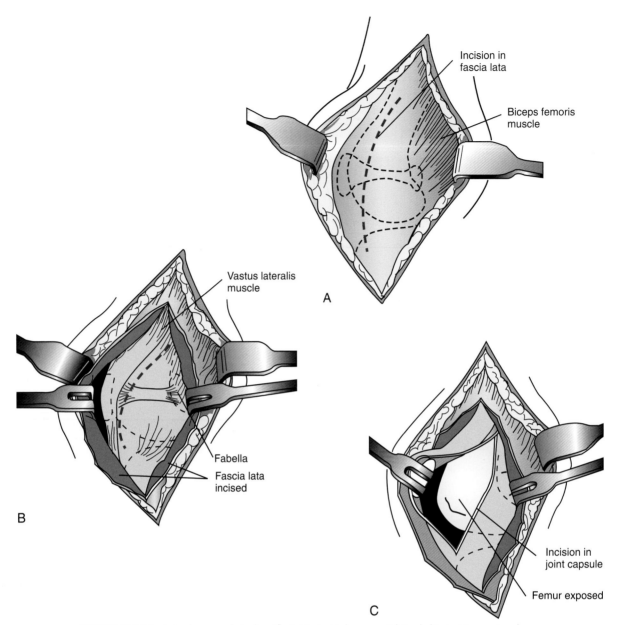

FIGURE 7-114 Lateral approach to the stifle joint. **A,** Make a craniolateral skin incision centered over the patella. Incise the subcutaneous tissues along the same line to visualize the septum between the superficial leaf of the fascia lata and the biceps femoris muscle proximally and then the lateral retinaculum distally. **B,** Make an incision through the fascia lata proximally, and carry the incision through the fascia lata and lateral retinaculum distally. **C,** Incise the joint capsule and continue the incision proximally, adjacent to the patellar tendon. Then incise along the border of the vastus lateralis toward the fabella. Displace the patella medially to expose the cranial surface of the joint. (From Fossum TW, Hedlund CS, Hulse DA, et al: Small animal surgery, ed 3, St Louis, 2007, Mosby.)

is passed around the fabella, then through the patellar ligament. A hole is drilled through the tibial crest with a Steinmann pin, and the suture is passed through the hole (Figure 7-115). The stifle is then flexed into a normal standing position, and the cranial drawer test is performed. Once the suture is under the appropriate tension, it is tied or crimped into place. The retinaculum should be closed with a vertical mattress pattern to provide appropriate imbrication of the joint capsule.

Both intracapsular and extracapsular reconstruction techniques rely on a recreation of the passive constraints of the stifle joint. In recent years a technique has been developed that recreates joint stability by altering the active constraints of the joint. CCL rupture causes the tibia to slide forward and the femur to fall back, creating a shear force referred to as *cranial tibial thrust*. The tibial plateau–leveling osteotomy (TPLO) functions to change the angle of the tibia, thereby directly altering joint

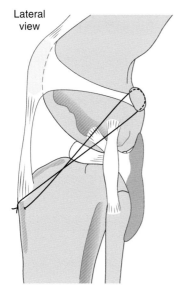

Lateral view

FIGURE 7-115 Extracapsular reconstruction using a heavy, nonabsorbable suture. The suture passes through the deep fascia surrounding the fabella and through a predrilled hole in the tibial crest. Tying or crimping the suture eliminates the cranial drawer. (From Fossum TW, Hedlund CS, Hulse DA, et al: Small animal surgery, ed 3, St Louis, 2007, Mosby.)

FIGURE 7-116 Three varieties of needle punch biopsy instruments.

mechanics and creating a new plateau that eliminates cranial tibial thrust. Currently, surgeons must be certified to perform the TPLO technique.

Postoperative Considerations and Instructions

A soft bandage should be placed on the limb for 48 hours after CCL repair to protect the surgical site and reduce swelling. The patient should return in 14 days for a recheck and suture removal.

The most important postoperative consideration is exercise restriction. Dogs should be restricted to short leash walks for at least 6 weeks after surgery. Activity can then be gradually increased over a 12-week period. Owners are discouraged from allowing their animals to run free, jump, climb stairs, and play rambunctiously with other animals. Failure to comply with strict exercise restriction may result in repair failure and the need for a second surgery.

Because CCL repairs are considered moderately painful, pain management is a major focus during the recovery period. Perioperative pain control involves injection of a local anesthetic directly into the joint. Animals are often treated immediately postoperatively with a variety of injectable pain medications, including opioids and NSAIDs. Animals are then often sent home with instructions for the owner to administer an oral NSAID (e.g., carprofen) for several days after surgery.

In recent years a rigorous rehabilitation program has been advocated as part of the standard postoperative care for patients with CCL repair. Rehabilitation programs promote wound healing and decrease muscle spasm,

adhesion formation, and edema while increasing muscle strength and joint range of motion (ROM). Typical programs include low-impact exercises (e.g., swimming), passive ROM exercises, heat, and whirlpool therapy.

Box 7-20 shows an example of a surgery report for a cranial cruciate ligament repair.

Minimally Invasive Surgery
Biopsy and Mass Removal

Biopsy and removal of a mass are important procedures in veterinary medicine. A biopsy is often recommended before mass removal. The biopsy is used to gather important information on the biologic and clinical behavior of the mass, allowing the formulation of an appropriate plan and prognosis. Current biopsy techniques include fine-needle aspiration, impression smear, punch, bone, excisional, and incisional biopsies.

Fine-Needle Aspiration Biopsy

Fine-needle aspiration (FNA) represents one of the simplest methods for cytologic evaluation of a mass. The technique is easy to perform, has minimal morbidity, and usually does not require sedation; however, FNA biopsy typically has a low diagnostic yield (Box 7-21).

Impression Smears

Impression smears are as simple to perform as FNA biopsy. This technique is especially useful for ulcerated surface tumors and is often performed on freshly cut surfaces. Impression smears of excised masses can also be easily made before the samples are placed into formalin (Box 7-22).

Needle Punch Biopsy

Needle punch biopsy instruments are currently manufactured by a variety of companies. Instruments are equipped with either a cutting or a core biopsy needle and are available as manual and automatic devices (Figure 7-116). These devices take a small piece of tissue (approximately the size of pencil lead) for histologic examination (Figures 7-117 and 7-118). These procedures are minimally invasive and generally are performed on sedated patients. Ultrasound-guided needle punch biopsies of various

BOX 7-20   Surgery Report: Cranial Cruciate Ligament Repair

Animal Hospital Name
Owner: John Doe
Address: 555 Sterling Lane
    Jupiter, NY 55555
Phone number: 555-5555
Animal Name: Sasha
Animal #: 65656501
Species: Canine
Breed: Labrador
DOB: 05/05/07
Date of Surgery: 12/03/2011
Primary Surgeon: Dr. Vet
Assistant: Nurse Scrub
Diagnosis or Preoperative Signs: Cranial cruciate ligament rupture.
Surgical Procedure: Right stifle arthrotomy, extracapsular cranial cruciate repair.
Implants: 80-lb-test fishing line, two SECUROS clamps.

Description of Surgical Procedure
Surgical Approach: An 8- to 10-cm parapatellar skin incision was made at the right stifle, and the underlying subcutaneous tissues were incised. The retinaculum and the joint capsule of the stifle were incised, and the interior of the stifle joint was visualized.
Surgical Pathology: Complete rupture of the cranial cruciate ligament.
Surgical Procedure: The remnants of the torn cranial cruciate ligament were removed and the joint was explored. No meniscal damage was evident at this time. The joint was lavaged with sterile saline, and the joint capsule was closed with 2-0 PDS in an interrupted suture pattern. Bupivacaine (10 mL) was injected into the joint capsule. A hole was then made in the tibial tuberosity with a Steinmann pin. A wire passer was used to pass 80-lb fishing line behind the lateral femoral fabellar ligament. The fishing line was then passed (medial to lateral) through the hole in the tibial tuberosity and then under the patellar ligament. A SECUROS clamp was then placed at the end of each line. A distractor was used to tighten the lines until the joint was stable. The joint was checked for drawer as well as range of motion. A SECUROS crimper was then used to crimp each of the clamps three times. The surgical site was lavaged with sterile saline and closed routinely.
Closure:
Joint capsule: 2-0 PDS in interrupted cruciate suture pattern.
Retinaculum: 2-0 PDS in interrupted suture pattern.
Subcutaneous tissue: 3-0 Monocryl in continuous suture pattern.
Skin: 3-0 nylon in interrupted suture pattern, followed by some skin staples.

BOX 7-21   Fine-Needle Aspiration Technique

1. Obtain a 22-gauge or 20-gauge needle and 5-mL syringe. Place the needle into the mass.
2. Apply negative pressure by pulling back on the hub of the syringe.
3. Withdraw the needle and syringe from the mass, and remove the needle from the syringe.
4. Fill the syringe with air, replace the needle, and gently blow the fluid and cells onto a glass slide.
   This method is generally performed several times to obtain representative samples.

BOX 7-22   Impression Smear Technique

1. Gently blot the surface of the mass with a paper towel to remove any excess blood and exudates.
2. Gently touch the surface of the mass to several areas of a glass slide. Take care not to twist or rub the slide against the mass, because doing so would crush cells and destroy the integrity of the sample.

larger surface sample; however, it does not penetrate deeply into the mass (Figure 7-119). Patients are generally placed under general anesthesia to undergo this procedure (Box 7-24).

Bone Biopsy
The most common instruments used to obtain bone biopsy samples are the Michele trephine (Figure 7-120) and Jamshidi bone biopsy needle (Figure 7-121). Bone biopsies are often painful and therefore are usually

internal organs, including the liver, spleen, and prostate, are also common procedures (Box 7-23).

Punch Biopsy
The punch biopsy technique is used primarily for external skin and oral masses. It has the advantage of providing a

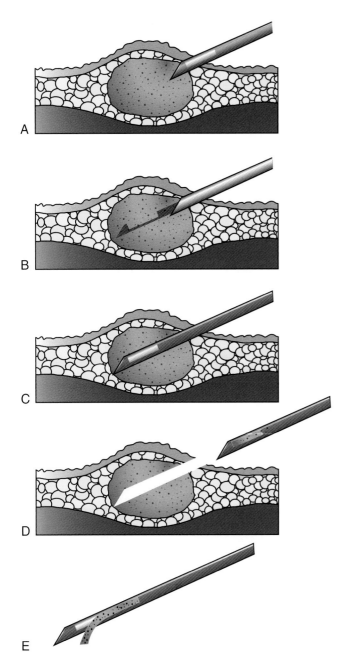

FIGURE 7-117 Use of the manual biopsy needle requires both hands and can be awkward, resulting in more discomfort for the patient and samples of lower quality. **A,** The tip of needle is inserted just into the tumor. **B,** The inner needle is advanced without advancing outer needle. **C,** Tissue from the tumor drops into the trough of the inner needle, and the outer needle is advanced to cover the inner needle, thereby cutting tissue within the trough free from the main mass. **D,** With the inner needle still completely within the outer needle, thus protecting the sample, the entire unit is removed. **E,** The inner needle is advanced beyond the end of the outer needle to allow the sample to be removed from the trough of the inner needle. (Modified from Mehler SJ, Bennet A: Surgical oncology of exotic animals. Vet Clin Exotic Anim Pract 7:783-805, 2004.)

FIGURE 7-118 Manual needle punch biopsy of the kidney during an exploratory laparotomy.

BOX 7-23	Needle Punch Biopsy Technique

1. Clip and aseptically scrub the area to be sampled.
2. Block the overlying skin and muscle with a local anesthetic.
3. Hold with one hand, and make a small stab incision into the overlying skin.
4. Insert the end of the needle through the stab incision (the instrument is fired; and the inner needle is advanced into the mass).
5. Withdraw the entire instrument from the mass
6. Gently remove the sample from the sample chamber with a cotton swab or needle (see Figures 7-117 and 7-118).

BOX 7-24	Punch Biopsy Technique

1. The area to be sampled is clipped and aseptically scrubbed.
2. The punch is rotated back and forth over the mass until the punch sits deeply in the lesion.
3. The punch is removed, and a scissors is used to detach the sample from its base (see Figure 7-119).

performed with the patient under general anesthesia. The Jamshidi needle biopsy is less invasive but provides a smaller sample size than other methods (Figure 7-122). The Michele trephine technique removes a larger sample of bone, increasing the diagnostic yield, but it also increases the likelihood of a pathologic fracture at the biopsy site (Box 7-25).

Incisional Biopsy
Incisional biopsies are generally used only after cytology or needle core biopsies have failed to provide a diagnostic

FIGURE 7-119 *Mechanism of punch biopsy.* **A,** *The punch is rotated back and forth over the suspect lesion until sufficient depth has been attained.* **B,** *The punch is removed or angled across the base to sever deep attachments.* **C,** *The specimen may be gently grasped with thumb forceps and cut off deeply.* (From Withrow SJ, MacEwen EG: Withrow and MacEwen's small animal clinical oncology, ed 4, St Louis, 2007, Saunders.)

FIGURE 7-120 *Michele trephine bone biopsy instrument.*

FIGURE 7-121 *Jamshidi bone biopsy needle.*

sample. A small wedge of the tumor is removed from the mass and submitted for histopathology (Figure 7-123).

Excisional Biopsy
An excisional biopsy involves the complete removal of a mass (see Figure 7-123). Excisional biopsies are generally performed only on benign skin tumors or when the removal of the organ is indicated.

Biopsy Sample Handling and Fixation
It is imperative that tissue samples are handled gently at all times. Improper handling can ruin the diagnostic value

---

BOX 7-25   Bone Biopsy Technique

1. A small incision is made over the center of the lesion.
2. The trephine or needle is pushed through the soft tissues until the bony cortex is reached.
3. The stylet is removed, and the cannula or trephine is advanced through the bony cortex.
4. Once an adequate sample has been obtained, the instrument is removed, and a wire is used to push the sample out of the hub of the needle (see Figure 7-122). It is extremely important to avoid pushing the sample out of the tip of the needle, because doing so would destroy the architecture of the sample.

FIGURE 7-122 **A,** Jamshidi bone biopsy needle: cannula and screw-on cap (a), tapered point (b), pointed stylet to advance cannula through soft tissues (c), and probe to expel specimen from cannula (d). **B,** With the stylet locked in place, the cannula is advanced through the soft tissue until bone is reached; *inset,* Close-up view showing stylet against bone cortex. **C,** The stylet is removed, and the bone cortex is penetrated with cannula. The cannula is withdrawn, and the procedure is repeated with redirection of the instrument to obtain multiple core samples. **D,** The robe is then inserted retrograde into the tip of the cannula to expel the specimen through the base (*inset*). (From Powers BE, LaRue SM, Withrow SJ, et al: Jamshidi needle biopsy for diagnosis of bone lesions in small animals. J Am Vet Med Assoc 193:206, 1988.)

of the sample. Impression smears should always be made before the sample is placed into fixative. It is often important to mark the margins of the surgical excision; this can be done by painting the outer edges of the excised mass with India ink or Alcian blue. The sample should then be allowed to dry for at least 20 minutes before it is placed into fixative.

All biopsy samples should be placed into a fixative before shipping. The most widely used fixative is 10% neutral buffered formalin. Proper fixation requires a ratio

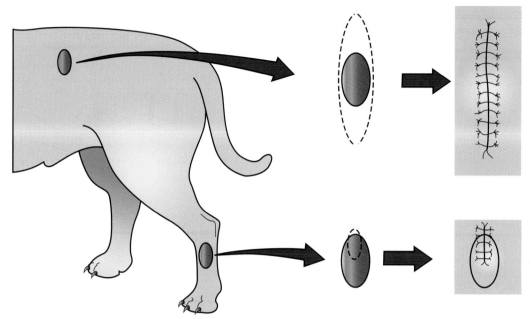

FIGURE 7-123 Excisional biopsy (*top*) contrasted with incisional biopsy (*bottom*). The top tumor may be as easy to remove as to biopsy, and removal may not negatively influence other possible treatments (e.g., additional surgery, irradiation). The bottom tumor, however, requires knowledge of the tumor type before excision, because inappropriate removal could compromise a subsequent aggressive excision (short of amputation). Note that the biopsy incision is in a plane that would be included in a subsequent resection. (From Withrow SJ, MacEwen EG: *Withrow and MacEwen's small animal clinical oncology*, ed 4, St Louis, 2007, Saunders.)

of 1 part tissue to 10 parts formalin. Tissue samples greater than 1 cm in thickness will not fix entirely; therefore, large masses should be sliced like a loaf of bread before they are placed into formalin. Multiple representative samples from a large mass can also be taken and preserved in the appropriate proportion of formalin. When multiple lesions or sites are sampled, each sample should be placed in a separate and appropriately labeled container.

All sample containers must be properly labeled. Important identification information includes the date, the patient's last name (and hospital ID number if applicable), and the site from which the sample was obtained. All cytology slides should be properly labeled with pencil or ink that will not smear when the slide is moistened. All appropriate documentation must be completed and should include history, signalment, clinical findings, and tentative diagnosis.

Laser Surgery

This section discusses the role of laser surgery in veterinary medicine, laser safety, and the advantages and disadvantages of using lasers as an alternative to traditional surgery.

How Does the Laser Work?

The word *laser* is used as an acronym for "light amplification by stimulated emission of radiation." Lasers are able to create light at distinct wavelengths and distinct delivery parameters. Laser light wavelength and frequency determine the color of the laser light and the way the laser light interacts with its target surface. When laser light hits its target, it may be reflected, absorbed, scattered, or transmitted through the tissues, depending on the type of laser light being used. The types of lasers most often used in veterinary medicine are the carbon dioxide (CO_2) laser, diode laser, and neodymium:yttrium-aluminum-garnet (Nd:YAG) laser. The CO_2 and diode lasers are discussed here.

The clinical functions of the CO_2 and diode lasers consist of ablation, incision, and excision of soft tissue. Both the CO_2 and the diode lasers operate through photothermal laser-tissue interaction. This means that the laser light is absorbed and transformed into heat within the tissue. Water, hemoglobin, melanin, and some proteins absorb different wavelengths of light, causing the tissue to heat. For example, the CO_2 laser is highly absorbed by water. The diode laser is highly absorbed by melanin and hemoglobin.

Heating of the tissue at different temperatures causes certain changes in the tissue. At 42° to 45° C, blood vessels are destroyed, resulting in necrosis of tissue. As tissue temperatures reach 50° to 100° C, proteins denature and coagulation occurs, causing irreversible tissue damage. Once tissue temperature surpasses 100° C, solid tissue becomes gaseous vapor and smoke plume. Increased heating of tissue can cause burning, resulting in carbonization of the tissue. This carbonization is called *char*. Charring occurs when tissue absorbs heat faster than it

FIGURE 7-124 Accuvet Novapulse LX-20SP CO₂ laser (Luxar Lumenis, Woodinville, WA).

FIGURE 7-125 Accu Vet V25 fiber-coupled diode laser system (Luxar Lumenis).

can be released. Heating to this extent results in damage to the surrounding tissue. Carbonization of the tissue also acts as a foreign substance and can hinder wound healing as well as cause inflammation at the site.

CO₂ Lasers versus Diode Lasers

CO_2 lasers are available at a wavelength of 10,600 nanometers (nm) (Figure 7-124). The CO_2 laser comes equipped with a selection of hand pieces and tips. Tips come in a variety of sizes (0.3-1.4 mm), and specific tips are used for specific surgical procedures. The CO_2 laser is considered a class IV laser system, as are most medical lasers. Lasers are separated into classes I to IV according to the degree of possible safety hazards to patients and users. The CO_2 laser is used predominantly to create surgical incisions, to excise after incision, or for ablation of tissue. Most CO_2 lasers use a noncontact mode in which the laser tip never comes in contact with the tissue.

The 10,600-nm wavelength of the CO_2 laser is perfect for incising and vaporization because it is highly absorbed by water. Because most tissues have high water content,

the laser energy is absorbed very close to the surface. The effect of the laser energy on tissue is determined by the laser wavelength, target tissue, spot size, power, and exposure (including exposure duration). Because laser wavelength (10,600 nm) and presumably the target tissue are known, the surgeon must choose the settings for the spot size, power, and exposure. *Spot size* refers to the diameter of the aperture. The distance of the tip from the tissue determines the exact spot size on the target tissue. Moving the tip away from the target tissue increases the spot size. Moving the tip closer to the target tissue decreases the spot size. The size of the tip also determines the spot size on the target tissue. Power settings are in watts (W), and the surgeon selects the appropriate wattage for a specific procedure. Power density depends on the set power, the spot size, and the distance of the tip from the tissue. The *exposure* refers to the duration of the laser beam, or how long the tissue is exposed to the laser beam. The clinician uses spot size, power, and exposure to control the interaction of the CO_2 laser beam and its effects on the tissue.

Available wavelengths for diode lasers in veterinary medicine range from 805 to 980 nm (Figure 7-125). The diode laser is also considered a class IV laser. Diode lasers are small, compact units that emit wavelengths that are easily transmitted through small, flexible optical fibers, allowing their use with most flexible and rigid endoscopes. Diode lasers also come equipped with a variety of hand pieces and tips. The diode laser can reach its target tissue using a contact mode or a noncontact mode, whereas most CO_2 lasers use a noncontact mode of light transmission. Noncontact fibers are available in squared, cleaved, or polished tips and are more appropriate for ablation procedures. Contact fibers tend to be sculpted and are more appropriate for incisional purposes. Diode laser light has better absorption in hemoglobin and melanin, whereas the CO_2 laser light has better absorption in water. More collateral thermal damage may occur with the diode laser because of the deeper penetration, unlike the absorption of water closer to the surface with the CO_2 laser. Because of the enhanced absorption of hemoglobin, the diode laser may provide more proficient incisions and better hemostasis, especially of larger vessels.

The CO_2 and diode lasers can be used in a continuous mode or a pulse mode. The mode, tip size, and settings chosen by the clinician vary according to the type of procedure performed. When using either the CO_2 or the diode laser, the clinician should start with low power settings and a short duration of exposure until becoming familiar with the effects of the laser on the target tissue. Also, the laser energy should be delivered perpendicularly from the hand piece to the target tissue. When incising tissue, the clinician should apply lateral tension perpendicular to the incision. This maneuver helps reduce the formation of char. A record or log should be kept of each procedure performed as well as the power and duration settings. This task will most likely be the technician's responsibility. A log of procedures will help the surgeon choose settings to use for future procedures.

Laser Procedures in Veterinary Medicine

Lasers may be used for surgical procedures ranging from minor elective procedures (e.g., feline declaw, lump removal) to more extensive procedures (e.g., celiotomy, thoracotomy). Other laser procedures include canine and feline castration, dewclaw removal, amputation, cystotomy, soft palate resection, oncologic procedures (e.g., neoplasia removal), and ophthalmic procedures. Whether to use laser energy or traditional surgery is ultimately the surgeon's decision. (See Box 7-26 for a list of advantages and disadvantages of laser surgery.)

BOX 7-26 | Advantages and Disadvantages of Laser Surgery

Advantages
- More rapid healing time of tissue
- Cauterization of blood vessels during incision
- Sterilization of tissue during incision (less risk of postoperative infection)
- Minimal risk of damage to underlying healthy tissue (CO_2 laser specifically)
- Less need for suturing
- Reduced postoperative discomfort or pain
- Reduced postoperative swelling
- Shorter surgery time in many cases

Disadvantages:
- Cost
- Safety
- Need for extensive training to prevent tissue damage

Laser Safety

Laser safety may be the technician's most important responsibility when assisting with laser surgery. It is imperative that precautions be taken to protect the clinical staff as well as the patient from the array of hazards associated with laser surgery. Many hospitals assign a laser safety officer, often the technician. The safety officer is responsible for following safety guidelines established by the manufacturer of the laser machine or by the American National Standards Institute (Standards ANSI Z136.3-1988 and Z136.1-1993). These guidelines give specific instructions to follow for laser safety and laser use. Most laser companies also provide user and safety training when a hospital purchases a laser machine. Laser surgery should never be performed by anyone who has not had proper training or education about laser use and safety. The ANSI Standards recommend that prospective laser users become knowledgeable about policies and procedures, review clinical literature, attend courses for a certain number of hours, consult with an experienced operator of laser surgery, and receive training on specific equipment before operating laser machines.

Laser Hazards

Laser warning signs should be posted in the surgery room as well as on all doors entering it. Figure 7-126 shows the warning sign for class IV lasers.

Dangers associated with class IV lasers include eye, skin, fire, and smoke plume hazards.

Eye hazards. Everyone in the laser surgery room must wear the eye protection goggles specific for the particular laser light (Figure 7-127). Different lasers emit different wavelengths, and the protection worn must coincide with the laser wavelength. Scattered reflections from the laser beam can cause serious corneal or retinal damage. The eyes of the patient should also be protected from scattered laser light. When a CO_2 laser is used, moistened sponges can be placed over the eyes for protection because the CO_2 laser beam is absorbed by water. Patient eye shields are also available.

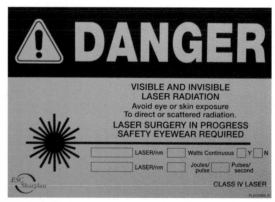

FIGURE 7-126 Laser warning signs should be posted on the doors to the surgery room as well as within the surgery room.

FIGURE 7-127 Wavelength-specific eye protection goggles for the diode laser.

Skin hazards. Skin hazards may occur from direct or scattered laser beams. It may be in the clinician's best interest to wear gloves and a gown for added protection.

Fire hazards. Possible fire hazards include the surgical drapes, anesthetic agents, oxygen, animal's fur, alcohol products used in surgical preparation, and methane from flatulence. With the CO_2 laser, wet sponges can be placed around the surgical area for protection of drapes. Any exposed fur around the surgical region can also be moistened with water. A nonalcohol surgical prep (e.g., chlorhexidine or povidone-iodine preparation) should always be used for all laser procedures. The anesthetist should always make sure the cuff of the endotracheal (ET) tube is inflated properly to decrease the chance that gaseous vapor or oxygen will escape. Standard polyvinyl chloride (PVC) tubes may be at risk for damage and ignition during a laser procedure. Laser-safe ET tubes can be purchased for procedures within the oral cavity. Another alternative is to lay moistened sponges around the standard ET tube to prevent a possible fire hazard when CO_2 lasers are used. Because methane is considered another possible source for fire ignition, moistened sponges can be placed within the rectum of the patient during perianal surgical procedures with the CO_2 laser. Fire extinguishers should be readily available in any laser surgery room in the event of unexpected ignition.

Smoke plume hazards. The smoke plume emitted from laser contact with tissue contains toxic and carcinogenic chemicals as well as bacteria and viral particles. An evacuator is usually purchased with the laser machines. Laser procedure should never be performed without an evacuation system. The smoke evacuator should be within 1 to 2 inches of the smoke's origin. Laser surgical masks are also available. Regular surgery room masks may not filter all toxic or infectious particles.

Laparoscopy

A *laparoscopy* is a minimally invasive abdominal procedure performed for the purpose of examining the peritoneal cavity and its viscera. A type of endoscope, called a laparoscope, is placed through a small midline incision or opening into the abdominal wall for inspection of the abdominal contents. Other incisions can be made into the abdominal wall (lateral to midline) for the insertion of laparoscopic instruments. These specialized instruments can be used for biopsy purposes as well as to perform specific procedures (e.g., spay, gastropexy) within the abdominal cavity. In many cases, laparoscopy can take the place of a full abdominal surgical procedure. In most cases, the procedure affords the patient a swift recovery with less potential for complications (Box 7-27). This section describes the equipment and procedures associated with laparoscopy.

Laparoscopic Equipment

The necessary equipment to perform a laparoscopy includes the laparoscope or telescope, trocar-cannula units, fiberoptic light cable, light source, Veress insufflation needle, gas insufflator, and camera/video system (optional).

Laparoscopes. Laparoscopes for small animals range in size from 1.7 to 10 mm in diameter. The most common size tends to be the 5-mm-diameter scope for dogs and cats (Figure 7-128). Laparoscopes are also designed with varying telescope angles. The scope with a 0-degree field of view allows the surgeon to observe the field precisely in front of the scope. Other angled scopes include the 30-degree and 45-degree fields of view. These angled telescopes enable the operator to look over the top of organs and examine small areas. Laparoscopes with an offset eyepiece that contains a channel for the introduction of accessory instruments are called *operating laparoscopes*. Trocar-cannula units are not needed with this type of scope.

FIGURE 7-128   A 5-mm laparoscope. (Courtesy Karl Storz.)

FIGURE 7-129   Smooth and threaded trocar-cannula units. (Courtesy Karl Storz.)

FIGURE 7-130   Fiberoptic light cable. (Courtesy Karl Storz.)

FIGURE 7-131   Veress insufflation needle. (Courtesy Karl Storz.)

Trocar-cannula units. Trocar-cannula units contain a trocar for puncturing through the abdominal wall and a cannula for the insertion of a telescope or laparoscopic instrument. These instruments are produced as threaded cannulas or smooth cannulas (Figure 7-129). The threaded cannulas screw into the abdominal wall, allowing for better gripping of the cannula. Threaded cannulas are less likely to slip or fall out of the abdomen. Laparoscopic cannulas also contain a trumpet valve that thwarts the escape of gas from the abdomen.

Fiberoptic light cable and light source. A fiberoptic cable emits light from the light source to the scope (Figure 7-130). The light from the scope illuminates the abdomen so that the operator can see the organs clearly. Light cables come in an assortment of diameters. A 4-mm to 5.5-mm cable is recommended for general use in dogs and cats.

Veress insufflation needle. The Veress insufflation needle is used for the original insufflation of the peritoneal cavity (Figure 7-131). This needle is composed of a sharp outer trocar and a blunt inner stylet. The stylet consists of a small opening to allow gas to insufflate into the abdomen. The outer trocar functions to puncture through the abdominal wall into the abdominal cavity. The trocar is then retracted, and the inner stylet with the small opening is exposed. Gas is then insufflated through the opening.

Gas insufflator. Gas insufflators are also referred to as *laparoflators*. Tubing is connected from the gas insufflator to the Veress needle. The gas insufflator pushes gas through the tube to the needle to inflate the abdomen. This inflation lifts the abdominal wall away from the abdominal viscera, allowing the surgeon to view the abdominal organs as well as to perform biopsies or surgical procedures. Gas insufflators include CO_2, nitrous oxide, and room air. CO_2 is recommended because of its rapid rate of absorption. The laparoflators allow the operator to control the volume of gas being emitted and regulate the intra-abdominal pressure. Excessive intra-abdominal pressure decreases venous return to the heart and reduces the ability to ventilate. Excessive pressure can also interfere with excursions of the diaphragm. The abdominal pressures should not exceed 15 mm Hg.

Camera/video system. A camera attached to a video system and monitor is mounted on top of the laparoscope (Figures 7-132 and 7-133). This system enables everyone in the surgery room to view the internal abdominal cavity on a monitor.

Special instruments. A general use soft tissue instrument pack should be available for laparoscopic procedures. The surgeon will require scalpel handles, blades, mosquito forceps, thumb forceps, needle holders, suture scissors, suture, and a bowl for saline. Laparoscopic instruments that should be available include biopsy instruments, cutting instruments, and palpation probe (Figures 7-134 and 7-135). These instruments can be passed through cannulas of accessory ports to aid in biopsy retrieval or to perform surgical procedures. Most laparoscopic instruments are insulated so that they can be used with electrocoagulation units.

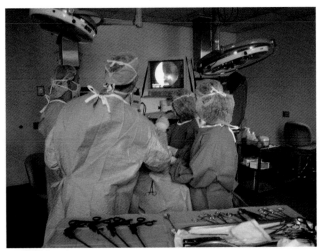

FIGURE 7-132 Laparoscopic video camera is used to allow viewing of the abdominal cavity on a monitor.

FIGURE 7-133 A 5-mm laparoscope with attached light cable. The camera is attached at the eyepiece of the laparoscope.

FIGURE 7-134 Various laparoscopic biopsy and grasping instruments.

FIGURE 7-135 Various laparoscopic biopsy and grasping instrument tips. *Left to right,* Atraumatic grasping forceps, biopsy forceps with teeth, bowel grasper, biopsy punch forceps.

Patient Positioning

A patient undergoing a laparoscopy should be fasted for 12 hours to prevent regurgitation during anesthesia and to keep the stomach from being distended. The bladder should be expressed before the patient enters the surgery room. An increased risk of traumatic puncture is present when these organs are distended. Distended organs can also make visualization of the target organs difficult. Most laparoscopic procedures are done with the patient under general anesthesia. The patient's abdomen should be clipped from the xiphoid process to the pubis as for any abdominal procedure. The clip should extend wide laterally for the placement of accessory ports. The animal may be placed in dorsal or left or right lateral recumbency. The positioning of the patient depends on the procedure. For purposes of this discussion, it is assumed that the patient has been placed in dorsal recumbency. The abdomen should be prepared routinely.

Patient Draping

A four-quarter draping method should be considered for laparoscopic procedures. Single fenestrated drapes are specifically not appropriate for this procedure.

Laparoscopic Procedure

Once the patient has been draped, the laparoscopic setup can begin. The surgeon should put on an extra pair of gloves for removing the scope and light cable from the glutaraldehyde solution in which it is stored after cleaning. A nonsterile technician pours sterile saline over the scope and light cable for rinsing purposes. The items should be rinsed thoroughly to remove all the glutaraldehyde from the cable and scope. The items should then be dried by a member of the sterile scrub team with a sterile towel, and the extra gloves removed. Next, a sterile sleeve is used to cover the camera, and the scope is placed on the head of the camera. The camera shows the images of the abdominal contents on a monitor to allow visualization of the abdomen by everyone in the surgery room. One end of the insufflation tubing is passed to a nonsterile technician and attached to the insufflator. The other end remains sterile and will be placed on the Veress needle.

FIGURE 7-136 After removal of the Veress needle, an 8-mm trocar-cannula unit is introduced at midline. The laparoscope will be introduced into the abdomen through this cannula. Note the attached tubing for insufflation of the abdomen.

FIGURE 7-137 Introduction of the laparoscope through the 8-mm cannula.

FIGURE 7-138 An accessory cannula has been introduced on the right side of this dog's abdomen. A blunt probing instrument has been inserted through the cannula to allow for manipulation of the abdominal organs.

The surgeon makes a 2 mm to 3 mm skin incision into the abdominal skin at midline for entry of the Veress needle. Once the Veress needle is placed, a drop of saline can be introduced at the hub of the needle. This will help the surgeon know when the abdominal cavity has been penetrated, because negative pressure in the abdominal cavity will draw the saline into the needle. Proper placement of the Veress needle is important. Subcutaneous emphysema can occur if the needle is placed between the muscle and subcutaneous tissue. Once proper placement is achieved, the outer trocar of the needle is retracted, and the blunt stylet with opening is uncovered. The insufflation tubing can then be connected to the needle, and insufflation can begin. Remember: Insufflation of the abdomen should never exceed 15 mm Hg. The insufflator or laparoflator can be regulated to stop at 15 mm Hg. If pressure in the abdomen should decrease, the insufflator will increase the volume of gas being released.

Once insufflation of the abdomen has been achieved, a trocar-cannula can be placed. A skin incision is made through the skin in the region of the Veress needle. The trocar aspect of the unit will puncture through the abdominal wall for introduction of the cannula (Figure 7-136). When the cannula has been sufficiently placed, the trocar is removed and the telescope (with camera) can be introduced through the cannula (Figure 7-137). The scrub team should now be able to view the abdominal contents on the monitor. In many cases the picture appears foggy at first because of the heat from the abdomen. The scope can be removed and wiped with a warm, moistened, sterile gauze sponge. The scope can then reenter the abdominal cavity through the cannula port.

If a surgical procedure or biopsy is to be performed, the introduction of a second and a third cannula may be required for instrumentation purposes. The same technique can be used as for the telescope cannula. These cannulas will most likely be placed lateral to midline (Figure 7-138). Placement of the cannulas will depend on the location of the organ requiring biopsy; Figure 7-139 shows an intraoperative laparoscopic liver biopsy. Box 7-28 shows an example of a surgery report for a laparoscopic procedure.

Endoscopy

Endoscopy is the technique of examining internal body structures using specialized optical instruments. Endoscopy is generally considered a high-yield and noninvasive or minimally invasive procedure. It is high yield in that it often results in diagnostic and therapeutic benefits for the patient. The body is entered ("invaded"), usually through an orifice (e.g., mouth, anus), but no incision (noninvasive) or a small incision (minimally invasive) is required

BOX 7-28 Surgery Report: Laparoscopic Procedure

Animal Hospital Name
Owner: John Doe
Address: 555 Sterling Lane
    Jupiter, NY 55555
Phone number: 555-5555
Animal Name: Sasha
Animal #: 65656501
Species: Canine
Breed: Doberman Pinscher
DOB: 05/05/07
Date of Surgery: 01/03/2011
Primary Surgeon: Dr. Vet
Assistant: Nurse Scrub
Diagnosis or Preoperative Signs: Liver disease.
Surgical Procedure: Laparoscopy.

Description of Surgical Procedure
Surgical Approach and Procedure: The patient was placed in dorsal recumbency, and a Veress needle was inserted at the level of the umbilicus. The abdomen was insufflated with CO_2 through this needle until the pressure was approximately 10 mm Hg. On conclusion of insufflation, a 5-mm laparoscopic cannula was inserted into the hole created by the Veress needle. The video laparoscope was directed into the abdomen through the cannula port, and the abdominal contents were examined. A second cannula was then placed approximately 7 cm lateral to the first site for the insertion of a laparoscopic biopsy instrument. A biopsy sample was retrieved from the left medial liver lobe. The region was observed for hemorrhage. Little hemorrhage occurred.
Surgical Pathology: All liver lobes were diffusely abnormal. Small nodules (1-2 mm in size) were observed throughout the liver lobes.
Closure:
3-0 PDS: Closure of the small incisions in the body wall and subcutaneous tissue in a simple interrupted suture pattern.
3-0 nylon: Closure of the skin incisions in a simple interrupted suture pattern.

FIGURE 7-139 Intraoperative laparoscopic liver biopsy. *Top left,* Laparoscopic view of diseased liver lobes. Note the many diffuse nodules throughout the liver lobes. *Top right,* A grasping instrument is placed through an accessory port to remove omentum away from the proposed biopsy site. *Bottom left,* A biopsy forceps is used to collect a piece of liver for diagnostic purposes. *Bottom right,* An absorbable gelatin sponge is placed at the biopsy site to control hemorrhage. This will stay in place and be absorbed by the body.

to enter the body. In the diagnostic evaluation of most cases, noninvasive tests (e.g., radiography, ultrasonography, some endoscopic procedures) are performed before minimally invasive procedures (e.g., other endoscopic procedures), which are performed before invasive procedures (e.g., exploratory celiotomy) (Box 7-29).

Endoscopy allows the clinician to examine tissues directly, obtain biopsy samples, and perform therapeutic procedures, such as the removal of foreign bodies. General anesthesia and proper fasting are required for all endoscopic procedures. For each procedure that requires passing the endoscope through the mouth, the patient should be intubated with an ET tube, and a mouth speculum should be used to prevent any damage to the endoscope. The cuffed ET tube will aid in preventing aspiration of reflux or regurgitated material from the oropharynx during the procedure.

Endoscope Selection

Endoscopy equipment is now affordable for private practices and not only for referral centers and educational institutions. When purchasing endoscopy equipment, veterinarians should primarily consider (1) the probable

Endoscopes can be used for the following noninvasive and minimally invasive procedures:

- Cystoscopy, to evaluate the bladder and lower urinary tract through the urethra.
- Gastrointestinal (GI) endoscopy, including:
  - Esophagoscopy, to examine the esophagus by way of the mouth.
  - Gastroscopy, to examine the stomach and upper small intestine (duodenoscopy) through the mouth.
  - Colonoscopy, to examine the colon by way of the anus.
- Rhinoscopy, to evaluate the nasal passages through the nares.
- Tracheobronchoscopy, to evaluate the trachea and bronchi by way of the mouth.

Endoscopes can also be used to examine the inside of a joint (arthroscopy) or the abdominal cavity (laparoscopy), but these procedures require incision of the tissues, whereas the procedures listed above do not require incisions.

FIGURE 7-141 Example of endoscope with the ability to retroflex 210 degrees. (Courtesy MJR-VHUP, Philadelphia.)

FIGURE 7-140 Pentax veterinary video endoscope for small animal procedures with an insertion tube length of 100 cm and diameter of 11 mm. (PENTAX Medical Company, Montvale, NJ.) (Courtesy MJR-VHUP, Philadelphia.)

frequency of use and the equipment's versatility, (2) the quality of the optical system, and (3) the ease of maneuvering the endoscope. Purchase price is important with many veterinarians, but purchasing a cheaper, low-quality endoscope instead of a higher quality scope can be a costly mistake; a thorough examination may be compromised by such an instrument, and a definitive diagnosis may not be achieved. High-quality endoscopes benefit hospitals because their cost can usually be recovered after 2 years, and if maintained properly, the endoscopes provide many more years of service than lower-quality models.

A standard flexible endoscope with a diameter of 8 to 11 mm and a working length of 100 cm is usually adequate for feline and canine upper GI examinations and colonoscopies (Figure 7-140). A new endoscope should

have these features and capabilities: (1) a four-way distal tip deflection with at least 180 degrees of upward deflection (for retroflexion), (2) water flushing, (3) air insufflation, (4) suctioning, (5) locking deflection controls, (6) an accessory channel with a diameter of 1.8 to 2.4 mm, and (7) forward-viewing optics.

Flexible Endoscopes

Because they are long and pliable, flexible endoscopes are better than rigid endoscopes for procedures that require bending or flexibility to examine areas such as the stomach, duodenum, and colon. Flexible endoscopes are used for noninvasive procedures and are available with either a two-way (up/down) or a four-way (up/down and left/right) distal tip deflection. The deflections are controlled by an angulation knob mounted on the control section of the endoscope. Older endoscopes have a maximum upward tip deflection of 180 degrees, whereas newer endoscopes have an upward tip deflection of 210 degrees (Figure 7-141). Endoscopes range in length from 50 cm to 170 cm, with insertion tube diameters ranging from 1 mm to 15 mm.

There are two types of flexible endoscopes: fiberoptic (Figure 7-142) and video (Figure 7-143).

Fiberoptic endoscope. With a fiberoptic endoscope, a light cable carries light by fiberoptic bundles from an external light source through the control section and to the insertion tube. The control section is protected by hard plastic and contains the viewing lens, angulation control knobs, biopsy ports, white balance, and camera controls. The control section also has an eyepiece. The insertion tube houses the fiberoptic light strands and channels for air insufflation and water flushing, biopsy and retrieval instruments, and suction. When the air/water valve is compressed, water flushes and rinses the lens on the distal tip of the endoscope. When the air/water valve port is covered, insufflation occurs and can be regulated (Figure 7-144).

The biopsy channel port is located at the base of the control section at the junction with the insertion tube. The insertion tube itself is protected by a waterproof

FIGURE 7-142 Control section for a Pentax fiberoptic endoscope. The angulation system is on the right side of the endoscope (right side of endoscope appears on left side of figure). The large inner knob deflects up and down, and the small outer knob deflects right and left. The top valve is for suctioning, and the bottom valve is for air insufflation and flushing water to clean a dirty lens. If any images are to be taken, a camera head can be attached from the eyepiece on the endoscope to the endoscopy unit. (Courtesy MJR-VHUP, Philadelphia.)

FIGURE 7-143 Control section for Pentax video endoscope. The angulation knobs and valves are the same as for the fiberoptic endoscope, except that images can be directly taken from the endoscope. The "F" button is to freeze an image, and the "C" button is to capture an image so it can be printed and stored in a computer. (Courtesy MJR-VHUP, Philadelphia.)

sleeve. Although the endoscope has three distinct sections (light guide plug, umbilical or universal cord, and control section), it is a one-piece unit that is sealed and watertight.

The distal tip of the insertion tube can bend more easily than the rest of the endoscope because a rubber insert covers the last few inches. Tip deflections can be fixed in any position by using the lock mechanisms situated next to the angulation knobs. This construction allows the endoscopist to control and maneuver the endoscope with ease. The umbilical cable or universal cord connects the light guide plug to the control section of the

endoscope. The light guide plug inserts into the light source. The plug has ports for the air/water and suction channels.

The fiberoptic endoscope is a direct viewing system. Fiberoptic bundles composed of thousands of individual fibers transmit light from the light guide plug to the distal tip of the insertion tube. The fibers' flexibility allows light to bend around corners and curves. Fiberoptic endoscopes also use a fiber bundle to transmit images from the objective lens at the distal tip, through the eyepiece, and to the endoscopist's eyes. The image guide bundles are set up so that each fiber carries a portion of the image and is in the same place at both ends of the bundle. Video cameras can be attached to the eyepiece of fiberoptic endoscopes to display images on a monitor. The final image is made up of the many small pieces of the whole image, so if a fiber breaks, a black or gray dot appears on the image.

The automatic brightness system in some fiberoptic endoscopes controls the light level. Illumination decreases as the object in view draws closer, and brightness increases as the object recedes farther away. The color, texture, and reflectivity of the tissue in view all affect the intensity of brightness. The auto-brightness control compensates for these differences.

Video endoscope. Video endoscopes are similar in construction to fiberoptic endoscopes, except they do not have a direct viewing lens aided by an eyepiece. Images are seen on a video screen. The image bundle in a fiberoptic endoscope is replaced in a video endoscope with a camera unit consisting of a lens assembly and an electronic chip known as a "charged coupled device" (CCD). The CCD chip is housed in the distal end of the insertion tube. The CCD chip is connected to an external video processor by approximately 16 small wires. The external video processor assembles the image and transmits it to a video monitor (Figure 7-145).

The automatic brightness system can control the light level in all video endoscopes as in some fiberoptic endoscopes. Video endoscope systems have the capability to freeze and capture images from recording-device buttons in the control section. Other media, such as videotapes, computer files, and prints, can aid in capturing information. The light guide plug in a video endoscope is heavier than that in a fiberoptic endoscope and needs to be handled with care. The terminals in the light guide plug are not waterproof and must be covered by soaking caps (supplied with the endoscope) before being immersed in solutions for cleaning.

Rigid Endoscopes
Rigid endoscopes are better than flexible endoscopes for procedures involving a direct pathway that are better viewed with a straight or a direct line of sight. Such areas include the ears, nose, urinary bladder, joint spaces, and abdominal or thoracic viscera. Rigid endoscopes are used for noninvasive to moderately invasive procedures that

Light guide connector section

Water container connector

Light guide

Air pipe

Suction connector

Venting connector

Universal cord
Contains light guide fiber bundle;
air, water, and suction channels;
and electric wiring for automatic
exposure system

Eyepiece

Up/down
angulation lock

Up/down angulation
control knob

Right/left angulation
control knob
(controls corresponding
tip deflection)

Right/left
angulation lock

Suction valve
(depress to activate suction)

Air/water valve
(cover for air insufflation;
depress to activate water
for lens washing)

Channel opening

Flexible
section

Bending
section

Distal end

Insertion tube

Light guides

Objective
lens

Air/water
nozzle

Instrument
channel

Distal end

FIGURE 7-144 Components of a typical fiberoptic endoscope. (From Stasi K, Melendez L: Care and cleaning of the endoscope. Vet Clin North Am Small Anim Pract 31:589, 2001.)

Light guide plug   **Umbilical cable**   **Control section**

Up/down
angulation lock

Waterproof cap

Suction port

Up/down angulation
control knob

Switches

Right/left angulation
control knob

Suction valve
Air/water valve

Leak tester
connection

Water bottle
(mouth piece)

Right/left
angulation lock

Air port
Light guide plug

Biopsy channel port

Light guides
Objective
lens

Instrument
channel

Air/water
nozzle

Bending
section

Distal end

Insertion tube

FIGURE 7-145 Components of a typical video endoscope. (From Schumway R, Broussard J: Maintenance of gastrointestinal endoscopes. Clin Tech Small Anim Pract 18:254, 2003.)

involve tissues that lie relatively close to the body surface and can be visualized with a straight line of sight. Procedures using rigid endoscopes include otoscopy and rhinoscopy. Some procedures, such as arthroscopy, laparoscopy, and thoracoscopy, require small incisions to allow access of the object lens into the specific area to be examined. (For more information on rigid endoscopy, see Bibliography and the previous section on laparoscopy.)

Endoscopy Preparation

A technician who works with the veterinarian performing endoscopy should also have the necessary training to assist with patient preparation, equipment setup, patient monitoring, obtaining biopsy specimens, freezing/ capturing and storing images, equipment breakdown, equipment cleaning, performing file backups, maintaining order of the endoscopy room, and ordering supplies.

The endoscopy technician is responsible for preparing and setting up the procedures. The endoscope of choice should be hooked up to the endoscopy machine with appropriate valves and biopsy channel covers. Before the procedure, the patient data should be ready in the computer. The machine is turned on when the endoscope is attached, and the light source is checked. The endoscope should be tested while the machine is warming up. First, the technician should confirm that an adequate amount of distilled water is available for flushing; the water valve can then be depressed to confirm that water comes out of the distal end. Water flushing is done to rinse off a soiled lens on the distal tip of the endoscope. Second, the air/ water valve should be gently covered, and the distal end of the insertion tube submerged in a bowl of water to check for bubbles; this is a test for insufflation. Third, the tip is left submerged in a bowl of water and tested for

suctioning. Any necessary accessory instruments or items, such as biopsy forceps, oral speculum, pathology request forms, water-soluble lubricant gel, gauze pads, and formalin cups or slides, should all be available and ready for use.

Endoscopy Work Area

The endoscopy room should be large enough to accommodate the cart or tower for the endoscopy unit (light source/suction unit, video printer/monitor, computer, keyboard), patient, anesthesia machine, endoscopy equipment (endoscopes, accessory instruments), a designated area to clean the endoscopy equipment, shelves and cabinets for miscellaneous storage needs, counter space, and a sink. Having the endoscope unit on a cart is convenient and allows portability to different areas of a hospital (Figures 7-146 and 7-147).

Ideally, a well-ventilated storage cabinet will be available in the endoscopy room to protect and store the endoscopes (Figure 7-148). If a cabinet is not available, wall mounts or cart pole mounts are acceptable (Figure 7-149). Storing endoscopes in their original custom-padded cases is not recommended; the hanging position rather than the coiled position is strongly advised. Also, endoscopes should never be placed on a flat surface (not even temporarily) because they could fall off or be knocked onto the floor, resulting in costly repair. After cleaning, endoscopes should be hung to dry either in a hanging storage cabinet or on a wall or cart pole mount, where they remain until required for another procedure. Hanging endoscopes allows any residual droplets of moisture in the insertion tube to drain. Residual moisture in the accessory channel may promote growth of bacteria and fungi and clogging of the air/water channel. This is why endoscopes should

FIGURE 7-146 Cart setup with Olympus endoscopy equipment (units for light source, air/suction/flushing, and brightness control), water bottle, TV monitor, biopsy forceps, and video endoscope (hanging on cart pole mount), with appropriate valves and biopsy channel cover. (Olympus America, Inc., Center Valley, PA.) (Courtesy MJR-VHUP, Philadelphia.)

FIGURE 7-147 Cart setup with Pentax endoscopy equipment (units for light source, air/suction/flushing, and brightness control), water bottle, TV monitor, computer (to store patient data and images), digital printer, biopsy forceps, and video endoscope (hanging on cart pole mount), with appropriate valves and biopsy channel cover. (Courtesy MJR-VHUP, Philadelphia.)

not be stored in their custom-padded case; if they are encased in a coiled fashion air cannot circulate through the channels, and problems are more likely to develop.

Handling the Endoscope

The control section of a flexible endoscope is the only area designed to bear its weight. During transport of an endoscope, one hand should hold the control section while the other hand holds the ends of the insertion tube and umbilical cable. The optics at the tip of the insertion tube are delicate, so extra care should be taken to protect them from damage.

There are basically two ways to hold the control section during endoscopy, described as the "two-finger grip" (Figure 7-150) and the "three-finger grip" (Figure 7-151). The straighter the endoscope can be maintained throughout a procedure, the more precisely it can be controlled and maneuvered. Practice and patience are required to obtain efficient and valuable endoscopic capabilities.

Biopsy Sampling

Endoscopic biopsy samples are obtained with flexible forceps. Samples obtained using forceps with a 1.8-mm cup are usually sufficient for diagnostic histopathology,

but cups of 2.4 mm or larger are always better because samples retrieved are substantially larger and deeper. The correct cup size is determined by the size of the endoscope's biopsy channel. Biopsy tissue samples obtained with flexible endoscopes may not always be deep enough to allow diagnosis of submucosal lesions, whereas using rigid endoscopes usually yields diagnostically sufficient amounts of tissue. It is ideal, but not always possible, to visualize the biopsy site. Depending on the difficulty in advancing the endoscope through areas of narrowing, such as the pyloric sphincter and ileocolic junction to obtain biopsies of the duodenum and ileum, respectively, the clinician may blindly lead the tip of the insertion tube to the site and carefully obtain "blind" tissue samples.

Any biopsy sample, especially an intestinal or gastric mucosa sample, must be handled carefully to minimize artifacts and distortion. If possible, tissue samples should be carefully removed from the biopsy forceps with a 25-gauge needle (Figure 7-152). Cytology can assist in making or confirming a diagnosis, but unremarkable cytology findings do not rule out specific disorders.

It is important that tissue samples from different locations be placed in different vials of formalin and properly

FIGURE 7-148 Cabinet for storage of endoscopes and accessory instruments. (From Tams T: Small animal endoscopy, ed 2, St Louis, 1999, Mosby.)

FIGURE 7-149 Typical wall mount for multiple endoscopes provides appropriate hanging position, especially after cleaning and disinfecting. (Courtesy MJR-VHUP, Philadelphia.)

FIGURE 7-150 Left-handed "two-finger" grip for holding an endoscope's control section using the fourth and fifth fingers. The index and middle fingers operate the suction and air/water valves, respectively. The thumb operates the angulation knobs. (Courtesy MJR-VHUP, Philadelphia.)

FIGURE 7-151 Left-handed "three-finger" grip for holding an endoscope's control section using the third, fourth, and fifth fingers. The index finger operates the suction and air/water valves, and the thumb operates the angulation knobs. (Courtesy MJR-VHUP, Philadelphia.)

FIGURE 7-152 A biopsy sample is carefully removed with a small-gauge needle. (From Tams T: Small animal endoscopy, ed 2, St Louis, 1999, Mosby.)

labeled so the pathologist can correctly identify the area sampled. Tissue samples should not be allowed to dry out or be damaged before placement in formalin.

Tissue samples that are too small and samples that have excessive artifact are common problems with endoscopy. For example, a lymphoma can be submucosal, and a superficial biopsy sample may only contain reactive cells above the tumor and may miss the neoplastic cells from the tumor. This finding could be misinterpreted as a diagnosis for inflammatory bowel disease. Three to five

FIGURE 7-153 Examples of biopsy forceps graspers and retrievers. (From Tams TR: Small animal endoscopy, ed 3, St Louis, 2012, Mosby.)

FIGURE 7-154 Normal-appearing canine lower esophageal sphincter. (Courtesy MJR-VHUP, Philadelphia.)

full-thickness biopsy samples are usually sufficient, but obtaining six to eight may be more helpful, especially with both mucosal and submucosal samples. The clinician should follow up with the pathologist to determine whether the quality of the tissue samples was adequate and whether the histologic findings are consistent with the patient's clinical signs.

Even though endoscopy is considered a minimally invasive procedure, one rare but significant complication is perforation. Therefore, when biopsy samples are obtained from diseased areas, extra caution and care should be taken to avoid applying too much force against mucosal walls.

Instrumentation

Many flexible instruments are available for use with endoscopes that have an accessory channel. Both flexible and rigid endoscopes can accommodate flexible instruments. Basic instrumentation includes biopsy forceps (e.g., oval/ellipsoid cups, serrated cups, alligator cups, serrated/nonserrated bayonets), instruments for grasping foreign bodies (e.g., "rat tooth" forceps, wired snares, wired baskets, meshed nets, two- or three-pronged grasping forceps), cytology brushes, aspiration tubes, injection needles, and coagulating electrodes (Figure 7-153).

Foreign bodies should not be retrieved through the accessory channel. Once the object has been visualized and firmly secured, the entire endoscope should be removed from the patient. Following this recommendation prevents costly damage to the accessory channel of the flexible endoscope. When removed, foreign bodies should be cleaned off as well as possible and placed in a secure bag or container for the animal's owner.

Disposable sheathed cytology brushes are recommended for obtaining brush samples, such as a gastric or duodenal mass or intestinal mucus. One cytology brush should be used per patient because cells from one sample may be transferred to the cytologic sample of another patient if the brush is used on more than one patient. This

transfer can happen because cytology brushes are difficult to clean thoroughly. Polyethylene tubing can be used to perform a duodenal wash through the endoscope to examine for evidence of giardiasis or to collect intestinal fluid for identification or quantification of bacteria.

Esophagoscopy

Esophagoscopy is the endoscopic technique of examining the esophagus. Esophagoscopy is a useful tool in the diagnosis and treatment of esophageal disease and is indicated for the evaluation of animals with signs of esophageal disease. These signs may include (but are not limited to) regurgitation, dysphagia, odynophagia, ptyalism, change in appetite, and weight loss. Esophagoscopy is the method of choice for diagnosing disorders that affect the mucosa or alterations affecting the lumen of the esophagus (Figure 7-154).

Esophageal foreign bodies, inflammation (esophagitis; Figures 7-155 and 7-156), esophageal strictures, ulcers, and neoplasia are conditions affecting the esophageal mucosa or lumen that can be definitively diagnosed by esophagoscopy. However, contrast radiography is more useful than esophagoscopy in diagnosing megaesophagus, hiatal hernias, vascular ring anomalies, and gastroesophageal intussusception. Whenever an esophagoscopy is performed, it is important for the endoscope to enter the stomach and for the surgeon to retroflex the scope's tip to view the gastroesophageal sphincter area to detect leiomyomas or other easily missed lesions (Box 7-30).

Canine mucosa differs from feline esophageal mucosa. A dog's esophageal mucosa is normally pale pink or grayish, and the surface is smooth and glistening. In dog breeds such as the Chow Chow and Shar-Pei, patches of pigmented mucosa may be observed. A cat's esophageal mucosa differs from that of a dog because of the presence of submucosal vessels and circular rings formed by circumferential mucosal folds, creating a characteristic pattern in the distal third of the cat's esophagus (Figures 7-157 and 7-158).

Gastroscopy

Gastroscopy is the endoscopic technique of examining the stomach. Gastroscopy is indicated for the evaluation of animals with signs of gastric disease. The signs may include (but are not limited to) nausea, salivation, vomiting, hematemesis, melena, unexplained abnormal changes in breathing, and anorexia. Gastroscopy identifies abnormalities of the mucosa and reveals distortion of the stomach's normal anatomic relationship to other abdominal organs by displacement or extrinsic compression. Many consider gastroscopy to be a more valuable diagnostic tool than radiography for disorders affecting the stomach.

FIGURE 7-155 Inflamed canine lower esophageal sphincter. (Courtesy MJR-VHUP, Philadelphia.)

BOX 7-30 Esophagoscopy Technique

1. The anesthetized and intubated patient should be placed in left lateral recumbency with a secured oral speculum.
2. The insertion tube should be prelubricated with a water-soluble gel to aid easy passage. The endoscope is then directed centrally through the oropharynx and guided dorsal to the endotracheal tube and larynx so that the cranial esophageal sphincter (CES) comes into view.
3. The CES is the entrance to the esophagus and is normally closed; it appears as a star-shaped area of folded mucosa dorsal to the larynx. The endoscope should meet minimal or no resistance as it is being advanced within the esophagus.
4. With insufflation, the scope should advance in a slow, continuous motion, only minor adjustments in tip deflection and torque being used to maintain a full view of the lumen and mucosal surfaces.
5. At the lumen of the thoracic esophagus, pulsations of the aorta can be seen at the level of the base of the heart.
6. When the endoscope is advanced through the gastroesophageal sphincter (GES), little or no resistance should be encountered.
7. To move the endoscope into the stomach, the tip of the insertion tube should be deflected approximately 30 degrees to the left (see note) while slight upward deflection is applied as the tip is advanced through the slitlike opening of the GES.
8. To examine the GES, the endoscope should be retroflexed. This is also known as the "J maneuver." The extent of retroflexion can be 180 or 210 degrees.
   NOTE: When one is referring to directional technique (i.e., left or right), the patient's orientation is the point of reference. Therefore, the instruction to turn the tip of the endoscope to the left refers to the patient's left. This principle applies to every endoscopic technique described in this chapter.

FIGURE 7-156 *Left,* Mild reflux esophagitis in 10-year-old male German Shepherd Dog. *Right,* Retroflexed view of gastroesophageal sphincter and cardia. (Courtesy MJR-VHUP, Philadelphia.)

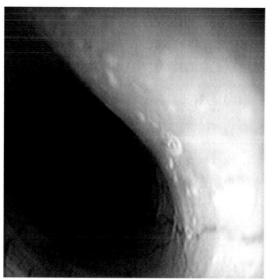

FIGURE 7-157 Distal third of feline esophagus with distinctive circular ring formation (herringbone pattern). This esophagus is mildly inflamed. (Courtesy MJR-VHUP, Philadelphia.)

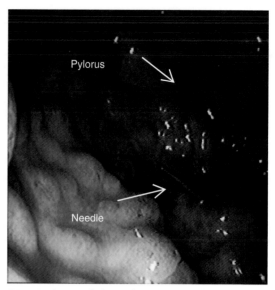

FIGURE 7-159 Needle located in the pylorus of a 3½-year-old male Labrador; it was retrieved without complications. (Courtesy MJR-VHUP, Philadelphia.)

FIGURE 7-158 Caudal thoracic feline esophagus with herringbone pattern not seen in canine esophagus. This esophagus is mildly inflamed. (Courtesy MJR-VHUP, Philadelphia.)

FIGURE 7-160 Steel nail in the stomach of a 6-month-old male Vizsla; it was retrieved without complications. (Courtesy MJR-VHUP, Philadelphia.)

The following conditions can be definitively diagnosed by gastroscopy or a combination of gastroscopy and associated diagnostic tests (cytology, histology): chronic inflammation (with or without overgrowth of *Helicobacter* organisms), superficial erosions, foreign bodies, motility disorders, ulcerations, and neoplasia. Gastroscopy can also be a therapeutic intervention when used to remove foreign bodies (Figures 7-159 to 7-161) and place feeding tubes (gastrostomy tubes and percutaneous endoscopy–guided [PEG] gastrostomy tubes).

Gastric biopsy is currently required for a diagnosis of *Helicobacter* infection. The bacteria are not uniformly distributed throughout the stomach; therefore, obtaining samples from various areas (body, fundus, antrum) is recommended. *Helicobacter* may be diagnosed by cytologic evaluation of the gastric mucosa or by examination for gastric mucosal urease activity (Box 7-31).

Biopsy sampling. Six to 10 gastric biopsy specimens should be collected even if the gastric mucosa appears normal (Figure 7-162). This is important because some patients with a histologic diagnosis of mild to moderate gastritis have no gross mucosal lesions; and patients with gastric motility disorders may have mucosal erythema but no histologic abnormalities. The gastric rugal folds are the best areas from which to obtain biopsy samples because they are easy to grasp with forceps. Biopsy specimens

FIGURE 7-161   *Left,* Article of clothing wedged in the pyloric sphincter of a 9-year-old female Alaskan Malamute. *Right,* Inflammation and swelling after minor complications in retrieving object. (Courtesy MJR-VHUP, Philadelphia.)

FIGURE 7-162   Normal-appearing gastric rugal folds. (Courtesy MJR-VHUP, Philadelphia.)

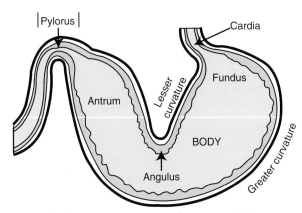

FIGURE 7-163   Five basic regions of the stomach. The areas indicated with *arrows* are the three most important landmarks for a gastroscopy. (From Tams T: Small animal endoscopy, ed 3, St Louis, 2011, Mosby.)

FIGURE 7-164   View of the gastroesophageal sphincter and cardia via retroflexion (J maneuver) of the endoscope. (Courtesy MJR-VHUP, Philadelphia.)

should be taken at various sites of the stomach, including the cardia, fundus, angulus, antrum, and pylorus (Figures 7-163 to 7-166).

If erosive or ulcerative lesions are present in the stomach, the biopsy samples should be collected from the upper wall where the lesions merge with the normal-appearing mucosa (Figures 7-167 and 7-168). Caution should be used in maneuvering the endoscope around the pit of an ulcer, because perforation could otherwise result. Obtaining biopsy specimens of superficial erosions is usually safer.

Biopsy samples from gastric masses should be taken as deeply as possible (Figure 7-169). If the samples are too superficial, fibrous or granulomatous tissue may be retrieved. Lymphosarcoma and benign gastric polyps can usually be diagnosed on biopsy. However, to diagnose

BOX 7-31 | **Gastroscopy Technique**

1. Fasting a patient for 12 to 18 hours and withholding water for 4 or more hours before a gastroscopy may be the key to a successful and a thorough examination.
2. The anesthetized and intubated patient should be placed in left lateral recumbency (LLR) with a secured oral speculum. With the patient in LLR, the antrum and pylorus are away from the tabletop, allowing the scope to traverse these structures more readily and the endoscopist to examine the stomach completely.
3. Because the esophagus is in a posterior plane in relation to the stomach, the tip of the insertion tube needs to be deflected in the distal esophagus before it can be advanced to the stomach.
4. The endoscope tip should be centered at the gastroesophageal (GE) orifice, and as the scope is advanced, the tip should be deflected to the left approximately 30 degrees with simultaneous slight upward deflection as the GE junction is passed. If the tip was properly directed, no resistance should be encountered as the scope advances to the stomach.
5. The endoscope tip should be positioned just through the GE junction to obtain an overview of the gastric lumen. As the tip enters the stomach, the rugal folds are seen, and the stomach is often partially or completely collapsed.
6. Gastric distension is required, so insufflation is used to the point that the rugal folds begin to separate. This step allows for spatial orientation and the identification of most gross abnormalities. In cats and small dogs, insufflation can be achieved within seconds, whereas large-breed dogs may require 30 to 120 seconds of constant insufflation for adequate distension.
7. The initial examination of the stomach should note the presence/absence of fluid or ingesta, the ease/difficulty with which the gastric walls distend with insufflation, and the gross appearance of the rugal folds and the mucosa.
8. The stomach should be empty in a properly fasted patient; however, a small pool of fluid in the fundus or at the proximal aspect of the greater curvature is considered normal. Aspiration should be performed, but with great care if a large pool of fluid is present and is obscuring the rugal folds.
9. As the scope is gradually advanced through the proximal stomach, the gastric body can be evaluated if the control knobs are used to deflect the tip.
10. With the patient in LLR, the smooth lesser curvature is on the endoscopist's right and the rugal folds of the greater curvature are seen below and to the left. The endoscope is then advanced along the greater curvature until the angulus, which extends from the lesser curvature, is identified.
11. The angulus separates the body of the stomach from the antrum. The insertion tube must be maneuvered around the angulus to the antrum in order to be advanced to the pylorus through the pyloric sphincter and to enter the duodenum.
12. During a gastroscopy, the cardia and fundus can be visualized only if the insertion tube is retroflexed (J maneuver).
13. The retroflexion maneuver allows a "face view" of the angulus, cardia, and fundus. This maneuver must be initiated at a point proximal to or opposite the angulus to provide a face view of the angulus.
14. The scope is advanced along the greater curvature to the level of the distal body.
15. The tip of the insertion tube is then deflected upward as far as possible as the scope advances farther. An upward tip deflection between 180 and 210 degrees is required to visualize the cardia.
16. Panoramic examination of the proximal stomach is completed by rotation of the insertion tube. The retroflexed scope tip should be reversed gradually to allow further examination of the gastric mucosa.

NOTE: Gastroscopy should follow esophagoscopy for a thorough upper GI examination, with the duodenum examined last and gastric biopsy specimens usually obtained after duodenal specimens.

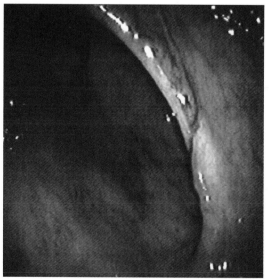

FIGURE 7-165 View of the angulus, which separates the body of the stomach from the antrum. (Courtesy MJR-VHUP, Philadelphia.)

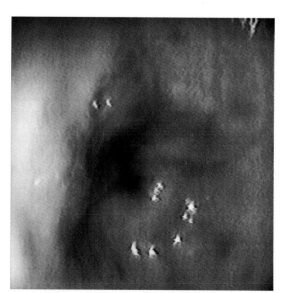

FIGURE 7-166 View of the pyloric sphincter. Once the sphincter opens, the duodenum can be entered by the endoscope. (Courtesy MJR-VHUP, Philadelphia.)

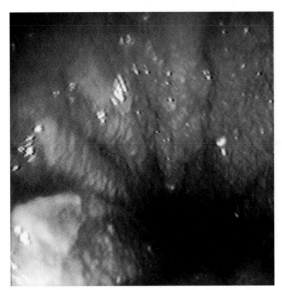

FIGURE 7-167 Ulcerated pylorus with irregular mucosa from a 9-year-old male Labrador. This dog was diagnosed with chronic gastritis and chronic duodenitis. (Courtesy MJR-VHUP, Philadelphia.)

FIGURE 7-169 Multifocal and diffuse, raised, pale circular lesions throughout regions of gastric mucosa from a 12-year-old male domestic shorthair cat. This cat was diagnosed with gastric and duodenal lymphosarcoma. (Courtesy MJR-VHUP, Philadelphia.)

FIGURE 7-168 Small gastric erosions from a 3-year-old female Australian Cattle Dog. (Courtesy MJR-VHUP, Philadelphia.)

adenocarcinoma and other neoplastic masses, deeper tissue samples are required.

Duodenoscopy

Duodenoscopy is the endoscopic technique of examining the duodenum. Duodenoscopy aids in the diagnosis and treatment of small intestine disease. Clinical signs of such disease may include (but are not limited to) vomiting, hematemesis, diarrhea, melena, change in appetite, and weight loss. Duodenoscopy identifies abnormalities of the mucosa and reveals distortion of the small intestine's normal anatomic relationships by displacement or extrinsic compression.

The following diagnoses and conditions can be identified with the use of duodenoscopy: intestinal parasites, inflammation (inflammatory bowel disease; Figures 7-170 to 7-172), lymphangiectasia, ulcerations, and neoplasia. Intestinal parasites (generally ascarids) are occasionally encountered on direct examination. These parasites can be easily removed, but biopsy specimens should still be obtained. If *Giardia* is suspected, a saline lavage can be performed to retrieve trophozoites. Partial-thickness specimens obtained by duodenoscopy may be preferable to full-thickness specimens obtained by abdominal exploratory surgery for patients in a protein-losing enteropathy. Duodenoscopy is preferred in hypoproteinemic patients, especially if the total protein value is 3.5 g/dL or less, because rate of healing is delayed once total protein falls to that level. The most common causes of protein-losing enteropathy in dogs are inflammatory bowel disease, lymphoma, and lymphangiectasia. Lymphoma is the most common intestinal neoplasia and is

FIGURE 7-170 Significant duodenal inflammation with mild ulceration from a 2-year-old female German Shepherd. This dog was diagnosed with a moderate form of chronic lymphoplasmacytic and neutrophilic enteritis. (Courtesy MJR-VHUP, Philadelphia.)

FIGURE 7-171 Edematous duodenum with dilated lacteals and pinpoint ulcerations from an 8½-year-old Bichon Frise. This dog was diagnosed with chronic duodenitis. (Courtesy MJR-VHUP, Philadelphia.)

believed to be more common in cats than in dogs (Box 7-32).

Biopsy sampling. It is best to obtain biopsy samples when the sites to be sampled can be visualized at the end of the endoscope. However, this may not be possible for collection of specimens from the small intestine, and samples may need to be collected "blindly." It is also important to note that the intestinal mucosa is more friable than the gastric mucosa. There are ways to obtain "blind" intestinal biopsy samples from the farthest regions of the small intestine (i.e., jejunum). However, some veterinarians are not comfortable with obtaining blind biopsy samples and attempt the same technique used for gastric biopsy.

Small intestinal biopsy samples can vary in size. Biopsy samples tend to be small with normal mucosa but invariably larger when the mucosa is compromised by some disorder. For example, a linear strip of tissue up to 1 inch long can be obtained with marked inflammatory

disease because the mucosal and submucosal integrity is altered.

Colonoscopy

Colonoscopy is the endoscopic technique used to examine the rectum, large intestine, and cecum. Colonoscopy aids in the diagnosis and treatment of large bowel disease. Clinical signs may include (but are not limited to) diarrhea, hematochezia, fecal mucus, tenesmus, dyschezia, constipation, and chronic vomiting (especially in cats). Hematochezia, fecal mucus, and tenesmus are signs of diarrhea in large bowel disease, and patients with these signs usually have self-limiting disease or a disorder that can be resolved with symptomatic treatment and supportive care. Chronic vomiting is usually more common in upper GI disease, although in cats this may indicate inflammation of the ascending colon or ileum, which is why every attempt should be made to enter the ileum during colonoscopy.

FIGURE 7-172 Friable, "cobblestone" duodenum with small, ulcerated areas from a 4-year-old male domestic short-hair cat. This cat was diagnosed with severe, chronic duodenitis. (Courtesy MJR-VHUP, Philadelphia.)

BOX 7-32 Duodenoscopy Technique

1. Fasting a patient for 12 to 18 hours and withholding water for 4 or more hours before a duodenoscopy may be the key to a successful and a thorough examination, as with gastroscopy.
2. The anesthetized and intubated patient should be placed in LLR with a secured oral speculum.
3. As the endoscope advances through the stomach until it reaches the pylorus, minor tip adjustments may be necessary to maintain the pyloric orifice in the center of the field of view.
4. Minimal forward pressure can be applied to advance the tip directly through the open pyloric orifice to reach the first segment of the duodenum; however, if the pyloric orifice is closed or slightly open, variable resistance may be encountered.
5. The insertion tube tip can be guided into the pyloric canal by application of leftward tip deflection alone or with slight to moderate upward tip deflection while the scope is advanced.
6. A blurred image will be seen once the insertion tube tip is in the pyloric canal, because the pyloric walls are usually pressed in around the tip of the insertion tube.
7. Turning both inner and outer control knobs on the endoscope in a clockwise direction as the scope advances provides a downward and rightward tip deflection that will aid entry into the proximal duodenum.
8. The color of the gastric mucosa is usually cream, and on entry into the duodenum, the color of the mucosa becomes pinkish red.
9. The tip of the insertion tube should then be directed into the descending duodenal lumen without the use of excessive force.
10. Because the tip of the insertion tube lies against the superior wall of the proximal duodenum, it should be angled acutely upward and sometimes also to the left. This maneuver with gentle advancement provides a tunneling view of the descending duodenum.
11. Air insufflation should be maintained to allow distension of the duodenal walls.
12. At times, minor forward or backward movements of the insertion tube may aid in freeing the endoscope tip.

NOTE: Air insufflation should be monitored carefully because excessive air may reflux into the stomach and cause unnecessary gastric distension. If this distension occurs, the endoscope should be withdrawn into the stomach and then air-suctioned.

Colonoscopy should be performed when clinical or laboratory findings (e.g., significant weight loss, hypoalbuminemia) suggest that a patient has a serious disorder (e.g., intussusception, histoplasmosis, adenocarcinoma) or when the clinical signs and symptoms of colonic disease do not respond to specific therapeutic trials. However, patients who have diarrhea with large bowel disease but are otherwise healthy should be tested for parasitic disease, dietary allergy or intolerance, fiber-responsive diarrhea, and clostridial colitis before colonoscopy is considered.

The most frequently diagnosed disorders include a variety of mucosal inflammatory disorders, with lymphocytic plasmacytic colitis the most common (Figures 7-173 and 7-174), and rectal polyps. Colonoscopy is much more accurate than contrast radiography in diagnosing large intestine disorders. Most patients with idiopathic colitis have grossly normal mucosa, so it is imperative that the colon be properly prepared for obtaining high-quality biopsy samples at various levels of the colon.

Strictured areas with relatively normal mucosa usually result from a submucosal lesion. In these cases, biopsying

FIGURE 7-173 *Left,* Moderately to severely inflamed duodenum with mild ulcerative areas. *Right,* Moderately inflamed ileocolic valve from a 2-year-old female German Shepherd. This dog was diagnosed with moderate to severe lymphoplasmacytic, neutrophilic, and erosive colitis. This dog was also diagnosed with enteritis (Courtesy MJR-VHUP, Philadelphia.)

FIGURE 7-174 *Left,* Rectal mass from 2-year-old male Brittany Spaniel. *Right,* Moderately inflamed colon from same patient. This dog was diagnosed with rectal papillary adenocarcinoma and moderate lymphoplasmacytic colitis. (Courtesy MJR-VHUP, Philadelphia.)

must be aggressive enough to ensure that submucosal tissue is obtained. Cytologic studies are sensitive in detecting histoplasmosis (*Histoplasma capsulatum* infection) and prototheocosis (*Prototheca* infection) and may be useful in detecting some neoplasms and eosinophilic colitis.

Patient preparation. Fecal examinations for parasites and ova (e.g., whipworms, *Giardia*), cultures for pathogens (e.g., *Salmonella, Campylobacter*), fecal cytology (e.g., for *Clostridium* spores), and assays (e.g., for *Clostridium perfringens* enterotoxin) should be done before enemas or lavage solutions are administered.

The patient should be fasted for 24 to 36 hours. The colon needs to be as thoroughly cleaned as possible. Lavage solutions are best for removing food and feces from the alimentary canal. These solutions are *isosmotic* (same osmotic pressure) and produce an osmotic

diarrhea that washes particulate matter out of the colon. One example of a lavage solution is GoLYTELY (Braintree Laboratories, Inc,. Braintree, MA), which is administered through a gastric or nasoesophageal tube if the patient does not consume the solution orally. GoLYTELY is a concentrated solution of polyethylene glycol and electrolytes that results in virtually no net absorption or excretions of ions or water. GoLYTELY can usually clean a bowel within 4 hours, although some patients may require more than one dosing. Large volumes can be given without causing significant changes in water or electrolyte balance. In addition to lavage solutions, an osmotic cathartic such as magnesium citrate may be used. This combination results in the best colonic preparation and minimizes artifacts induced by enema tubes.

Problems associated with lavage solutions include (1) they are more expensive than enemas, (2) large volumes are needed for some patients, and (3) orogastric intubation administration can be difficult in aggressive animals.

Colonic lavages such as a warm-water enema are helpful but may need to be repeated multiple times. Improper technique can easily result in an inadequately prepared patient with possible mucosal artifacts. For this reason, it is best to fast a patient for 36 hours rather than 24 hours. When performing an enema with a well-lubricated enema tube, the tube should not be forced if resistance is encountered because traumatic mucosal hemorrhages will likely occur. If the colon has been lavaged properly, clear water should be evacuated after the last enema. Enemas are helpful for cleaning the descending colon but are inadequate for cleaning the ascending and transverse colon and the ileocolic valve (Box 7-33).

Biopsy sampling. Biopsy samples from the ileum, cecum, ascending colon, transverse colon, and descending colon should all be obtained if possible, regardless of how normal the tissues appear. These mucosal biopsy samples are for histopathologic evaluation. However, *Salmonella* organisms sometimes can be cultured from tissue samples if none can be grown from feces.

Attempting to put more distance between the distal tip of the endoscope and the ileocolic valve allows a panoramic view of structures rather than a close-up

view. Having the distal tip of the endoscope withdrawn into the descending colon and then re-inserted into the ascending colon allows visualization of the ileocolic valve (Figure 7-175). With this technique, flexible biopsy

FIGURE 7-175 View of the ileocolic valve (top opening), but dilated; bottom opening is the cecocolic valve. (Courtesy MJR-VHUP, Philadelphia.)

BOX 7-33 Colonoscopy Technique

1. After the patient has been fasted properly (ideally 36 hours) and the colon adequately cleaned, the patient can be anesthetized and intubated and placed in left lateral recumbency (LLR).
2. The flexible endoscope tip is inserted into the rectum, followed by insufflation.
3. As the tip of the scope is advanced central to the lumen, the mucosa and lumen are examined. The endoscope is advanced to its most orad (toward the mouth) limit and then slowly withdrawn so that the mucosa can be thoroughly examined.
4. The splenic flexure, the most orad part of the descending colon, is the area where the descending colon turns and becomes the transverse colon.
5. To enter the transverse colon, the distal tip of the endoscope must be diverted in the direction of the lumen, and then the tip must be carefully advanced using a blind "slide-by" technique. With this technique the distal tip usually pushes lightly against the colonic wall, and visualization is lost for 1 to 2 cm because the lens is too close to the mucosa.
6. In cats the transverse and ascending sections of the colon usually merge. It is difficult to examine the mucosa of this section because the tight bend makes it impossible for the distal tip to stay in the center of the lumen.
7. The blind slide-by technique is used from the descending colon up to the ascending colon, which leads to the cecum and ileocolic valve.
8. When the ileocolic valve is approached, careful observation is necessary, or the valve may be bypassed and the distal tip may enter the cecum.

9. If the area is adequately clean, the ileocolic valve and the cecocolic valve can both be seen (see Figure 7-175). In some cases the ileocolic valve appears as another opening adjacent to the cecocolic valve. However, this area tends to be less well prepared because mucus and debris entering from the ileum may cover and hide the ileocolic valve.
10. As the distal tip reaches the ileocolic valve, minor tip adjustments may be necessary to maintain the ileocolic orifice in the center of the field of view.
11. Minimal forward pressure can be applied to advance the tip directly through the open ileocolic orifice to access the ileum; however, if the ileocolic orifice is closed or slightly open, variable resistance may be encountered.
12. If the cecum is entered and was thought to be the colon, the lumen will make additional bends that cannot be negotiated with the distal tip. No force should be applied to push the distal tip past one of these bends, or the cecum may be perforated.
13. If the working length of the scope has been exhausted in the process of entering the cecum, the endoscope should be retracted slightly and air aspirated to partially collapse the lumen. This maneuver should shorten the distance to the cecocolic or ileocolic valve.
14. If rectal lesions are present, a retroflexed view is necessary. This can usually be achieved in dogs that are medium to large breeds. However, a rigid proctoscope is often the better scope for examining rectal lesions.

forceps can be passed through the valve, and blind ileal samples obtained.

It is often helpful for the colonic lumen to be partially collapsed before the mucosa is grasped with biopsy forceps. This maneuver allows the forceps to take a larger,

deeper sample that should include the submucosa. It is safe to re-inflate the colon after biopsy samples are obtained with flexible forceps. The risk of perforation with flexible biopsy instruments is much less than with rigid instruments.

KEY POINTS

1. To be a competent surgical assistant, the veterinary technician must have proficient knowledge of the surgical procedure, surgical instruments, and aseptic and sterile technique.
2. The intraoperative duties of the surgical assistant include retraction of tissue, bone reduction, wound sponging, suction of the surgical site, and providing hemostasis. Responsibilities also include anticipation of the surgeon's needs and sponge counts before surgery and before closure of the cavity.
3. Preoperative blood tests should be performed for any animal undergoing anesthesia and surgery. An animal more than 5 years old should have a more extensive blood analysis (CBC and chemistry) than a younger patient (CBC).
4. The patient's bladder should be expressed before it enters the surgery room.
5. The bladder of a traumatic injury patient should not be expressed before it enters the sugery room.
6. Patients undergoing abdominal procedures should be clipped from the xiphoid process to the pubis. This allows the surgeon to extend the incision as needed.
7. The use of Balfour retractors during abdominal surgical procedures allows for enhanced exposure to the abdominal cavity.
8. Laparotomy (lap) sponges should be used to isolate organs during hollow-organ surgery. The use of laparotomy sponges helps reduce contaminants that may enter the abdominal cavity.
9. Lap sponges can also be used to keep exteriorized tissue moist and protected during surgery.
10. Stay sutures should be placed during hollow-organ surgeries (e.g., cystotomy, gastrotomy) to allow for manipulation of the organ as well as to prevent leakage of contaminants within the abdominal cavity. The sterile surgical assistant should also take care when handling the exposed viscera; gloves or sponges used should be moistened to reduce tissue damage.
11. Abdominal lavage with warm sterile saline before closure of the abdomen helps dilute any pollutants and to warm the patient.
12. A barium contrast study should never be performed if perforations of the gastrointestinal tract are suspected.
13. During an enterotomy procedure, Doyen clamps or the fingers of an assistant should be used to occlude the intestines to avoid leakage of chyme within the abdomen.
14. Abdominal incisions should be monitored daily for swelling, discharge, or malodor. Many postoperative complications are related to the incision site.
15. Patients with gastric dilatation and volvulus (GDV) are considered true surgical emergencies. The immediate treatment includes decompression of the stomach, correction of fluid and electrolyte imbalances, treatment for shock, and surgery to derotate the stomach and gastropexy.
16. An orogastric tube should never be forced down the esophagus during placement. Gentle placement is necessary to avoid damage to the esophagus.
17. A roll of hospital tape can be placed between the upper and lower jaws of the patient receiving an orogastric tube. The tube can be placed through the hole in the roll of tape. This will keep the jaws of the animal from biting down on the tube or the assistant's hand during placement.
18. The stomach of a dog with a GDV generally rotates in a clockwise direction.
19. Animals should be spayed before their first ovarian cycle to decrease the incidence of mammary tumors.
20. The most common complication reported after an ovariohysterectomy is hemorrhage.
21. Pyometra is a potentially life-threatening condition. A complete ovariohysterectomy should be performed to remove the uterus; medical management is not recommended.
22. Care should be taken when removing an infected uterus. The organ is damaged and in many cases friable; purulent contents could leak out into the peritoneal cavity, leading to an increased chance of peritonitis.
23. Indications for performing a feline or canine castration include eliminating reproductive function, preventing roaming, preventing urine spraying, treating scrotal neoplasia, and treating endocrine abnormalities.
24. Before placing a dog or cat under anesthesia for castration, the testicles are examined to be sure both have descended into the scrotum. If they have not, an inguinal or abdominal procedure may be necessary for testicle retrieval.

25. For cats undergoing castration, the hair of the scrotum should be gently plucked before it enters the surgery room.

26. Scrotal bleeding is the most common complication associated with canine and feline castration.

27. Lateral ear canal resection involves lateralization and exposure of the horizontal ear canal for drainage purposes, generally in patients with chronic ear infections. Medical management is usually required even after resection.

28. *Entropion* refers to "rolling in" of the eyelid. Surgery is usually done to alleviate ocular irritation.

29. A meibomian (sebaceous) adenoma is the most common eyelid neoplasm in the dog.

30. Squamous cell carcinoma is the most common feline eyelid tumor and is often found in cats with white or pink eyelids.

31. A wedge resection procedure is the most common procedure performed for eyelid neoplasia.

32. Orthopedics involves injuries or diseases of the skeletal system.

33. Orthopedic injuries are usually not considered life threatening unless they involve the skull or spine or unless a long-bone fracture has resulted in great loss of blood.

34. Fracture assessment should include a history, thorough physical examination, and radiographs.

35. When radiographs of a long-bone fracture are taken, the joint below and above the fracture site should be included in the film.

36. Open fractures are classified according to mechanism of puncture and the severity of the soft tissue damage.

37. Surgical options for fracture repair include internal fixation and external fixation. Internal fixation includes plates, screws, nails, pins, and wire. External fixation includes casts, rigid splints, and custom-made devices.

38. Casts and splints must be kept dry and clean and should be observed for slippage, self-mutilation, and toe swelling.

39. Hindlimb and forelimb amputations are considered major procedures and should be performed only with a thorough knowledge of the patient's physical status.

40. Local nerve blocks contribute significantly to postoperative pain control in amputation patients.

41. Cranial cruciate ligament (CCL) ruptures are also referred to as anterior cruciate ligament (ACL) injury or "football player's knee" in humans.

42. The major diagnostic tests for CCL injury include the cranial drawer test and the tibial compression test. Palpation of the affected leg often reveals muscle atrophy, pain, joint effusion, and asymmetry.

43. Biopsy techniques for diagnostic purposes include fine-needle aspiration, impression smears, needle punch, punch, bone, incisional, and excisional.

44. Minimally invasive procedures include laser surgery, laparoscopy, and endoscopy.

45. The technician's most important role in laser surgery is laser safety. Most practices using laser surgery appoint a laser safety officer, most likely the technician.

46. Many hazards are associated with laser surgery, including eye, skin, fire, and smoke plume hazards. All safety steps should be taken to avoid potential hazards.

47. Advantages to laser surgery over traditional surgery include more rapid healing time of tissue, less risk of postoperative infection, reduced postoperative pain and swelling, and decreased surgery time.

48. Laparoscopic procedures are performed to examine and obtain biopsy specimens of the internal organs or tumors of the abdominal cavity. Laparoscopy can also be used to perform specific surgical procedures, such as a spay and gastropexy.

49. Some advantages to laparoscopic procedures include improved patient recovery, smaller surgical sites, lower postoperative infection rate, and decreased postoperative pain.

50. The patient undergoing laparoscopy should be fasted for 12 hours and the bladder should be expressed before it enters the surgery room.

51. When performing endoscopy, an insertion tube should always be handled carefully. Sharp bends, tight coiling, and striking of the tube against hard surfaces should be avoided.

52. Maintaining endoscopes involves proper cleaning and disinfection, leak testing and inspection, microbial monitoring, and storage.

53. In dogs and cats, gastric and duodenal disorders are more common than esophageal disorders. Because clinical signs of these diseases can overlap, endoscopic examination of the esophagus should extend to the stomach and duodenum for a thorough upper gastrointestinal examination.

54. Patient preparation for colonoscopies is crucial because the whole colon needs to be visualized, and it is more difficult to clean the ileocolic valve area than the descending colon. Also, large debris cannot be aspirated as well with flexible scopes as with rigid scopes.

55. Narcotics (fentanyl, morphine, hydromorphone) should not be used for gastroduodenoscopies because they may cause spasms, and entering the duodenum will be more difficult because of an increase in pyloric tone.

56. Appropriate analgesics should be administered for every surgical patient postoperatively.

57. A surgical patient may need to be sent home with Elizabethan collars if the pet attempts to mutilate the incision site.

REVIEW QUESTIONS

1. What position is the patient placed in for an abdominal exploratory surgery?
   a. Sternal recumbency.
   b. Dorsal recumbency.
   c. Right or left lateral recumbency.
   d. Ventral recumbency.
   e. It is the surgeon's preference.

2. Which of the following are considered abdominal surgical procedures?
   a. Ovariohysterectomy.
   b. Routine, closed castration.
   c. Incisional gastropexy.
   d. All of the above.
   e. Both a and c.

3. What is the primary indication for an ovariohysterectomy?
   a. To prevent mammary carcinoma.
   b. To prevent pyometra.
   c. Dystocia.
   d. Reproductive sterilization.
   e. Uterine torsion.

4. Why is it beneficial to spay a dog before her first heat cycle?
   a. To decrease the chance of unwanted litters.
   b. To decrease the chance of the development of mammary gland tumors.
   c. To decrease weight gain.
   d. Both a and b.

5. Which of the following breeds of dogs have an increased risk of dystocia?
   a. Golden Retrievers.
   b. Pugs.
   c. Bulldogs.
   d. Both b and c.

6. During which of the following procedures is the uterus removed?
   a. Routine ovariohysterectomy.
   b. Cesarean section without an ovariohysterectomy.
   c. En bloc resection.
   d. All of the above.
   e. Both a and c.

7. Which of the following is an indication for abdominal exploratory surgery?
   a. Routine ovariohysterectomy.
   b. Splenic tumor.
   c. Ruptured bladder.
   d. All of the above.
   e. Both b and c.

8. Which of the following retractors is routinely used in abdominal exploratory surgeries?
   a. Gelpi.
   b. Senn.
   c. Weitlaner.
   d. Balfour.
   e. None of the above.

9. Which of the following procedures involves making an incision into the stomach?
   a. Abdominal exploratory.
   b. Gastrotomy.
   c. Enterotomy.
   d. Splenectomy.
   e. Laparotomy.

10. Which of the following intestinal surgeries involves removing a piece of the intestine and suturing the ends of the remaining intestines back together?
   a. Enterotomy.
   b. Resection and anastomosis.
   c. Gastropexy.
   d. a and b.

11. *True or False:* Sterile saline can be injected into the surgical site to check for any leakage after the anastomosis site has been closed.

12. Which of the following should be performed before closing the abdomen if peritonitis is suspected?
   a. Bacterial culture swab.
   b. Gastropexy.
   c. Urinalysis.
   d. All of the above.
   e. None of the above.

13. Which of the following refers to surgically attaching the stomach to the body wall?
   a. Gastric dilatation and volvulus (GDV).
   b. Gastropexy.
   c. Splenectomy.
   d. Enterotomy.
   e. Celiotomy.

14. *True or False:* A gastropexy procedure prevents further bloat occurrences.

15. *True or False:* A patient that needs to have an abdominal exploratory for internal hemorrhage resulting after having been hit by a car (HBC), should have his/her bladder expressed before being moved into the surgery room.

16. Which of the following terms refers to a joint?
    a. Malunion.
    b. Comminuted.
    c. Articular.
    d. Interfragmentary.
    e. None of the above.

17. *True or False:* Neonatal kittens should be placed with the dam to allow nursing as soon as possible.

18. *True or False:* Purulent discharge from the vulva is present in all cases of pyometra.

19. Which term refers to a fracture that is on an incline or slanting in relation to the long axis of the bone?
    a. Transverse.
    b. Oblique.
    c. Spiral.
    d. Comminuted nonreducible.

20. Which term refers to a fracture that curves around a center point or axis?
    a. Transverse.
    b. Oblique.
    c. Spiral.
    d. Comminuted nonreducible.

21. Which of the following are devices used in internal fixation of fractured bones?
    a. Intramedullary (IM) pins.
    b. Ring fixation.
    c. Bone plates.
    d. Both a and c.
    e. All of the above.

22. Which of the following devices are used in external fixation of fractured bones?
    a. IM pins.
    b. Ring fixation.
    c. Bone plates.
    d. Both a and c.
    e. All of the above.

23. Which of the following are possible complications associated with internal fixation of fracture repair?
    a. Non-union.
    b. Malunion.
    c. Delayed union.
    d. Aseptic loosening.
    e. All of the above.

24. *True or False:* Splints are appropriate only for fractures that are distal to the elbow and stifle.

25. Which of the following diagnostic tests may aid in diagnosing a torn cranial cruciate ligament?
    a. Cranial drawer test.
    b. Palpation of the hock joint.
    c. Tibial compression test.
    d. Both a and c.
    e. All of the above.

26. Which of the following diagnostic tests used to evaluate masses does not usually require sedation or anesthesia, is easy to perform, has minimal morbidity associated with it, but has a low diagnostic yield?
    a. Needle punch biopsy.
    b. Fine-needle aspiration.
    c. Excisional biopsy.
    e. All of the above.

27. For what condition is a lateral ear canal resection indicated?
    a. Chronic otitis externa.
    b. Neoplasia of the ear canal.
    c. Deafness.
    d. Both a and b.

28. *True or False:* Baby shampoo diluted 1:3 with water is both effective and safe in cleansing the periocular area before ophthalmic surgery.

29. Which of the following breeds are predisposed to protrusion of the gland of the third eyelid, also known as "cherry eye"?
    a. Cocker Spaniel.
    b. Boston Terrier.
    c. Great Dane.
    d. All of the above.

30. Which of the following procedures is/are considered minimally invasive?
    a. Laser surgery.
    b. Laparoscopy.
    c. Endoscopy.
    d. All of the above.

31. What are some of the workplace hazards associated with laser surgery?
    a. Eye and skin damage.
    b. Smoke plume hazard.
    c. Fire hazard.
    d. All of the above.

32. What advantage does laparoscopy have over traditional laparotomy?
    a. None; the procedures are essentially the same.
    b. Smaller surgical incisions.
    c. Lower postoperative morbidity.
    d. Both b and c.

33. *True or False:* A flexible endoscope with a diameter of 8 to 11 mm and a working length of 100 cm is usually adequate for most feline and canine upper gastrointestinal examinations and colonoscopies.

34. *True or False:* When the endoscope is not being used, it should be set on the examination table.

35. Which of the following can be diagnosed by gastroscopy?
    a. *Helicobacter* infection.
    b. Foreign bodies in the stomach.
    c. Gastric ulceration.
    d. All of the above.

36. How long should a patient be fasted before gastroscopy?
    a. 12-hour to 18-hour food fast, 4-hour water fast.
    b. 6-hour to 8-hour food fast, 4-hour water fast.
    c. 24-hour to 36-hour food fast, 8-hour water fast.
    d. 10-hour food fast; water fast unnecessary.
    e. None of the above.

37. *True or False:* Duodenoscopy aids in the diagnosis and treatment of small intestine disease.

38. *True or False:* Lymphoma is the most common intestinal neoplasia.

39. Colonoscopy refers to the endoscopic technique of examining the:
    a. Rectum.
    b. Large intestine.
    c. Cecum.
    d. All of the above.
    e. None of the above.

40. Which of the following applies to the patient about to undergo colonoscopy?
    a. He/she needs to be fasted 24 to 36 hours.
    b. He/she will receive an enema.
    c. Both a and b.
    d. None of the above.

41. In addition to rendering a male cat unable to reproduce, which of the following is an indication for castrating a male cat?
    a. Prevent aggressive behavior.
    b. Prevent urine spraying.
    c. Prevent roaming.
    d. All of the above.
    e. None of the above.

ANSWERS

1. b	12. a	23. e	34. False
2. e	13. b	24. True	35. d
3. d	14. False	25. d	36. b
4. d	15. False	26. b	37. True
5. d	16. c	27. d	38. True
6. e	17. True	28. True	39. d
7. e	18. False	29. d	40. c
8. d	19. b	30. d	41. d
9. b	20. c	31. d	
10. b	21. d	32. d	
11. True	22. b	33. True	

BIBLIOGRAPHY

American National Standards Institute: Safe Use of Lasers. (ANSI Z136.1-1993.) New York, 1993.

Bassert JM, McCurnin DM, editors: McCurnin's Clinical textbook for veterinary technicians, ed 7, St Louis, 2010, Elsevier.

Bessler M, et al: Is immune function better preserved after laparoscopic versus open colon resection? Surg Endosc 8:881, 1994.

Bjorab MJ, Ellison GW, Slocum B: Current techniques in small animal surgery, Philadelphia, 1998, Williams & Wilkins.

Blood DC, Studdert VP: Saunders comprehensive veterinary dictionary, ed 3. London, 2007, Saunders.

Brockman DJ, Washabau RJ, Drobatz KJ: Canine gastric dilatation/ volvulus syndrome in a veterinary critical care unit: 295 cases (1986-1992). J Am Vet Med Assoc 207:460, 1995.

Burrows CF, Bright RM, Spencer CP: Influence of dietary composition on gastric emptying and motility in dogs: potential involvement in acute gastric dilatation. Am J Vet Res 46:2609, 1985.

Darvelid AW, Linde-Forsberg C: Dystocia in the bitch. J Small Anim Pract 35:402, 1994.

Doverspike M, et al: Contralateral cranial cruciate ligament rupture: incidence in 114 dogs. J Am Anim Hosp Assoc 29:275, 1993.

Flanders JA, Harvey HJ: Results of tube gastrostomy as treatment for gastric torsion in the dog. J Am Vet Med Assoc 185:74, 1984.

Fossum TW, Hedlund CS, Hulse DA, et al: Small animal surgery, ed 3, St Louis, 2007, Mosby.

Gaudet DA: Retrospective study of 128 cases of canine dystocia. J Small Anim Pract 21:813, 1985.

Gelatt KN: Essentials of veterinary ophthalmology, Philadelphia, 2000, Lippincott Williams & Wilkins.

Glickman LT, Lantz GC, Schellenberg DB, et al: Analysis of risk factors for gastric dilatation and dilatation volvulus in dogs: a practitioner/owner case-control study. J Am Anim Hosp Assoc 34:253-259, 1997.

Glickman LT, Glickman NW, Schellenberg DB, et al: Multiple risk factors for the gastric dilatation-volvulus syndrome in dogs. J Am Vet Med Assoc 216:40, 2000.

Gross ME, Jones BD, Bergstresser DR, et al: Effects of abdominal insufflation with nitrous oxide on cardiorespiratory measurements in spontaneously breathing isoflurane-anesthetized dogs. Am J Vet Res 54:1352, 1993.

Gualtieri M: Esophagoscopy. Vet Clin North Am Small Anim Pract 31:605, 2001.

Harvey CE: The ear and nose. In Harvey CE, Newton CD, Schwartz A, et al, editors: Small animal surgery, Philadelphia, 1990, Lippincott.

Hitz CB: An overview of laser technology. In Understanding laser technology: an intuitive introduction to basic and advanced laser concepts, ed 2, Tulsa, OK, 1991, Pennwell.

Holt TL, Mann FA: Soft tissue applications of lasers. Vet Clin North Am 32:569, 2002.

Jacques SL: Laser-tissue interactions: photochemical, photothermal, and photomechanical. Surg Clin North Am 72:531, 1992.

Johanningmeier JP: TPLO repair method for CCL tears. Vet Tech 682, October 2003.

Johnson JA, Austin C, Bruer GJ: Incidence of appendicular musculoskeletal disorders in veterinary teaching hospitals from 1980-1989. Vet Comp Orthop Trauma 7:56, 1994.

Johnson JM, Johnson AL: Cranial cruciate ligament rupture: pathogenesis, diagnosis and postoperative rehabilitation, Vet Clin North Am 23:717, 1993.

Katzir A: Medical lasers. In Lasers and optical fibers in medicine, San Diego, 1993, Academic Press.

Katzir A: Single optical fibers. In Lasers and optical fibers in medicine, San Diego, 1993, Academic Press.

Lettow E: Laparoscopic examinations in liver diseases in dogs. Vet Med Rev 2:159, 1972.

Leib MS, Konde LJ, Wingfield WE, et al: Circumcostal gastropexy for preventing recurrence of gastric dilatation-volvulus in the dog: an evaluation of 30 cases. J Am Vet Med Assoc 187:245, 1985.

Lucroy MD, Bartels KE: Using biomedical lasers in veterinary practice. Vet Med 95:4, 2000.

Lumenis LX-20SP NovaPulse Laser System Operator's Manual, Lumenis, 2002, Santa Clara, CA.

Macoy DM, et al: A gastropexy technique for permanent fixation of the pyloric antrum. J Am Anim Hosp Assoc 18:763, 1982.

Maggs D: Fundamentals of veterinary ophthalmology, ed 4, Philadelphia, 2008, Saunders.

Magne ML, Tams TR: Laparoscopy: instrumentation and technique. In Tams TR, editor: Small animal endoscopy, ed 3, St Louis, 2011, Mosby.

Marsolais GS, Dvorak G, Conzemius MG: Effects of postoperative rehabilitation on limb function after cranial cruciate ligament repair in dogs. J Am Vet Med Assoc 220:1325, 2002.

Matthiesen DT: Partial gastrectomy as treatment for gastric volvulus. Vet Surg 14:185, 1985.

Mehler SJ, Bennett A: Surgical oncology of exotic animals. Vet Clin Exotic Anim Pract 7:783-805, 2004.

Monnet E, Twedt DC: Laparoscopy. Vet Clin North Am 33:1147, 2003.

Moore CP, Constantinescu GM: Surgery of the adnexa. Vet Clin North Am 27:1011, 1997.

Moore KW, Read RA: Rupture of the cranial cruciate ligament in dogs. Compend Contin Educ Pract Vet 18:223, 1996.

Morrison WB: Cancer in dogs and cats, Baltimore, 1998, Williams & Wilkins.

Muir WW: Gastric dilatation-volvulus in the dog, with emphasis on cardiac arrhythmias. J Am Vet Med Assoc 180:739, 1982.

Nelson R, Couto C: Small animal internal medicine, ed 4, St Louis, 2009, Mosby.

Osborne CA et al: Analysis of 77,000 canine uroliths. Vet Clin North Am Small Anim Pract 29:1, 1999.

Pearce J, Thomsen R: Rate process analysis of thermal damage. In Welch AJ, van Gamert MJC, editors: Optical-thermal response of laser irradiated tissue, New York, 1995, Plenum.

Pearson H: The complications of ovariohysterectomy in the bitch. J Small Anim Pract 14:257, 1973.

Phillips BS: Bladder tumors in dogs and cats. Compend Contin Educ Pract Vet 21:540, 1999.

Piermattie DL, Flo GL, DeCam CE: Brinker, Piermattei and Flo's handbook of small animal orthopedics and fracture repair, ed 4, St Louis, 2006, Elsevier.

Richter KP: Laparoscopy in dogs and cats. Vet Clin North Am 31:707, 2001.

Robben JR, Stokhof AA, van Sluisjs FJ: Arrhythmias after surgery of gastric dilatation volvulus in dogs. Tijdschr Diergenneeskd 118(Suppl):67S, 1993.

Roberts SM, Severin GA, Lavach JD: Prevalence and treatment of palpebral neoplasms in the dog: 200 cases (1975-1983), J Am Vet Med Assoc 189:1355, 1986.

Rothuizen J: Laparoscopy in small animal medicine. Vet Q 3:225, 1985.

Sammarco JL, et al: Postoperative analgesia for stifle surgery: a comparison of intraarticular bupivacaine, morphine or saline. Vet Surg 25:59, 1996.

Schneider R, et al: Factors influencing canine mammary cancer development and post surgical survival. J Natl Cancer Inst 43:1249, 1969.

Schumway R, Broussard J: Maintenance of gastrointestinal endoscopes. Clin Tech Small Anim Pract 18:254, 2003.

Sirois, M: Principles and practice of veterinary technology, ed 3, St Louis, 2011, Mosby.

Slatter D: Textbook of small animal surgery, ed 3, Philadelphia, 2003, Saunders.

Smeak DD: The Chinese finger trap suture technique for fastening tubes and catheters. J Am Anim Hosp Assoc 26:215, 1990.

Smith GK, Torg JS: Fibula head transposition for repair of cruciate-deficient stifle in the dog. J Am Vet Med Assoc 187:375, 1985.

Stasi K, Melendez L: Care and cleaning of the endoscope. Vet Clin North Am Small Anim Pract 31:589, 2001.

Sullins KE: Diode laser and endoscopic laser surgery. Vet Clin North Am 32:639, 2002.

Tams T: Handbook of small animal gastroenterology, ed 2, St Louis, 2003, Saunders.

Tams T, editor: Small animal endoscopy, ed 3, St Louis, 2011, Mosby.

Theran P: Early-age neutering of dogs and cats. J Am Vet Med Assoc 202:914, 1993.

Tobias KM, Johnston SA: Veterinary surgery: small animal, St Louis, 2012, Saunders.

Troncy E et al: Results of preemptive epidural administration of morphine with or without bupivacaine in dogs and cats undergoing surgery: 265 cases (1997-1999). J Am Vet Med Assoc 221:666, 2002.

Welch AJ, van Gemert MJC: Introduction to medical applications. In Welch AJ, van Gamert MJC, editors: Optical-thermal response of laser irradiated tissue, New York, 1995, Plenum.

Welch AJ, et al: Definitions and overview of tissue optics. In Welch AJ, van Gamert MJC, editors: Optical-thermal response of laser irradiated tissue, New York, 1995, Plenum.

Whittick WG: Canine orthopedics, ed 2, Philadelphia, 1990, Lea & Febiger.

Willard MD: Small animal clinical diagnosis by laboratory methods, St Louis, 2004, Saunders.

Withrow SJ, MacEwen EG: Withrow and MacEwen's Small animal clinical oncology, ed 4, St Louis, 2007, Saunders.

Withrow SJ, Postorino NC, Straw RC: Tumors of the gastrointestinal system. In Clinical veterinary oncology, Philadelphia, 1989, Lippincott.

Witney WO et al: Belt-loop gastropexy: technique and surgical results in 20 dogs. J Am Anim Hosp Assoc 25:75, 1989.

Young WP: Feline onychectomy and elective procedures. Vet Clin North Am 32:601, 2002.

Zepp CP: Surgical technique to establish drainage of the external ear canal and correction of hematoma of the dog and cat. J Am Vet Med Assoc 115:91, 1949.

The Postoperative Patient

Marianne Tear and Ann Wortinger

KEY TERMS

Active drains
Autotransfusion
Brachycephalic
Cryotherapy
Debridement
Dehiscence
Dissociative anesthetic
Emergence delirium
Fenestrated
Hypoglycemia
Hypothermia
Lavage
Normothermia
Occlusive wound
  dressing
Passive drains
Pétrissage
Semiocclusive wound
  dressing
Seroma
Thermoregulatory
Wind-up

OUTLINE

Recovery from Anesthesia and Extubation, 230
Postoperative Monitoring, 231
Complications Related to Anesthesia, 231
  Hypothermia, 231
  Emergence Delirium, 232
  Prolonged Recovery, 233
Complications Related to Surgery, 234
  Hemorrhage, 234
  Seroma, 235
  Dehiscence, 235
  Self-Trauma, 236
  Infection, 239
Postoperative Nursing Care, 239
  Wound Management, 239
  Wound Classification, 239
  Wound Cleansing, 240
  Wound Closure, 243
  Intravenous Catheter Maintenance, 245
  Urinary Catheter Maintenance, 246
  Nutritional Support, 246
  Physical Therapy, 248
Postoperative Analgesia, 249
  Common Analgesic Classes, 250
  Wind-Up, 250
  Dispensed Analgesia, 250
Key Points, 250
Review Questions, 251

LEARNING OBJECTIVES

After completion of this chapter, the reader will be able to:
- Monitor the patient during the anesthesia recovery period:
  - Identify the proper time to extubate the patient.
  - Safely extubate the patient.
  - Recognize and administer prescribed treatments for postanesthesia complications, such as hypothermia, emergence delirium, and prolonged recovery.
- Recognize and administer prescribed treatments for postsurgical complications, such as hemorrhage, seroma, dehiscence, self-trauma, and infection.
- Thoroughly and properly cleanse wounds, understanding the principles of lavage and débridement.
- Maintain and monitor bandages, casts, splints, and slings.
- Maintain and monitor surgical drains.
- Maintain and monitor indwelling venous and urinary catheters.
- Provide nutritional support for postoperative patients through the techniques of force-feeding and tube feeding.
- Understand the basic forms of physical therapy.
- Provide effective postoperative analgesia.
- Understand the importance of preemptive, presurgical analgesia on the success of postoperative analgesia.
- Safely combine different classes of analgesics to provide effective postoperative pain management.

The work of the veterinary technician is still far from complete even when the last suture is placed and the surgeon leaves the surgical table. The patient still needs to recover from the anesthesia. The surgical wounds need to heal. The surgical procedure has yet to be

BOX 8-1   Sequence of Events for Endotracheal Extubation

1. Turn off the anesthetic vaporizer and leave the patient on oxygen for 5 minutes, if possible.
2. Find an empty syringe with the plunger depressed completely. Attach a syringe to the cuff if using a silicone tube with a spring valve in the pilot tube (non–red rubber tube), and deflate the cuff. Leaving the cuff inflated without having it securely fastened can lead to tracheal trauma, necrosis, and/or tearing. It is imperative to monitor the patient for any signs of vomiting or regurgitation once the cuff is deflated to prevent aspiration.*
3. Untie the endotracheal (ET) tube attachment from the patient's head or muzzle.*
4. Check the patient's reflexes. Not every patient will stay under for the full 5 minutes. The anesthetist must know whether or not the patient is close to jumping off the table.
5. Untie the patient from the table, detach all monitoring devices, and decrease fluid administration to a maintenance rate. Remove the V-trough or sandbags and place the patient in lateral recumbency. When rotating the patient into lateral recumbency, guard the tube and do not let it rotate in the patient's trachea. It is important to prevent twisting injury to the trachea. Small patients are especially prone to this injury.
6. Take the immediate postoperative temperature at this point. Continue anesthetic monitoring of the vital signs every 5 minutes until the patient is sufficiently recovered to be returned to the cage.
7. Once the 5 minutes of oxygen administration are completed, disconnect the patient from the anesthesia machine while the oxygen is flowing. This will ensure that the patient always has a source of oxygen in case of an emergency. Place a hand over the end of the Y-piece and squeeze the reservoir bag. This will empty the circuit of most of the gas through the exhaust system.
8. Now shut of the oxygen at the flowmeter.
9. Recheck the reflexes and determine the patient's stage of anesthesia. If the patient is still "asleep," stimulate the patient by rubbing its thorax, stroking the neck, and gently

pulling the tongue or ears. It may also help to gently rotate the animal form side to side.
10. Once the patient has swallowed two or three times, gently pull the ET tube down and out of the mouth. (See exception for brachycephalic breeds noted on page 230.)*
11. Check the end of the ET tube for blood, regurgitated stomach contents, and food. If the animal has regurgitated material in the mouth, hang the head down off the surgical table to allow the material to drip out of the mouth. Quickly determine whether the patient needs to be re-intubated or the pharynx needs to be suctioned. Carefully rinsing the mouth gently with water may suffice, provided that it does not cause the patient to gag and choke from the rinsing process.
12. Take the patient to the recovery cage.
13. Continue to monitor the patient every 5 to 10 minutes to ensure that recovery is a safe and smooth event until complete. At this point, give postoperative pain medications as instructed. Generally, if the patient's temperature is below 98°F postoperatively, opioid drugs will not be given. Hypothermia concerns are discussed later.

Alternative Steps
If the ET tube cuff is not deflated prior to being untied, extreme care must be taken to ensure tracheal trauma does not occur; the following alternative steps should be used:
*2. Untie the endotracheal (ET) tube attachment from the patient's head or muzzle.
*3. Find an empty syringe with the plunger depressed completely. Attach the syringe to the cuff if using a silicone tube with a spring valve in the pilot tube (non–red rubber tube). Do not deflate the ET tube cuff yet.
*10. Once the patient swallows two or three times, deflate the cuff and gently pull the ET tube down and out of the mouth. (See exception for brachycephalic breeds noted on page 230.) The ET tube cuff should never be deflated before the patient regains the ability to swallow. A patient that cannot swallow is vulnerable to aspiration of material that has pooled in the pharynx. A properly inflated ET tube cuff prevents such aspiration.

proved successful. The patient and the owner need help and guidance during the recuperation period. Careful patient monitoring and owner mentoring are important responsibilities of the veterinary technician.

Compassion, caring, and concern are the hallmarks of an excellent technician. All hospitalized patients need an advocate. The observant technician who advocates for the patient's needs and points out changes in the patient's physical status to the attending veterinarian is an invaluable asset to both the patient and the veterinarian.

Recovery from Anesthesia and Extubation

Shepherding the patient from the surgical plane of anesthesia back to consciousness is the first step in the recovery process. The recovery period starts with the cessation of anesthesia and continues until the patient's

vital signs and level of consciousness have returned to normal.

First, the patient must be safely extubated. The steps in the process of extubation are outlined in Box 8-1.

Brachycephalic breeds of dogs, such as English Bulldogs, Pugs, and Pekingese, are prone to developing complications while recovering from anesthesia. These short-headed dogs frequently have stenotic nares and elongated soft palates and are predisposed to laryngeal obstruction during sedation. An elongated soft palate can occlude the larynx and prevent the passage of air through the mouth. The stenotic nares do not allow sufficient air to pass through the nasal passages (Figure 8-1). When managing a brachycephalic dog under anesthesia, the best course of action is to delay extubation as long as possible. Many anesthetists will extubate brachycephalic dogs only after they can lift their heads by themselves. Allow these patients to recover as fully as possible before pulling the ET tube. Once the ET tube is out, closely monitor the patient for any signs of dyspnea and cyanosis (blue mucous membranes).

Postoperative Monitoring

Close monitoring and documentation of vital sign values are usually discontinued after the patient is extubated and placed in the recovery cage. Although the recovery period technically begins when the animal is disconnected from anesthesia, the patient is not completely recovered until all physiologic parameters, including neurologic responses, are normal. This period lasts for hours. Potential complications include airway obstruction, hypotension, thermoregulatory problems (primarily hypothermia), and cardiac arrhythmia. Although patient monitoring may not need to be as frequent, regular monitoring should continue.

The recovery area should be a separate and quiet area in the animal hospital dedicated to recovery from anesthesia. The recovery area should be constantly staffed with one or more technicians. The area should be fully stocked with drugs and equipment necessary to handle any

FIGURE 8-1 Brachycephalic breeds of dogs and cats frequently have nasal openings that are extremely small. Breathing through the nose is difficult. This condition is known as stenotic nares.

emergency. In small hospitals with limited personnel, the recovering patients should be placed in a staffed area where they will be observed frequently. Patients should never be left unattended, because many accidents can occur during this time.

At-risk patients should be monitored closely while recovering. A charting system should be used to help the recovery technicians identify trends and initiate appropriate treatments. The vital signs may be plotted on a graph similar to the anesthesia form, or the vital sign readings may be written in a chart (Figure 8-2).

Complications Related to Anesthesia
Hypothermia

Most patients lose body heat while they are anesthetized. Mild hypothermia, or body temperature no lower than 97° F (about 36° C), is expected and is usually well tolerated by the patient. A body temperature below 93° F (about 34° C) is worrisome and can affect the patient's recovery adversely. As the body temperature decreases, the amount of anesthetic required decreases. The metabolism of the body cells functions best at normal body temperature. As the body temperature drops, normal metabolism slows down, adversely affecting the functioning of all organs of the body. The brain and heart are particularly sensitive to hypothermia.

Hypothermia results when body heat loss exceeds heat production. Causes of hypothermia are related to the effects of anesthesia and the consequences of surgery. Preanesthetic and analgesic drugs can alter the thermoregulatory center in the brain, thus interfering with the maintenance of a constant, optimum body temperature. As the body cools, the anesthetized animal cannot compensate by shivering or seeking a warmer environment. Muscular activity involved with shivering increases body heat. The anesthetized patient is lying still, so body heat production from muscular activity is absent.

All animals undergoing a surgical procedure are at risk for development of hypothermia. Neonates, very lean

Time				
Temperature				
Pulse				
Respiration				
Blood tests				
PVC/TS				
Electrolytes				
Blood gases				
Other				
Blood pressure				

FIGURE 8-2 Postanesthesia monitoring form. *PCV/TS,* Packed cell volume/total solids.

FIGURE 8-3 Gaymar convection-air patient-warming system blanket is placed over cat recovering from anesthesia. The warm air diffuses around the patient, providing a warm microenvironment.

animals (Body Condition Score < 2/5 or 4/9), and geriatric animals are at greatest risk for hypothermia. Numerous procedures are performed on the surgical patient that increase the loss of body heat (Box 8-2).

Various means to prevent hypothermia during surgery are discussed in Chapter 2. Treatment of hypothermia is discussed here. Many of the treatment measures are similar to the measures used to prevent hypothermia. The hypothermic patient needs to be monitored closely and frequently. Placing pads or blankets with circulating warm water or air under, over, and around the patient is a first step (Figure 8-3). SnuggleSafe Microwave Heat Pad (SnuggleSafe, Lenric C21 Ltd., Littlehampton, West Sussex, UK), sacks of rice or lentils heated in a microwave oven, and warm water bottles or bags can supplement other measures. The patient, including his/her head, can be placed under a "tent" made by blankets and warming objects. The air under the blankets is warmer than the room air; breathing in the warmed air helps warm the body. Fluids administered subcutaneously or

intravenously should be warmed to approximately 98° to 99° F. The fluid temperature can be tested on the technician's wrist, as in testing for the proper temperature of baby formula before feeding. Warming devices for intravenous (IV) fluids are also available.

Water-filled balloons or latex gloves can be used instead of bottles. Expired fluid bags can be heated in a microwave oven and are effective in warming the patient. These are softer than bottles and mold to the contours of the patient's body. Towels or blankets can be warmed in the dryer and then wrapped around the patient with an outer blanket to help trap the heat.

Uncooked rice or lentils can substitute for the water in bottles, balloons, or gloves. The rice-filled containers are placed in a microwave oven for several minutes. The time required depends on the power level used, the oven's wattage, and the size of the bottle or bag. The technician must experiment beforehand to determine the proper heating time needed. These containers tend to remain warmer for a longer time than water bottles. Care must be taken not to leave plastic containers in the microwave too long; overheating could melt the plastic. The technician must ensure that none of these warming devices is in direct contact with the skin, which might cause thermal burns. Either the patient or the warming device should be wrapped in at least a single layer of cloth to protect the skin. The patient is unable to move away from these heat sources if they are too warm or if damage to the skin is occurring.

As the warm water bottle cools and its temperature falls below the temperature of the hypothermic patient, the bottle that was warming the patient will now be cooling the patient. The water bottles should be rewarmed frequently. Also, leaking of the warm water on to the patient is a concern. A wet patient is at risk of becoming a colder patient.

Electric heating pads should not be used. They can become too hot for the recumbent patient, and severe thermal burns of the skin may occur. Such burns usually do not become evident until several days later. Large areas of skin that were in contact with the electric heating pad may be affected. Significant skin sloughing can be a serious complication.

Emergence Delirium

Occasionally when recovering from general anesthesia, the animal exhibits signs of excitement, possibly with exaggerated and uncontrollable movements. The patient may thrash around in the cage, cry out, or "paddle" all four legs. This phenomenon is called *emergence delirium* (Figure 8-4).

Emergence delirium occurs for several reasons. During the recovery process the animal travels back through the stages of anesthesia. Stage II is the "excitement" stage of anesthesia. In some cases the patient passes slowly through stage II and spends several minutes exhibiting signs of excitement. Analgesic and anesthetic side effects

FIGURE 8-4 Dog exhibiting emergence delirium. Between periods of thrashing in the cage, the dog presses its nose against the cage door.

contribute to the development of emergence delirium. Opioids are given for their analgesic effects, but these drugs can sensitize the patient to loud auditory stimuli and bright visual stimuli. When stimulated, these patients may be aroused and may exhibit erratic behavior. Dissociative anesthetic agents are known to cause hallucinations in humans, so animals also may undergo hallucinations when given these agents.

If the patient thrashes violently in the cage, problems may arise. The surgical site may undergo severe trauma and possibly dehiscence. The animal may smash its head against the hard side of the cage, causing bruising, scraped skin, and even fractured teeth. Toes can become wedged into the bars of the cage, causing skin damage or even broken bones. The patient that is wildly thrashing in the cage may also become hyperthermic, so a body temperature reading should be taken as soon as possible. Howling and screeching may become loud and may disturb other patients, hospital personnel, and clients.

The animal undergoing emergence delirium needs to be approached carefully. This animal is capable of hurting itself as well as the staff. Nevertheless, this patient needs to be calmed down; in some cases, "tincture of time" and holding the animal are sufficient. Some animals benefit from administration of a tranquilizer. The technician should notify the veterinarian in charge of the case for a consultation if the animal has injured or may injure itself or if the delirium lasts several minutes.

Prolonged Recovery

Some animals may take an unexpectedly long time to recover from the anesthesia. Most animals are able to maintain sternal recumbency and lift their head within several minutes after extubation. The patient that is unable to raise its head or to be aroused while recovering in its cage is a concern for the recovery room nurse. There are many reasons why a patient may have a prolonged recovery from anesthesia.

Anesthesia-Related Causes

Excessive depth of anesthesia. If the patient was maintained for a long time under anesthesia (>1 hour) and the depth of anesthesia was maintained at a deep level (stage III, plane 3), the patient will have a high concentration of the anesthetic in the body tissues. Gas anesthetics must pass out of the body tissues into the bloodstream and be eliminated by the lungs. A small percentage of a gas anesthetic is metabolized by the liver.

Breed predisposition. "Sight hounds" are sensitive to barbiturate anesthetics. In most dogs, barbiturates are redistributed from the vessel-rich tissues of the brain and muscles to the fat stores. Once in the fat stores, the barbiturate slowly reenters the bloodstream and is eventually metabolized in the liver. Sight hounds do not typically have as much fat on their bodies as most other breeds. Therefore, when the muscles become saturated, the barbiturate has no place for storage and is recirculated back to the brain, thus prolonging anesthesia recovery.

Patient-Related Causes

Hypotension, poor perfusion, or shock. The patient that is in shock or has hypotension is not effectively perfusing the organs and tissues. The anesthetic is therefore not being delivered to the organs that will eliminate it.

Liver or kidney disease. Many anesthetics are metabolized and eliminated through the liver or kidneys. Patients with compromised liver or kidney function eliminate these anesthetic agents more slowly than patients with healthy organs. Preanesthetic blood tests help identify such patients. The dose of anesthetic should then be reduced for these patients, or that anesthetic should not be used.

Intracranial disease. Patients with an altered level of consciousness caused by central nervous system (CNS) disease are especially sensitive to the side effects of certain anesthetics. Some anesthetics increase intracranial pressure. Patients with a history of head trauma or seizures may not be able to tolerate anesthetic agents that lower the seizure threshold. In these patients a different anesthetic protocol should be used.

Hypoglycemia. Neonatal patients are extremely susceptible to development of hypoglycemia. Glucose is stored in the form of glycogen in the liver for use between periods of eating. Because of their small size and immature livers, these animals tend to not have as much stored glycogen and will become hypoglycemic much sooner than one would expect. These patients should not be fasted, or fasted for only 1 to 2 hours, before anesthesia. Hypoglycemia adversely affects the patient's recovery from anesthesia and predisposes the patient to seizures. Food should also be offered as soon after anesthesia recovery as possible. Once they are swallowing, normothermic, and have had their pain managed, the patients can be offered food.

Hypothermia. The cells of the body function best at normal body temperature. The cellular enzymes involved in metabolizing anesthetic drugs are less active when the body temperature falls. Bradycardia and subsequent perfusion abnormalities are other consequences associated with hypothermia. If perfusion and circulation are adversely affected, the anesthetic cannot be redistributed to the organs that will eliminate it.

Therapeutic Measures

The patient recovering slowly from anesthesia needs to be assessed by the veterinarian, who may order laboratory tests to be run. Additional nursing care measures may be instituted as well. Close monitoring is important because this is a fragile patient in which a life-threatening complication could develop. Several methods can be used to hasten the patient's recovery from anesthesia.

Physical stimulation. Physical stimulation by rubbing, massaging, and turning is a simple way to increase the patient's level of consciousness. Talking to or whistling to the animal can help speed up the recovery.

Ventilation. The patient that is still intubated can be manually ventilated with pure oxygen. Gas anesthetic agents are mainly eliminated through the lungs. Ventilating the patient with pure oxygen and increasing the frequency of respirations raises the rate at which the gas anesthetic leaves the body. Care must be taken not to overventilate the patient and cause apnea. The pure oxygen in the system triggers the respiratory center to decrease respirations, causing a decrease or cessation of respirations.

Fluid therapy. A bolus of IV fluids can help increase the blood pressure of the hypotensive patient and improve perfusion of internal organs such as the lungs, liver, and kidneys. Warmed fluids can help raise the core body temperature.

Reversal agents. Some injectable anesthetic agents have reversal agents. The technician should consult with the veterinarian before administering a reversal agent. Giving an opioid antagonist, such as naloxone, reverses all the effects of the opioid, including its analgesic effects. The loss of analgesic effects could be detrimental to the patient. Doxapram is a respiratory stimulant that helps to arouse the deeply anesthetized patient; it is not a specific reversal agent.

Warming measures. The hypothermic patient recovers slowly from anesthesia and will benefit from warming measures (see earlier discussion).

Dextrose. Hypoglycemia may be documented through a blood test or may be suspected from the patient's symptoms and risk factors. Clinically, patients with hypoglycemia may appear disoriented, may gaze blankly off into space, may be slow to respond to noxious stimuli, and may have either a prolonged recovery from anesthesia or seizures.

Dextrose solution administered intravenously is the preferred treatment. For IV administration of sterile 50% dextrose, diluted 1:1 with sterile water. The solution should be administered slowly to patients with marked hypoglycemia. The desired effect includes increased awareness and consciousness. A constant-rate infusion (CRI) of 2.5% to 5% dextrose solution may be required to maintain blood glucose levels high enough to eliminate signs of hypoglycemia (see the Appendix for instructions).

Dextrose should not be given orally. Oral administration may lead to aspiration if the gag reflex is diminished or absent. Dextrose should also not be given by intramuscular (IM) or subcutaneous (SC) injection. The dextrose solution is hypertonic and will draw fluid into the subcutaneous space, causing cellular dehydration and cell death, and the dextrose will not be efficiently absorbed into the bloodstream because of poor peripheral perfusion.

Complications Related to Surgery

Hemorrhage

The surgical incision should be routinely inspected during postoperative monitoring. Any bleeding at the surgical site should be attended to (Figure 8-5). If direct pressure applied to the site for 5 to 10 minutes does not stop the bleeding, a bandage should be applied if possible, and the surgeon notified. Excessive bleeding at the surgical site that does not stop may indicate that bleeding is also occurring internally.

Internal bleeding can manifest as the following clinical signs: pale mucous membranes, slowed capillary refill time (>2 seconds), rapid respiratory rate, abdominal bloating, swelling at or around the surgical site, and hypotension, ultimately culminating in hypovolemic shock. An abdominocentesis (abdominal tap, "belly tap") can be performed using a 22-gauge needle and syringe. Collecting frank blood from the abdominocentesis is a positive diagnosis for internal bleeding into the peritoneal cavity. A thoracocentesis ("chest tap") is performed if internal bleeding is suspected after thoracic surgery.

FIGURE 8-5 Bleeding at the surgical site is often seen when drains are placed. It is important to clean the blood from the surgical site or cover the site with a bandage temporarily. Dogs and cats otherwise are driven to lick at the surgical site covered with blood.

Excessive postsurgical bleeding occurs for several reasons. The patient may have a coagulation disorder. A surgical ligature around a major vessel may have dislodged. Smaller arteries that were not bleeding intraoperatively because of hypotension may begin to bleed as the patient regains normal blood pressure and the effects of anesthesia wear off.

Coagulation disorders may predispose the patient to hemorrhage. Certain breeds, such as Doberman Pinschers, may have a genetic disorder called von Willebrand's disease, which manifests as a primary coagulation problem. Animals with chronic liver disease may have secondary coagulation problems caused by a clotting factor deficiency. Clotting factors are produced primarily in the liver, and when it is not functioning properly, these may not be synthesized normally or in sufficient amounts to allow formation of a stable blood clot. Preanesthetic assessment of animals with chronic liver disease usually includes a coagulation profile. This usually consists of a complete platelet count, prothrombin time (PT), and an activated partial thromboplastin time (aPTT). Certain toxins, such as rodenticides, can cause coagulation disorders. Platelet disorders caused by immune-mediated disease (e.g., immune-mediated thrombocytopenia) or infectious disease (e.g., Rocky Mountain spotted fever) predispose the patient to hemorrhage.

In some cases the surgeon may decide to re-anesthetize the patient and "go back in." The patient may need to be surgically explored to find the bleeding vessel or vessels. This patient is at high risk. Fluid therapy should be maintained, and colloid fluids may replace the crystalloid fluids. It is important to be prepared for emergency situations and to work efficiently. An additional venous access site may be needed for administering a blood transfusion or blood component therapy. In general, a "blood transfusion" refers to administering whole blood (fresh or stored) from one patient to another. Depending on how recently the whole blood was collected from the donor and when it is administered to the recipient, it may contain red blood cells (RBCs), white blood cells (WBCs), platelets, plasma proteins, and functional coagulation factors. Blood component therapy involves separating out the parts of whole blood and administering only those parts that the patient needs (e.g., plasma, packed RBCs) and that will extend the usefulness of the blood collected from the donor (Table 8-1).

The blood pooling in the abdomen or thorax can be aseptically collected, passed through a blood transfusion micropore filter, and re-administered to the patient. This procedure is called an *autotransfusion*. If an exogenous source of blood is needed, ideally crossmatched units of blood are administered. Whole blood increases the colloid pressure and oxygen delivery to the tissues. Administering blood rich in clotting factors improves coagulation. Some practices have blood products such as fresh plasma, fresh frozen plasma, and platelet-rich plasma available for administration.

Another manifestation of excessive bleeding is the formation of a hematoma at the surgical site, such as in the scrotal sac after a castration procedure (Figure 8-6). The surgical site may be traumatized if the patient has a difficult recovery (e.g., emergence delirium). Clots covering the cut ends of small subcutaneous blood vessels can become dislodged, allowing blood to pool under the skin at the suture site. Initially, a soft, fluctuant swelling is observed. Aspirating the lump with a 22-gauge needle and syringe shows the lump to be filled with blood. The presence of the hematoma impedes the healing process.

The surgeon may order application of warm, moist compresses to the area multiple times daily. This helps speed up the flow of blood into the area allowing quicker reabsorption of the hematoma. The surgeon may choose to suction the blood with a needle and syringe, followed by application of a pressure bandage. Alternatively, a Penrose drain can be surgically placed for continuous drainage.

Seroma

A *seroma* is a collection of tissue fluid in a pocket under the skin that forms at an area of excessive movement. A seroma may develop at the surgical site in a patient that is overactive postoperatively. The irritation from the scraping of rough sutures causes inflammation. When tissues are inflamed, serum leaks from the capillaries. The serum collects in the potential space between the skin and muscle layers (Figure 8-7). This seroma interferes with the normal healing process. If the serum leaks through the skin suture line, bacteria from the skin may contaminate the serum in the pocket, and an abscess may form.

Seromas appear as lumps at the surgical site. An abscess, hematoma, or hernia can resemble a seroma. Aseptically aspirating the mass with a 22-gauge needle and syringe allows a differential diagnosis. A straw-colored or light red fluid is seen if the mass is a seroma. Hematomas are filled with blood. Purulent fluid fills the syringe when the swelling is caused by an abscess. The syringe appears empty or has a small drop of liquefied fat if the lump results from herniation of omentum.

Seromas are treated much like hematomas. Small seromas can be managed by warm, moist compresses applied multiple times during the day. The pocket can be drained using a syringe and needle, followed by a pressure bandage. Large seromas need to be drained surgically (Figure 8-8). Surgical drainage also allows the surgeon to explore the surgical site to ensure that all the muscle-layer sutures are intact.

Dehiscence

Postoperative dehiscence is the premature loss of sutures that allows the surgical site to open. Dehiscence exposes underlying tissues to contamination. Any or all layers of the surgical closure may undergo dehiscence. If a thoracic surgical site dehisces, pneumothorax can follow. Dehiscence can have serious and even fatal consequences.

TABLE 8-1	Blood and Fluid Products: Indications for Use and Doses	
Product	Indications	Infusion Rate
Isotonic crystalloid solutions*	Shock Dehydration Maintenance	Dogs: Up to 90 mL/kg (to effect) Cats: Up to 60 mL/kg (to effect) Maintenance rate is approximately 66 mL/kg/day for a 10-kg dog; larger dogs need less (e.g., 44 mL/kg/day for a 40-kg dog), whereas smaller dogs need more (e.g., 81 mL/kg/day for a 5-kg dog)
Hetastarch	Shock Hypoalbuminemia	Dogs: 10–20 mL/kg/hr (shock) Cats: 10–15 mL/kg/hr over 10–15 min (shock) 5–10 mL/kg (can repeat) or constant-rate infusion (1–2 mL/kg/hr) up to 20 mL/kg/day (hypoalbuminemia)
Dextran 70	Shock Hypoalbuminemia	Dogs: 10–20 mL/kg/hr (shock) Cats: 10–15 mL/kg/hr (shock) 5–10 mL/kg (can repeat) or constant-rate infusion (1–2 mL/kg/hr) up to 20 mL/kg/day (hypoalbuminemia)
25% Human serum albumin	Shock Hypoalbuminemia	5–25 mL/kg; maximal volume 2–4 mL/kg (bolus or slow push) 0.1–1.7 mL/kg/hr as a constant-rate infusion[‡]
7% Hypertonic saline[†]	Shock Hypoalbuminemia	4 mL/kg over 5 min, then isotonic crystalloids (10–20 mL/kg/hr) to effect
Fresh whole blood	Anemia Hemorrhage Coagulopathy Shock	10–22 mL/kg; in general, 2 mL/kg will raise the PCV by 1% For shock: 22 mL/kg/hr maximum
Stored whole blood	Anemia Hemorrhage	10–22 mL/kg; in general, 2 mL/kg will raise the PCV by 1%
Packed red blood cells	Anemia Hemorrhage	6–10 mL/kg and then reassess the patient's PCV to determine if more is necessary; in general, 1 mL/kg will raise the PCV by 1%
Platelet-rich plasma	Thrombocytopenia Coagulopathy	1 unit/3–10 kg
Fresh-frozen plasma	Coagulopathy Hypoproteinemia Disseminated intravascular coagulation	10–20 mL/kg; then reassess serum albumin or antithrombin III concentration to determine if more is necessary
Cryoprecipitate	Von Willebrand's disease Hemophilia	1 unit/5–15 kg
Oxyglobin	Anemia Shock	Dogs: 15–30 mL/kg at a maximum rate of 10 mL/kg/hr Cats: 5–10 mL/kg at a maximum rate of 5 mL/kg/hr

Modified from Fossum TW, Hedlund CS, Hulse DA, et al: Small animal surgery, ed 3, St Louis, 2007, Mosby.

PCV, Packed cell volume.

*Monitor central venous pressure to prevent fluid overload.

[†]To prolong the effect of hypertonic saline, hetastarch or other colloid may be administered simultaneously. Do not exceed the maximum rate for either fluid.

[‡]Data from Mathews KA, Barry M: The use of 25% human serum albumin: outcome and efficacy in raising serum albumin and systemic blood pressure in critically ill dogs and cats, J Vet Emerg Crit Care 15:110, 2005.

The animal can cause dehiscence by excessively licking the surgical site. Infection of the site can also weaken the tissues, and the suture can tear through the skin and muscles. Blunt trauma to the surgical site can cause sutures to rip through healthy tissue. Active playing with other dogs or falls while climbing steps postoperatively can create blunt trauma extensive enough to lead to dehiscence.

Self-Trauma

Self-trauma may be a problem in the postoperative patient. Excessive licking, scratching, or rubbing of the surgical site slows the healing process and can lead to dehiscence.

Animals instinctually lick their wounds. Sutures are at risk of being removed by the animal before healing is

FIGURE 8-6 Postoperative scrotal hematoma: Bleeding into the scrotal sac has occurred. This picture was taken 18 hours after the castration surgery.

FIGURE 8-7 Formation of large seroma around the surgical site caused when dog scratched at the site over a 24-hour period.

FIGURE 8-8 Postoperative seroma drainage. Penrose drains were placed on each side of the surgical incision to allow drainage of the seroma fluid.

FIGURE 8-9 Elizabethan collar is applied to prevent licking and chewing on a drain.

complete. When licking occurs, bacteria from the mouth can be deposited deep into the surgical incision. The surgical site becomes contaminated, and the animal runs the risk of infection.

Preventive Measures

Prevention of self-trauma is essential. The strategy for keeping the postoperative patient free of self-trauma requires two tactics: (1) preventing the animal from reaching the surgical site and (2) preventing the animal from wanting to reach the surgical site.

Block access to surgical site

Elizabethan collar. The flat, plastic Elizabethan collar, or "E-collar," is placed around the neck. It is attached to the animal's collar, or a gauze strip is threaded through the collar stays. The plastic shield blocks the patient from licking surgical sites caudal to the neck (Figure 8-9). The animal can still scratch or rub the site. It is important to make sure that the patient can eat and drink with the E-collar. The pet is awkward and has no peripheral vision while wearing the collar. The pet should never be loose outside while wearing an E-collar. The pet will probably knock things over and collide with door frames. It is also imperative to ensure that the animal can still eat and drink with the E-collar in place. In some instances, the E-collar makes contact with the floor around the bowl, preventing the animal's mouth or tongue from reaching the bowl.

BiteNot collar. While fitted with The BiteNot Collar (BiteNot Products, Inc., San Francisco), the patient is unable to bend its neck to reach any part of its body and lick. As with an E-collar, the pet wearing the BiteNot Collar can still scratch or rub at the site (Figure 8-10).

Bandaging the area. A bandage may be enough to block the patient from licking the area. Surgical sites are not always in areas that can be easily bandaged. A pet may find a way to remove the bandage or may even eat the bandage. Thus it is essential that the bandage be monitored closely for signs of slipping or wetness and for tooth marks (Figure 8-11).

FIGURE 8-10 A and B, The BiteNot Collar (BiteNot Products, Inc., San Francisco) properly placed.

FIGURE 8-11 This pet had a bandage that encircled the chest. The bandage covered Penrose drains that had been placed to drain a seroma. The bandage also helped to keep the dog clean during the first 12 hours postoperatively. The hind legs are taped together ("hobbled") to prevent scratching at the chest area with the rear paws.

Basket muzzle. A dog can be fitted with a basket muzzle, which prevents the patient from chewing at the site. The dog may rub the site with the muzzle and may also be able to lick. However, this type of muzzle may act as an effective psychological barrier.

Hobbles. Taping the hind legs together can prevent the patient from scratching at the surgical site (Figure 8-12).

Block desire to reach surgical site

Foul-tasting product applied around the site. Bitter-apple liquid and Yuk2e or YukForte ointments (Vet Planet LLC, Boyds, MD) are examples of bitter-tasting applications that can be placed on the skin around the surgical site. The foul taste may deter the patient from licking the area.

Sedation. "Chemical restraint" can be very effective. Chronic tranquilization during the recuperative period may be necessary to prevent licking as well as overactivity.

FIGURE 8-12 Hobbles. **A,** Adhesive tape wide enough to cover half of the metatarsal region is placed loosely around the metatarsal region. **B,** The tape is then adhered together between the legs and placed around the opposite metatarsus. The hind limbs are positioned apart at a distance equal to the width of the pelvis. (From Bassert JM, McCurnin DM, editors: McCurnin's clinical textbook for veterinary technicians, ed 7, St Louis, 2010, Saunders.)

Stainless steel suture or staples. The surgeon may anticipate a problem with licking and elect to place staples in the skin rather than to close with sutures. Stainless steel sutures prick the tongue when licked. Staples can withstand more licking than sutures or tissue adhesive ("skin glue").

BOX 8-3   Phases of Wound Healing

Inflammatory
Begins immediately after injury; characterized by formation of blood clot; platelets stimulate other stages by release of growth factors.

Débridement
Part of inflammatory phase; characterized by influx of white blood cells (macrophages, monocytes) into wound; occurs approximately 6 hours after injury; wound healing is sustained by release of growth factors from multiple cell types.

Repair (Fibroblastic)
Begins 3 to 5 days after wounding; characterized by invasion of fibroblasts and development of granulation tissue; wound strength increases exponentially.

Maturation
Characterized by remodeling of the collagen of the scar and slow gain in wound strength; begins approximately 3 weeks after injury and may take weeks to years to complete.

From Bassert JM, McCurnin DM, editors: McCurnin's clinical textbook for veterinary technicians, ed 7, St Louis, 2010, Saunders.

BOX 8-4   Factors Affecting Wound Healing

Host Factors
- Geriatric patients: Debilitated state decreases wound healing.
- Malnourishment: Decreased protein levels delay wound healing.
- Hepatic disease: Clotting factor deficiency.
- Underlying disease: Hyperadrenocorticism or diabetes mellitus.

Wound Characteristics
- Foreign material: Drains, implants, sutures, etc., can cause inflammatory responses that interfere with healing, and soil, gravel, or plant material can introduce infection-causing agents.
- Type of incision: Electroscalpel or electrocoagulation cause more necrosis than a conventional scalpel.
- Infection of any kind.

External Factors
- Drugs: Corticosteroids depress wound healing and increase the chance of infection. Chemotherapeutic agents and radiation therapy can also delay wound healing.

Infection

When the surgical site becomes infected, healing is delayed. The patient is in pain and may have a fever. The surgical site is swollen, red, and draining, and the sutures are at risk of falling out.

Surgical débridement and resuturing may be necessary. Some animals may have an allergic reaction to the absorbable sutures that has the appearance of an infected wound. In either instance, the surgeon will cut away the dead tissue and suture healthy tissue together using less reactive suture material. The patient will most likely receive systemic antibiotic therapy. Warm, moist compresses and cleaning of the site with dilute antiseptic solution also may be prescribed.

Postoperative Nursing Care
Wound Management

A wound occurs whenever there is an interruption in the normal integrity of the tissue. Wounds can be purposeful, such as a surgical incision, or incidental, such as a traumatic injury. Wound healing begins directly after the injury occurs and is a dynamic process, with more than one phase of wound healing occurring at the same time (Box 8-3).

Wound healing can be influenced by many factors, including host factors, wound characteristics, and external factors (Box 8-4). Successful management of the wound requires accurate assessment and planning.

Wound Classification

Wounds are classified by several means. One method of classification is by etiology, or cause. In this scheme a surgical wound is called an incisional wound, because the soft tissue damage (or wound) is caused by the surgeon's scalpel. Another method of classification is based on the duration and degree of wound contamination. Class 1 wounds are 0 to 6 hours old with minimal contamination; most surgical wounds fall into this class. Class 2 wounds are 6 to 12 hours old with significant contamination. Class 3 wounds are more than 12 hours old with profound (gross) contamination. However, this system fails to address the contaminated wounds that are new or a few hours old, such as traumatic wounds sustained in animal fights or automobile accidents.

A more useful classification scheme is based only on the degree of contamination. Age of the wound is not part of this system. Using degree of contamination to classify wounds guides the veterinarian in making decisions regarding wound management. There are four classes: clean, clean-contaminated, contaminated, and infected (Box 8-5).

Clean Wound
Surgical wounds made under aseptic conditions are considered "clean." Surgical sites of castration or ovariohysterectomy are considered examples of "clean" wounds (Figure 8-13).

Clean-Contaminated Wound
Surgical wounds that are contaminated with contents from the gastrointestinal (GI), respiratory, or urinary tract are considered clean-contaminated wounds. The contamination is minimal and easy to remove. Traumatic

BOX 8-5   Wound Contamination Classifications with Examples

Clean
Created under sterile conditions. Does not enter into the gastrointestinal tract, respiratory tract, or the urogenital or oropharyngeal areas.

   Examples: Surgical wound.

Clean-Contaminated
Minimal contamination; the level of contamination can be removed or reduced.

   Examples: Surgical incision into the gastrointestinal tract, respiratory tract, urogenital or oropharyngeal areas.

Contaminated
Heavy contamination present.

   Examples: Leakage of intestinal contents into the peritoneum during an enterotomy. Traumatic wounds that are presented shortly after they occur, e.g., road rash after animal is hit by a motor vehicle.

Dirty
Old traumatic wound; active infection with purulent exudate.

   Examples: Laceration that was left unattended and became infected.

FIGURE 8-14 After flushing and débridement, this lacerated paw was sutured closed; clean contaminated wound.

FIGURE 8-15 The wound in this dog's mouth was caused by a spider bite. Dark red tissue is necrotic. Wound was flushed with sterile saline, and dog received a regimen of broad-spectrum antibiotics. Because the wound was located in a contaminated area, in this case the mouth, the wound was initially classified as a "contaminated" wound.

FIGURE 8-13 Surgical wound 24 hours after completion of procedure; clean wound.

wounds can be considered clean-contaminated wounds after lavage and débridement (Figure 8-14).

Contaminated Wound
These types of wounds have heavy contamination. Foreign material (e.g., grass, asphalt) and compromised tissue are incorporated in the wound. The wound can become contaminated when there is major spillage from the GI tract. Wounds sustained in fights are another example of contaminated wounds. Wounds located within the mouth cavity are immediately contaminated by oral cavity flora (Figure 8-15).

Infected Wound
Infected wounds are inflamed, contaminated with many bacterial organisms (by definition more than 100,000/gram of tissue), purulent discharge (pus), and varying amounts of necrotic (dead) tissue. Traumatic or surgical wounds can progress to become infected if treatment is inadequate or nonexistent (Figure 8-16).

Wound Cleansing
Regardless of the wound classification, it must be managed properly in order to facilitate healing. Box 8-6 lists the fundamentals of wound management. Surgical site preparation, sterile gloving, sterile draping, use of sterile instruments, and adherence to aseptic technique all minimize initial contamination of the surgical wound. Circumstances such as immunosuppressed patient status, self-mutilation, or unavoidable intraoperative contamination can render the surgical wound contaminated. Cleansing of contaminated wounds facilitates healing. Whether

FIGURE 8-16 This open, "infected" wound was covered with a thick layer of dried, purulent fluid, blood, and fur.

FIGURE 8-17 Lavage procedure. Syringe with dilute chlorhexidine solution (1:40 dilution) is flushed around the wound to rinse debris and blood from the area.

BOX 8-6	Fundamentals of Wound Management

1. Temporarily cover the wound to prevent further trauma and contamination.
2. Assess the traumatized animal and stabilize its condition.
3. Clip and aseptically prepare the area around the wound.
4. Culture the wound.
5. Debride dead tissue and remove foreign debris from the wound.
6. Lavage the wound thoroughly.
7. Provide wound drainage.
8. Promote healing by stabilizing and protecting the cleaned wound.
9. Perform appropriate wound closure.

From Fossum TW, Hedlund CS, Hulse DA, et al: Small animal surgery, ed 3, St. Louis, 2007, Mosby.

caused by surgery or trauma, contaminated wounds are cleansed of debris and protected from microorganisms through numerous means, including lavage, débridement, dressings, and antimicrobial agents.

Lavage

Lavage is the procedure of forceful rinsing of a wound (Figure 8-17). Anesthesia may be necessary if the patient is in pain and struggles. Thorough lavage flushes out foreign debris, purulent fluid, and microorganisms from a wound. The goal of a successful lavage is to reduce the number of microorganisms in the wound to a level that the immune system can handle. As the criticalists say, "the solution to pollution is dilution."

Solutions used to lavage external wounds include tap water, sterile saline, lactated Ringer's solution, diluted chlorhexidine, and diluted povidone-iodine. Although tap water is not sterile, it is still a safe and effective lavage agent for external wounds that do not penetrate a body cavity (thorax or abdomen) or joint. Two percent chlorhexidine solution is diluted 1:40 with water to make a 0.05% concentrated solution for lavage.

Povidone-iodine (10% stock solution) is diluted 1:10. These diluted solutions should be prepared fresh daily; their potency diminishes with time. (See Table 8-2 for a list of lavage solutions with their advantages and disadvantages.)

Débridement

Débridement is the removal of adhered debris and dead tissue from the wound. Surgical débridement is the cutting away of dead tissue from the living tissue until fresh bleeding edges are exposed. Dead tissue or foreign material left in a wound will delay healing. After the area is debrided, the fresh skin edges are sutured together. Usually, surgical débridement is performed with the patient under anesthesia. General anesthesia is used if the animal is stable and the involved area is large. Local anesthesia is often administered for debilitated animals and smaller wounds (see anesthesia texts for specific techniques).

During the early phase of wound healing, débridement may need to occur. The primary layer of bandage material can provide a means of débridement. Dry mesh gauze directly applied to an open wound with embedded foreign material or necrotic tissue is called a *dry-to-dry bandage*. Removal of the dry-to-dry bandage can be painful.

Mechanical débridement can also be accomplished on a daily basis through the use of wet-to-dry bandaging techniques. The *wet-to-dry bandage* is used with open wounds that have embedded foreign material, devitalized tissue, and viscous exudates. A primary layer of sterile, saline-soaked gauze sponges is applied directly to the wound. A secondary layer of dry gauze sponges and rolled-cotton batting is layered onto the primary layer and then secured to the animal with rolled gauze and tape. The dressing is changed two or three times daily. When the primary layer is removed, the foreign matter and necrotic debris that have dried to the gauze are pulled off

TABLE 8-2	**Lavage Solutions**	
Cleanser	Advantage	Disadvantage
Tap water	Availability Inexpensive Ease of application	Hypotonic Cytotoxic trace elements Not antimicrobial
Balanced electrolyte solution: Lactated Ringer's solution (LRS) Normosol	Isotonic Least cytotoxic	Not antimicrobial
Normal (0.9%) solution	Isotonic	Slightly more acidic than LRS Not antimicrobial
0.05% Chlorhexidine (1 part stock solution to 40 parts sterile water or LRS) or (≈25 mL stock solution per liter)	Wide antimicrobial spectrum Good residual activity Not inactivated by organic matter	Precipitates in electrolyte solutions More concentrated solutions are cytotoxic and may slow granulation tissue formation *Proteus, Pseudomonas,* and *Candida* are resistant Corneal toxicity
0.1% Povidone-iodine (1 part stock to 100 parts LRS) or (≈10 mL stock to 100 mL LRS)	Wide antimicrobial spectrum	Inactivated by organic matter Limited residual activity Cytotoxic at concentrations greater than 1% Contact hypersensitivity Thyroid disorders if absorbed

Modified from Fossum TW, Hedlund CS, Hulse DA, et al: Small animal surgery, ed 3, St Louis, 2007, Mosby.

the wound. As with dry-to-dry bandaging, the patient may need to be sedated for bandage changes because this procedure tends to be painful.

Wet-to-dry and wet-to-wet bandages have the disadvantage of possible bacterial growth in the bandage. A moist environment at the wound surface dilutes the viscous exudates, allowing the secondary layer to absorb the fluid more readily.

Enzymatic preparations of trypsin or chymotrypsin can be applied to wounds to digest and remove necrotic tissue. This technique is indicated when (1) further surgical débridement may damage important nerves and blood vessels, (2) deeper fistulas exist, or (3) the patient is a poor anesthesia risk.

Wound Dressings
Wound dressings are categorized as two types, semi-occlusive and occlusive. Wound dressings are the contact, or primary, layer of a bandage. Semi-occlusive dressings include the wet-to-dry bandages used to debride wounds mechanically. Cotton and polyester gauze pads, petroleum jelly–coated gauze pads, antibiotic ointment–coated polyethylene glycol sponges, and polyurethane foam sponges are examples of nonadherent, semi-occlusive dressings. Semi-occlusive dressings allow excess fluid to be absorbed by the secondary layer.

Occlusive wound dressings are impermeable to air and produce a moist environment that facilitates wound healing. These dressings are used in the later stages of wound healing, when the bandage needs less frequent changing. Examples of occlusive dressings are natural cellulose and gelatin, as well as polyethylene polymers attached to a synthetic film. These occlusive wound dressings do not adhere to the wound.

Antimicrobial Agents
Antimicrobial agents may be applied topically to superficial wounds. However, the use of antimicrobial agents is not a substitute for appropriate and careful débridement and lavage. Large multiuse tubs of antimicrobial agents may be a source of patient-to-patient contamination through introduction of bacteria unless aseptic technique is used to retrieve the contents. Just because the product contains an antibiotic does not ensure that there is no bacterial growth in the tub. A better option is the use of single-dose packets of antibiotic ointment. Topical treatment can be discontinued once granulation tissue appears in the wound.

Drains
A *drain* is a surgically placed implant that is temporarily affixed in the wound. The drain provides a channel through which unwanted fluid or gas may leave the wound. When surgery or other trauma to the skin disrupts the hypodermis, the skin may no longer adhere to the underlying fascia. This creates a potential space that the body will try to fill with tissue fluid. Healing occurs most rapidly if the fluid is evacuated. Drawing the fluid out through a needle is only effective temporarily. Continuous drainage needs to be provided.

The two basic categories of drains are passive and active. *Passive drains* use gravity and overflow gradients to evacuate the fluid or gas. *Active drains* create negative-pressure gradients to the area and suck the fluid and gas from the wound.

Passive drains are typically made of soft, pliable latex tubing. Red rubber tubes and silicone tubes are stiff, less compliant, and potentially more irritating. "Teat cannulas," originally made to drain purulent fluid from infected

FIGURE 8-18 Plastic "teat cannulas" are also used to drain aural hematomas in dogs. **A,** Teat cannula has two small prongs that help keep it in place. **B,** Cannula is sutured into place at the most dependent aspect of the hematoma pocket to allow gravity to assist in drainage.

FIGURE 8-19 Each end of the drain is sutured to the skin to keep it in place.

mammary glands in cows, are also used to drain aural hematomas in dogs. Teat cannulas are made of polyethylene plastic and are quite hard (Figure 8-18).

The passive drain exits the skin at the most ventral (gravity-dependent) spot possible. The drain does not exit from the primary surgical incision. A small stab incision is made through the skin adjacent to the surgical incision. The drain is secured to the skin by one or two sutures. The opposite end of the drain may remain buried below the skin or may exit at the opposite end of the wound. Whether the end of the drain is buried or exits to the surface, a suture secures the end of the drain (Figure 8-19).

An *active drain* is usually made out of polymeric silicone (Silastic), red rubber, polyethylene, or polypropylene plastic. The drain is fenestrated (has holes) in multiple places. The fenestrated section of the drain is placed in the area that requires draining. Many commercial suction devices are available. Attaching a syringe to the tube can make a simple, homemade suction device. The plunger of the syringe is pulled back and secured by a pin placed through a predrilled hole in the plunger's shaft to hold the plunger in place.

All drains must be kept clean. Dried fluid accumulates around the drain where it exits the skin. Placing a warm, moist cloth over the drain loosens the dried material. The cloth is soaked in a bowl of water or dilute solution of an antiseptic such as chlorhexidine (1:40 dilution). This procedure may need to be repeated several times daily. The skin surrounding the drain may become raw and irritated from contact with the serous or purulent fluid. Petrolatum-based ointments applied to the skin can facilitate cleaning and protect the skin from further damage.

The veterinary surgeon determines the best time to remove the drain. Usually, the drain is removed 3 to 5 days after surgery. Any dried fluid is cleaned out, and all sutures securing the drain are cut. The drain is firmly grasped and pulled out with one swift motion. If the proximal end of the drain is not buried, one end is freed and pulled as much as possible from the incision and then cut. The other end is then freed, and the remainder of the drain removed.

If the patient has removed the drain prematurely, the owner should be asked to bring the drain in for inspection. It is important to determine that the pet has removed the entire drain. A piece of drain left under the skin will fester. The immune system will treat the piece of drain as a foreign invader, surrounding it with fluid and inflammatory cells. This drain piece will have to be surgically removed.

Wound Closure

The choice of wound closure will be based on the nature of the wound. They may be closed immediately, primary closure, several days after the injury, delayed primary closure, after the formation of granulation tissue forms,

BOX 8-7 Methods of Wound Closure

Primary Closure
Closed immediately. Used for clean, new wounds with little to no contamination.

Delayed Primary Closure
Closed within 1 to 5 days after the injury occurs. Used for moderately contaminated or traumatized wounds. The wound should be free of infection, and granulation tissue has not formed.

Secondary Closure
Closed after 5 days. Granulation tissue has formed. Used for severely contaminated or traumatized wounds that require extended wound management.

Secondary Intention
Wound is not closed. It is allowed to heal by contraction and epithelialization.

FIGURE 8-20 These wounds were left unsutured. They healed as open wounds.

secondary closure, or they may not be surgically closed, secondary intention or contraction or epithelialization (Box 8-7).

Wounds heal quickest when sutured closed. Depending on the level of contamination, however, the wound may not be sutured closed immediately. If a wound is sutured closed immediately, it has received *primary closure*. If a wound is left open for a few days, protected with dressings, and sutured closed later, *delayed primary closure* has been performed. Leaving the wound open for a longer period (5-7 days) and then suturing it closed is known as *secondary closure*. It is important to appose healthy skin edges that have an adequate blood supply with sutures or staples. Apposing necrotic skin edges or compromised skin edges (rather than healthy skin edges) together will result in dehiscence (sutures pull apart) and delayed healing.

Some wounds may be left to heal closed without suturing. This method is known as *second-intention healing* (Figure 8-20). Scarring is most likely to occur in second-intention healing.

Bandages, Splints, Casts, and Slings
Bandages, splints, casts, and slings are frequently applied after surgical procedures or trauma to a limb. The purposes of these applications are to protect wounds, speed the healing process, and immobilize the extremities. Immobilization helps the patient by decreasing pain and facilitates healing by securing bone fragments and soft tissue pieces close together to allow healing.

Bandages have three basic layers: primary (contact) layer, secondary (padded) layer, and tertiary (outer) layer (Table 8-3). The primary layer is in contact with the wound. This contact layer may adhere to the open wound or may be nonadherent. Adherent materials such as cotton gauze are usually applied early in the healing process and

allow débridement when the bandage is changed. Nonadherent dressings are used later in the healing process or to cover wounds closed by sutures.

The secondary layer secures the contact layer to the wound and provides an absorptive layer for blood, serum, and purulent fluid. This padded layer also provides support to the extremity. It applies pressure to the wound, thus compressing any dead space and preventing hemorrhage. Rolled cotton, synthetic polyester batting, multilayer absorbent pads, or cast padding may be used. Rolled gauze is used to hold the layer in place, with pressure applied to compress the padding underneath. It is important not to use too much pressure and occlude the blood supply to the extremity. Mastering the technique of applying the proper pressure and placing a comfortable, supporting bandage on a patient requires practice. Thus, an experienced technician or veterinarian should supervise the first few bandage wrappings attempted by newer personnel.

When a bandage, cast, or sling is applied immediately after trauma to an extremity, swelling of the limb is expected. When the limb is confined by such a stabilizing measure, swelling may result in cessation of blood flow to the extremity. Toes can be left exposed at the distal end of the bandage or cast to monitor the amount of swelling under the bandage. The nails of the two middle toes should be only a few millimeters apart. If the nails are farther apart, the toes are swollen. If the toes look swollen, the bandage should be removed immediately.

The tertiary layer of the bandage is made of porous adhesive tape or elasticized tape, such as Vetrap (3M, St Paul, MN) or Elastikon (Tyco Healthcare/Kendall, Mansfield, MA). This layer provides protection to the secondary layer. If this outer layer becomes wet, either from moisture on the outside (e.g., soiled by rainwater) or seepage from the inside, the entire bandage must be changed immediately.

It is important to keep these bandages intact, secure (no slipping down the leg), and dry. The animal may try to remove the wrappings by gnawing, violently shaking

TABLE 8-3 Characteristics of Primary, Secondary, and Tertiary Bandage Layers

Type	Indication and Purpose	Example
PRIMARY		
Adherent	No longer indicated in wound care	Dry gauze (dry-to-dry) Wet gauze (wet-to-dry)
Hypertonic	Contaminated and infected wounds; hypertonicity is antimicrobial and draws fluid and tissue debris from wound	Hypertonic Sodium Chloride Dressing (20%) (e.g., CURASALT*)
Nonadherent semiocclusive	Moderately or copiously exudative wounds; keeps wound surface moist, draws fluid and tissue debris from wound	Transparent polyurethane film—Polyskin II* With hydrophilic properties: Hydrogel (e.g., Curagel*), Absorptive foam (e.g., Hydrasorb*) Hydrocolloid (e.g., Ultec Hydrocolloid Dressing*)
Nonadherent occlusive	Minimally exudative wounds; partial-thickness wounds (abrasions); keeps wound surface moist and promotes epithelialization; protects new epithelium	Without hydrophilic properties: OpSite,* Tegaderm Transparent Dressing,* BIOCLUSIVE Transparent Dressing† With hydrophilic properties: Hydrogel (e.g., NU-GEL†); Hydrocolloid (e.g., Hydrocol Dressing†)
Nonadherent without occlusive properties	Intact wound surface (e.g., surgical wound, recently epithelialized wound)	Petrolatum-impregnated gauze (e.g., Adaptic†); rayon or Teflon pads (e.g., Telfa pads†)
SECONDARY		
Padding	Absorbs exudate, pads and supports the wound	Cast padding—Specialist Cast Padding‡ Roll cotton
TERTIARY		
Conforming gauze	Conforming and holding layer	Conforming gauze (e.g., Kling*)
Nonocclusive elastic adhesive tape	Holding and protective layer, permeable to moisture	Elastikon*
Nonocclusive elastic bandage	Holding and protective layer, permeable to moisture	Vetrap§
Occlusive tape	Contraindicated	Waterproof tape
Occlusive wrap	Contraindicated	Plastic wrap

From Bassert JM, McCurnin DM, editors: McCurnin's clinical textbook for veterinary technicians, ed 7, St Louis, 2010, Saunders.
*Tyco Healthcare/Kendall, Mansfield, MA.
†Johnson & Johnson Medical, Arlington, TX.
‡Johnson & Johnson Orthopaedics, Raynham, MA.
§3M Animal Products, St. Paul.

the extremity, or prying off the bandage. After several days, stretching of the outer layer and compression of the inner padding will loosen the bandage, which may slip or shift position. Also, the skin adjacent to the edges of the bandage, sling, splint, or cast may become abraded. Wetness, staining, and odor may also be noted. If any of these problems occurs, the bandage, cast, or splint should be changed.

Intravenous Catheter Maintenance

IV catheters are placed and maintained for extended periods in some surgical patients. Common veins used for peripheral catheter placement include the left and right cephalic, left and right lateral saphenous (dogs), and left and right medial saphenous (cats). The left and right jugular veins are generally used for central catheters. Central catheters ("central lines") allow the technician to measure central venous pressures and collect blood

samples for frequent blood glucose checks without a separate venipuncture for each sample collected.

All IV catheters provide direct access to the patient's vascular system, and therefore all catheters should be placed using aseptic technique. (See Chapter 2 for more information on IV catheterization techniques.) All connections among the catheter, connector sets, and IV lines need to be left untaped but secure. Access to these connections must be available at all times without untaping the connections. The patient often attempts to pull or chew out the catheter. Sufficient taping and restraint devices (e.g., E-collar) can prevent many problems. Figure 8-21 shows a cage that was occupied by a cat that pulled off the catheter cap (catheter remained intact).

A peripheral IV catheter requires replacement every 3 days (72 hours) with a new catheter placed in a different vein. A catheter placed into a central vein may remain in place for 5 to 7 days if there is no indication of phlebitis

FIGURE 8-21 Consequence of a lost catheter cap.

FIGURE 8-22 Hand-feeding a highly palatable food.

and the catheter remains patent. The old catheter is removed only after the new catheter is secured in place. If no continuous infusion is being administered through the catheter, the catheter is flushed with 1 to 5 mL of heparinized saline every 6 to 8 hours. This procedure helps ensure that the catheter remains patent the entire 72 hours. Bandages securing catheters in place should be changed if they become soiled with vomitus or other contaminants.

Each time the catheter is flushed, the insertion site and all connections should be checked. If the tape is soiled, it should be retaped. If swelling is noted in the paw, the tape may be wrapped too tightly, and it should be replaced. If swelling is noted proximal to the catheter, the catheter may be perivascular (not in the vein). If the catheter bandage is soaked, the entire catheter should be replaced at a different site. The old catheter site is covered for a few minutes with a piece of gauze. A spot of antibiotic ointment can be applied to the gauze, which is secured by adhesive tape.

When administering medication through the catheter, the technician should check for patency using a heparinized saline flush prior to drug administration. After the medication is administered, the catheter is flushed again with heparinized saline. Blood samples are often collected through the IV catheter, but the clinician must keep in mind that residues from medications administered through the catheter could interfere with test results. A three-syringe technique can be used to help decrease the incidence of contaminants in a blood sample collected from an IV catheter. A 3-mL syringe is half filled with heparinized saline, and blood is withdrawn into the syringe from the catheter. This helps clean any contaminants from the catheter. Then the second syringe is used to withdraw the appropriate sample and place it in the desired collection tubes. Lastly, the original syringe is used to replace the withdrawn blood and flush the catheter with the remaining heparinized saline.

Urinary Catheter Maintenance

Patients recovering from back surgery, urinary tract surgery, and orthopedic procedures may have a urinary catheter. The urinary catheter helps ensure urethral patency, allows for quantification of urine production, and helps keep the patient clean.

The catheter is placed aseptically. The distal end is secured to the patient with tape and sutures. An empty, sterile IV fluid bag and administration set are connected to the distal end of the catheter. The bag is suspended below the level of the bladder for urine flow by gravity.

It is important to check the patency of the urine collection system regularly. The tubing may become kinked. As the patient turns in the cage, the collection tubing may become twisted and cause the tube's lumen to collapse. The collection tube can be pinched in the cage door as it is closed. Blood clots can be passed and form obstructions in the tubing. The catheter and tubing should be checked for leaks. Often the patient attempts to pull out the catheter, and tooth marks may be detected. Leaking systems are replaced, and the patient is fitted with an Elizabethan collar to prevent further problems. Replacement of the entire collection system every 24 hours is recommended to decrease the incidence of opportunistic bacterial infections.

Nutritional Support

All animals need to maintain appropriate levels of nutrient intake, but this need is especially important in patients recuperating from surgery and serious illness. Inadequate nutrition can negatively affect the animal through decreased wound healing, suppression of the immune system, decreased cardiac and respiratory function, and increased bacterial translocation from the gut. Voluntary oral intake is the preferred route for food administration but may be insufficient to meet the animal's energy requirements. The animal needs to be able to consume at least 85% of the calculated resting energy requirements (RER) to be able to feed orally. Feeding a calorically dense, highly palatable food may help increase voluntary oral intake (Figure 8-22). If needed, oral intake can be supplemented with the use of assisted feeding techniques, pharmacologic appetite stimulants, and tube feedings.

Assisted feeding is best accomplished with pureed or liquid diets and a catheter tip syringe. The food needs to be of a consistency that can be easily administered through the syringe. If necessary, small amounts of water can be added to commercial gruel diets to increase their ease of passage through the syringe and catheter. The food may be smeared on the animal's lips to initiate licking and cleaning. A lump of food may be applied to the roof of the mouth. A liquid diet may be squirted through a syringe into the cheek pouch. Assisted feeding is a labor-intensive and time-consuming process and frequently falls short of the required caloric goal. Additionally, calculating the actual amount of food that the animal consumed can be very tricky. The animal often fights the feedings and may become stressed. Aspiration of the food into the lungs from the mouth during the struggle is a major concern. No patient should be allowed to have a decreased nutrient intake for longer than 3 days, which includes the time prior to surgery. Metabolic changes will start occurring within this time that can have a significantly negative impact on recovery.

Animals should be offered food as soon after anesthesia recovery as possible. They need to be able to protect their airway, to be normothermic, and to be able to swallow prior to being fed. There is no nutritional reason to delay postoperative feeding and numerous reasons why the animals should be fed. Delayed wound healing has been demonstrated in animals from which food has been withheld in the first 24 hours postoperatively. With small and neonatal animals, feeding is even more important as their functional reserves are significantly less than older, larger animals.

Several pharmacologic agents are thought to increase the appetite of dogs and cats. The benzodiazepine tranquilizer diazepam has been shown to stimulate the appetite of cats. An IV injection generally induces the cat immediately to eat any palatable food within reach. The food should be in place and warmed to body temperature before the cat is returned to the cage after the injection. Cyproheptadine is a serotonin antagonist that stimulates the appetite of both dogs and cats. It is typically given orally. It is not unusual for a cat or dog to "pout" his/her way through any appetite stimulation. Corticosteroids and progestational steroids (e.g., megestrol) work well in humans but are seldom used in dogs and cats because of potential adverse side effects, such as diabetes mellitus, immunosuppression, and delayed healing. When these medications are given as treatment for a disease, increased appetite may be a beneficial side effect of treatment.

Acupuncture also may stimulate a surgical patient's appetite postoperatively, in addition to providing some pain relief. A veterinary acupuncturist should be consulted for these cases.

Effective pain management is also important; many animals have suppressed appetite secondary to unrecognized or untreated pain. Nausea caused by therapeutic medications such as narcotics and antibiotics can also suppress appetite. If it is seen, a decision to change medications may need to be made if possible to allow increased food intake.

The initial amount of food that the patient will need per day is calculated in the following way:

$$\text{Resting energy requirement (RER)} = 70\,(\text{Body weight in kg})^{0.75}$$

For those who do not have calculators that can do logarithms, the following formula can also be used:

$$\text{Dogs weighing 2 to 50 kg:} (\text{wt [kg]} \times 30) + 70 = \text{RER}$$
$$\text{Cats: wt [kg]} \times 40 = \text{RER}$$
$$\text{Estimated food intake} = \text{Resting energy requirement}$$

Calculate food intake by finding RER and then determine the caloric density of the food being used. Divide the caloric density by the RER to determine the quantity that should be fed every 24 hours. If the animal has not eaten in more than 3 days, start the initial food intake at 30% to 50% of RER for the first 24 hours. Small frequent meals also help to decrease food-related discomfort as well as nausea.

Enteral tube feeding may be necessary to meet nutritional needs. Neonatal animals adapt well to repeated orogastric tubing. Juvenile and adult animals deal better with the placement of a semipermanent, indwelling feeding tube. The feeding tube may be placed through the nose, esophagus, or stomach. A tube placed through the abdominal wall into the stomach, known as a gastric tube, is the easiest of all feeding tubes to maintain but does require more anesthesia and equipment than some of the other types of tubes available.

Using an indwelling feeding tube is convenient and less time-consuming, and less stressful to the patient than force-feeding, but indwelling tubes are not without problems. A nasoesophageal or esophagostomy tube (Figure 8-23) that passes down the esophagus may irritate the

FIGURE 8-23 Esophagostomy tube.

esophagus or, if passed through the cardiac sphincter into the stomach and irritate the stomach wall, cause gastro-esophageal reflux and may initiate vomiting. The tube can be vomited up, displacing it from the esophagus so that it instead comes out of the mouth, and the patient may then chew through it. A nasogastric tube must be very small in diameter to pass through the nasal turbinates and therefore can easily become obstructed when food is administered through it. The nasogastric tube can cause nosebleeds, sneezing, and inflammation of the nasal passage with mucous discharge. Premature removal of the tube by the patient is a complication inherent in all types of feeding tubes.

The gruel or liquid diet may be homemade or commercially purchased. The benefit of commercially prepared recovery diets is that their nutrient content and caloric density are known, making food administration calculations easier. Any food that can be blenderized can be fed through a feeding tube. Feeding of a raw or uncooked diet through a feeding tube is not recommended because of the possibility of bacterial contamination of the food. When the tube feedings are initiated, the amounts should be small (2-10 mL, depending on animal's size) and administered frequently (about every 2 hours). The desired amount to be fed is based on the RER. For the first day, 50% of the RER is divided up into multiple equal-sized feedings administered every 2 to 4 hours. Use of a gastrostomy tube should be delayed for 24 hours after it is placed to allow a temporary stoma to form internally between the visceral peritoneum and the parietal peritoneum (Figure 8-24).

Vomiting of food occurs most frequently in the first or second day. Once the feedings are tolerated, larger amounts and less frequent feedings can be done. After the first day, 75% to 100% of RER can be given divided up into four to six equal feedings throughout the day. The

FIGURE 8-24 Gastrotomy (percutaneous endoscopic gastrostomy [PEG]) tube.

food is slowly administered over 10 to 20 minutes through the feeding tube with use of either an infusion pump or a catheter-tipped syringe to allow the stomach to accommodate gradually to the presence of the food. After the food is injected, 10 to 15 mL of water is slowly administered through the catheter to rinse the inside of the tube and remove any food that may have remained in the tube. This step helps prevent tube obstruction. The tube is closed with a Luer-Slip adapter plug. How the tube is managed externally depends on which type of feeding tube is placed, the condition of the animal, and the desires of the veterinarian. Some tubes are not secured at all to the animal, and others are glued or sutured in place.

Depending on type selected, the feeding tube may remain in place for a period of 3 to 5 days to the remainder of the animal's life. Tube removal also depends on which tube is selected.

Physical Therapy

Physical therapy techniques can benefit most patients. Immobility resulting from sickness, trauma, or surgical procedures can complicate recuperation. Physical therapy techniques enhance patient comfort, prevent complications from disuse, and hasten healing. The success of many orthopedic procedures rests on the rehabilitation of the patient. Veterinarians, veterinary technicians, and owners can perform many physical rehabilitation techniques to improve surgical outcomes and ensure client satisfaction. Some states have limited the practice of physical therapy on animals to licensed physical therapists. Therefore, many veterinarians prefer to use the term "physical rehabilitation" when referring to the following techniques.

Massage, application of heat or cold, bandaging, range-of-motion (ROM) exercises, and physical exercise are all therapeutic techniques that may be prescribed. Under the supervision of the attending veterinarian, the veterinary technician or owner may perform the techniques with the patient. Detailed descriptions of these techniques are found in other texts and articles; this section briefly describes the various types of physical therapy that may be used postoperatively.

In the first 72 hours after surgery, opioid analgesics, anti-inflammatory drugs, passive ROM exercises, and cryotherapy are used to decrease pain, prevent edema formation, and gradually improve range of motion. Pain management is discussed later. *Cryotherapy* is the application of cold, such as ice packs wrapped in a towel, to the affected limb. The packs can be affixed to the limb with elastic wraps. The cold packs are applied for up to 30 minutes two to four times a day. The cold causes vasoconstriction, which decreases blood flow and limits edema formation. The cold temperature of the tissue also reduces nerve conduction, producing analgesia.

Passive ROM exercises are exercises that support a joint while moving it to the extent of its limitations (Figure 8-25). The best time to perform passive ROM exercises is

FIGURE 8-25 Physical therapist demonstrating passive range-of-motion movements.

FIGURE 8-26 Massage can relax the pet as well as increase blood and lymph flow, relieve pain, and break down adhesions.

shortly after administration of analgesic drugs. This procedure should be performed slowly with the muscles relaxed, as follows: While supporting the limb, slowly and gently flex and extend each joint one at a time, taking care to keep all the joints in the working extremity in their normal anatomic alignment throughout the exercise. Flex and extend each joint only to the extent that the joint just begins to resist the degree of flexion or extension applied to it. Passive ROM helps prevent contracture, improve blood and lymph flow, maintain normal range of joint movement, and stimulate sensory awareness. Ten to 15 repetitions should be performed two or three times daily. Treat every joint of the affected limb, starting with the joint distal to the injury or surgical site.

Between 3 and 5 days after surgery, other physical therapy procedures may be added. Cryotherapy is replaced with *thermotherapy*. Warm, moist heat is applied to the injured area. The heat causes vasodilation, increases local circulation, and provides mild pain relief. Thermotherapy should be applied for 10 to 20 minutes before passive ROM, massage, or exercise. Massage therapy relaxes muscles, breaks down adhesions, improves blood and lymph flow, and relieves pain. The massage session starts with gentle running of the hands over the surface of the animal's skin (effleurage, frottage). The stroking movements should start distally and move proximally. The second massage method kneads the muscles in small circles with the pads of the fingers (not the fingertips) or the heel of the hand with a gradual increase in pressure (pétrissage). The massage session lasts about 20 minutes and is done every 24 to 48 hours (Figure 8-26).

Exercise that elevates the heart rate and increases muscle tone can be initiated about 2 weeks after surgery. Initial exercise is assisted by slings and harnesses. Swimming is also a good initial exercise; the buoyancy of the water helps support the patient. This low-impact exercise is replaced in a few weeks with unassisted exercise, such as leash walks. As the patient's stamina increases, the length of time spent exercising also increases.

Although physical therapy has many benefits, contraindications to it do exist. Massage should not be performed over open wounds, infected areas, or malignant tumors. Animals with thromboembolic disease and those receiving anticoagulants should not be massaged. Cryotherapy is avoided in patients with ischemic injury, diabetes mellitus, vasculitis, or indolent pressure sores. ROM procedures should not be performed on nonstabilized legs after a severe orthopedic injury (e.g., fracture, ligament rupture). Bandaging to prevent or reduce edema needs to be performed carefully to prevent vascular compromise of the limb. Exercise regimens and active ROM procedures must start slowly and increase gradually in length and frequency.

Postoperative Analgesia

The ease and success of managing postoperative pain are directly related to preoperative analgesia. That is, the more successful the attempts to preempt surgical pain, the easier it is to control postoperative pain with minimal additional analgesics. Assuming adequate preemptive analgesia, the overall goal of postoperative pain management should be to maintain the analgesic plane achieved throughout the procedure.

The patient should recover quietly and calmly without displays of overt signs of pain (e.g., vocalization, excessive movement, abnormal body posturing). At no time should the patient be required to return to a painful state and "request" additional analgesics during the immediate postoperative period. Some patients experience pain that persists or develops despite adequate doses of analgesics and must be treated with additional analgesia or analgesic techniques. This type of pain is termed *breakthrough pain* because it has "broken through" the usual analgesic barriers.

Postoperative pain management also includes medications dispensed for home use. This is a service and level of care that veterinary medicine has not sufficiently advocated until recently. Now, with veterinarians' increased awareness of the options available for take-home pain medication and the benefits to the patient, effective pain management can continue throughout the at-home recovery period.

Common Analgesic Classes

The two classes of analgesia most often used postoperatively are opioids and nonsteroidal anti-inflammatory drugs (NSAIDs). These two classes of agents can be used individually, but the drugs may be most efficacious when used in combination with each other. Postsurgical pain should be managed aggressively for anywhere from 24 hours up to a full week or more, depending on its severity. In general, experts agree that most patients with soft tissue elective surgery should receive opioids for 24 hours and NSAIDs for 3 to 4 days postoperatively. Patients that have emergency or nonroutine soft tissue procedures (e.g., thoracotomy, gastric dilatation–volvulus repair) may be managed initially with opioids alone until their cardiovascular health is restored. A major concern is the effect of opioids on GI motility. Although morphine may slow GI motility, the benefit of opioids outweighs the risk of altered GI function, because stress and pain are likely to play a larger role in decreasing GI motility than short-term postoperative opioid administration. Patients with severe GI disease may benefit from the addition of a CRI of lidocaine for systemic analgesia, provided that the patient does not have cardiovascular disease (see the Appendix).

Patients may also benefit from postoperative local anesthetics, such as bupivacaine, which can be instilled through indwelling chest tubes or by soaker catheter.

Patients undergoing orthopedic procedures should receive postoperative opioids for 24 to 72 hours of and NSAIDs for at least 1 week. The exact type of opioid is matched to the expected level of pain. The appendix provides specific protocols for postoperative pain management, including take-home medications.

Wind-Up

Patients who do not respond satisfactorily to maximum dose and frequency of opioids and require additional analgesia may have experienced the phenomenon known as *wind-up*. In this condition the spinal cord has become hypersensitized to incoming pain signals as a result of constant bombardment. Once hypersensitization occurs,

traditional analgesia may no longer be adequate. There are several effective techniques for managing wind-up, including CRI of morphine, ketamine, or lidocaine. Ketamine blocks sensitization of neurons in the spinal cord, essentially "unwinding" it, and may allow the patient to become responsive to usual dosing regimens, as described earlier.

Dispensed Analgesia

Nonsteroidal Anti-inflammatory Drugs

The availability of veterinary NSAIDs has greatly improved outpatient pain management. These relatively inexpensive analgesics provide long-lasting perioperative and chronic pain relief in convenient oral formulations. Once-daily administration tends to improve owner compliance. NSAIDs provide adequate pain relief to many patients during the at-home recovery period, especially if therapy was instituted preoperatively. Some patients require additional take-home medications, most often opioids.

Opioids

Several oral opioids are available for take-home use; however, because of the potential for human abuse of these controlled drugs, care must be taken in prescribing them. Sustained-release morphine is available and can be used in dogs, but morphine is difficult to obtain in sufficiently small doses to administer safely to cats. On the basis of research at the University of Florida, buprenorphine can be safely and efficaciously administered to cats by the transbuccal (sublingual) route. Small, single-dose aliquots can be prepared for administration by owners at home. The opioid fentanyl is available in a transdermal patch (Duragesic, Janssen Pharmaceuticals), which can be applied in the hospital to provide up to 3 days of postoperative analgesia for hospitalized as well as discharged patients. A fentanyl patch does require up to 24 hours to become fully effective, so additional forms of pain relief may be necessary to cover this period adequately.

Butorphanol tablets are not recommended for take-home analgesia because of butorphanol's extremely short duration of action. Just because an animal is sedated does not mean that its pain has been addressed.

The synthetic opioid tramadol is available in tablet form. Tramadol is gaining popularity for long-term use in dogs and cats as an effective nonscheduled take-home analgesic. Tramadol can be used as an adjunct to NSAIDs for the treatment of moderate to severe pain.

KEY POINTS

1. When monitoring recovery of a patient intubated with an ET tube, the technician must be prepared for the animal to awaken quickly. The ET tube is untied from the head or muzzle. All limbs should be untied and the patient placed in lateral recumbency. A syringe is at hand if needed to deflate the ET tube cuff. The technician should never leave the patient unattended on the table, and it is best to have a hand on the patient at all times.
2. The ET tube should not be removed until the patient has regained the ability to swallow.

3. Extubation of a brachycephalic breed should be delayed until the patient can raise its head without assistance.
4. All patients should be closely monitored until fully recovered.
5. When the body temperature is below 97° F, immediate and active measures should be taken to warm the patient. Additional postoperative opioid analgesics should not be given until the patient's temperature is above 98° F.
6. When treating an animal for hypothermia, do not assume that the measures are successful. Monitor the patient's body temperature, and confirm that the body temperature is rising.
7. A patient thrashing in a cage during recovery must be protected from injury, but the staff should ensure that the animal does not cause injury to itself or others.
8. The technician who thinks a patient is not recovering as expected should notify the attending veterinarian. The cause of the delayed recovery needs to be identified and corrected.
9. Attention to the surgical wound is an important part of the recovery process. Any change in the wound's condition should be reported immediately to the surgeon.
10. Débridement and lavage are important steps in the wound cleansing process.
11. Bandages, casts, splints, and slings must be monitored closely for displacement, patient mutilation, wetness, and odor.
12. A drain must be kept clean so that drainage can continue as long as needed and the skin around the exit wound for the drain does not become irritated by draining fluid.
13. Indwelling IV and urinary catheters need regular inspections to ensure that they are functional and have not been disturbed by the patient.
14. A patient that will not eat will not heal quickly and is predisposed to development of complications.
15. Enteral tube feeding may be necessary to meet nutritional needs.
16. Any food that can be blenderized can be fed through a feeding tube.
17. Feeding of a raw or uncooked diet through a feeding tube is not recommended because of the possibility of bacterial contamination of the food.
18. Use of a gastrostomy tube should be delayed for 24 hours after it is placed to allow a temporary stoma to form internally between the visceral peritoneum and parietal peritoneum.
19. Physical therapy techniques used during the recuperative period can greatly improve patient outcome and enhance client satisfaction.
20. Providing adequate preoperative analgesia ("preemptive analgesia") makes it easier to achieve successful postoperative pain management.
21. Postoperative pain management should continue at home. Oral analgesics and transdermal analgesic patches can provide continued pain relief after the patient leaves the veterinary hospital.
22. The best pain relief is achieved by combining different classes of analgesics that block or prevent pain by different mechanisms of action. Postoperatively, these typically include oral opioids and NSAIDs.

REVIEW QUESTIONS

1. When does the postoperative recovery period begin for the surgical patient?
   a. As soon as the surgeon begins closing the incision.
   b. On discontinuation of anesthesia.
   c. On regaining full mental capacity.
   d. On return of normal vital signs (temperature, pulse, respiration) and consciousness.
   e. None of the above.

2. *True or False:* Brachycephalic breeds should have the endotracheal tube removed at the first sign of return of the ability to swallow.

3. *True or False:* Once the patient is extubated, the anesthetist can relax because all risks associated with anesthesia immediately cease on extubation.

4. *True or False:* All animals that undergo an anesthetic/surgical procedure are at risk for hypothermia.

5. What phrase is used to describe the excitement and exaggerated and uncontrollable movements some patients exhibit during the recovery phase of anesthesia?
   a. Drug-induced dysphoria.
   b. Endorphin euphoria.
   c. Emergence delirium.
   d. Reverse induction.
   e. None of the above.

6. Which of the following conditions can contribute to a prolonged recovery from anesthesia?
   a. Hypoglycemia.
   b. Liver disease.
   c. Kidney disease.
   d. All of the above.
   e. Both b and c.

7. Which of the following methods can hasten a patient's recovery from anesthesia?
   a. Physical stimulation.
   b. Oxygen supplementation with or without manual ventilation.
   c. Warming measures.
   d. Reversal agents.
   e. All of the above.

8. Which of the following postoperative complications involves premature suture loss and surgical site opening?
   a. Dehiscence.
   b. Hemorrhage.
   c. Seroma.
   d. Hematoma.
   e. Both c and d.

9. Débridement is:
   a. The process of removing dead tissue and debris from a wound.
   b. The name given to a divorce caused by a household of too many dogs.
   c. A way to check for a fluid wave in the abdomen of animals with suspected ascites or hemoabdomen.
   d. Necessary in all cases of neoplastic surgery.
   e. None of the above.

10. Topical antimicrobial medications are usually:
    a. Not used on wounds.
    b. Discontinued once granulation tissue appears in the wound.
    c. Only used once granulation tissue appears in a wound.
    d. Only applied to anesthetized patients with wounds.
    e. None of the above.

11. Which of the following statements is true?
    a. Bandages, splints, and casts are used to immobilize bones and joints.
    b. Immobilization helps decrease pain associated with fractures.
    c. Immobilization facilitates healing by securing bone fragments close together.
    d. All of the above.

12. With a bandaged limb, leaving the toes exposed:
    a. Is useful to monitor the amount of swelling that may occur under the bandage.
    b. Is an example of a poorly placed bandage.
    c. Allows the animal's caregiver to compare the toes on the bandaged limb with the toes on the other limb.
    d. Both a and c.
    e. None of the above.

13. Which of the following statements regarding drains is true?
    a. Drains are usually removed 3 to 5 days after surgery.
    b. Petrolatum-based ointments applied to the skin around the drain's exit site help prevent exudates from accumulating and clogging the drain's exit site.
    c. All types of drains have hollow lumens to allow for the fluid to drain out of the wound through them.
    d. All of the above.
    e. Both a and b.

14. Which of the following statements regarding urinary catheters is true?
    a. Catheters help ensure urethral patency.
    b. Catheters allow measurement of urine production, which reflects the condition of the kidneys.
    c. Urinary catheters help keep the patient clean and dry.
    d. Both a and c.
    e. All of the above.

15. *True or False:* Physical therapy should be performed shortly after analgesics have been administered to the surgical patient.

16. *True or False:* Cold generally is applied to recent wounds and heat to wounds at least 3 to 5 days old.

17. Massage provides which of the following benefits to the surgery patient?
    a. Muscle relaxation.
    b. Improved blood and lymph flow.
    c. Pain relief.
    d. Both a and b.
    e. All of the above.

18. The terms effleurage and pétrissage refer to which physical therapy modality?
    a. Cryotherapy.
    b. Passive range-of-motion exercises.
    c. Massage.
    d. All of the above.
    e. None of the above.

19. What is the minimum amount that an animal should consume orally before assisted feeding is needed?
    a. 25%.
    b. 45%.
    c. 65%.
    d. 85%.
    e. 100%.

20. How long should an animal be allowed to not eat before intervention is sought?
    a. 1 day.
    b. 2 days.
    c. 3 days.
    d. 4 days.
    e. 5 days.

21. How can a veterinary technician determine whether a patient's pain was successfully managed through surgery and into the postoperative phase?
    a. Recovery from anesthesia is smooth.
    b. The patient is calm and quiet postoperatively.
    c. Signs of overt pain (e.g., vocalization, excessive movement) are absent.
    d. All of the above.
    e. Both a and c.

22. Which of the following statements regarding postoperative analgesia is true?
    a. Patients undergoing soft tissue elective surgery should receive opioids for 24 hours and NSAIDs for 3 to 4 days postoperatively.
    b. Patients undergoing emergency or nonroutine soft tissue surgery should never receive opioids.
    c. Patients undergoing surgery of the gastrointestinal tract should never receive NSAIDs.
    d. Patients undergoing orthopedic surgery should receive opioids and NSAIDs only for the first 24 to 72 hours postoperatively.
    e. None of the above.

23. True or False: NSAIDs are the only class of analgesics that may safely be sent home with the owner for at-home pain management following surgery.

ANSWERS

1. b	7. e	13. e	19. d
2. False	8. a	14. e	20. c
3. False	9. a	15. True	21. d
4. True	10. b	16. True	22. a
5. c	11. d	17. e	23. False
6. d	12. d	18. c	

BIBLIOGRAPHY

Bassert JM, McCurnin DM, editors: McCurnin's clinical textbook for veterinary technicians, ed 7, St Louis, 2010, Saunders.

Clark B, McLaughlin RM: Physical rehabilitation in small-animal orthopedic patients, Vet Med 96:3, 2001.

Davidson EB: Managing bite wounds in dogs and cats. Part II, Compend Contin Educ Pract Vet 20:9, 1998.

Fossum TW, Theresa W: Small animal surgery, ed 3, St. Louis, 2007, Mosby.

Fowler D, Williams JM: Manual of canine and feline wound management and reconstruction, Shurdington, 1999, British Small Animal Veterinary Association.

Manning AM, Rush J, Rudnick D: Physical therapy for critically ill veterinary patients. Part II. The musculoskeletal system. Compend Contin Educ Pract Vet 19:7, 1997.

Simpson AM, Radlinsky M, Beale BS: Bandaging in dogs and cats: basic principles. Compend Contin Educ Pract Vet 23:1, 2001.

Slatter D: Textbook of small animal surgery, ed 3, Philadelphia, 2003, Saunders.

Taylor R, McGehee R: Manual of small animal postoperative care, Baltimore, 1995, Williams & Wilkins.

Wortinger A: Nutrition for the veterinary technician and nurse, Ames, Iowa, 2007, Wiley-Blackwell.

9

Postoperative Surgery Room and Equipment

Paige A. Allen

LEARNING OBJECTIVES

After completion of this chapter, the reader will be able to:
- Describe the ideal cleaning procedure for a surgery room.
- Identify the different types of disinfectants and the microorganisms they target.
- Describe the steps to prepare instruments for use in surgery.
- Describe the cleaning methods used for preparing instruments for sterilization.
- Identify which method is best for sterilizing particular instruments.
- Demonstrate how to wrap a pack for sterilization.
- Describe the types of expiration dating.
- Explain the different types of sterilization indicators.
- Identify the supplies that should be stocked in a surgery room.
- Explain supply rotation in the surgery room.

Cleaning of the Surgery Room

Ideally, the equipment used to clean the surgery room should be used only in the surgery room to prevent cross-contamination from other areas of the veterinary facility. Various agencies or organizations that evaluate human medical facilities provide recommendations that the veterinary facility can use when setting up a protocol for the cleaning and maintenance of the surgery room.

The Association of periOperative Room Nurses (AORN) publishes recommended practices for environmental cleaning in the surgical setting. Although these recommendations may be difficult to meet in all veterinary practices, it is important to the veterinary patient's health that guidelines for cleanliness and disinfection of the surgical area include as many recommended practices as possible.

The U.S. Centers for Disease Control and Prevention (CDC) has no recommendation for disinfecting the surgery room after each procedure in the absence of visible soiling and contamination. However, wet vacuuming the surgery room floor is recommended at the end of the day. The CDC also states that the actual physical removal of microorganisms and soil by scrubbing is more important than the antimicrobial effect of the cleaning agent used.

AORN recommends cleaning a 3-foot to 4-foot perimeter around the surgical field when it is visibly soiled, with the cleaning area extended as necessary. Also, the entire floor should be cleaned each day. The following AORN recommendations, including a rationale (purpose) to clarify some practices, may be useful as a protocol for the cleaning of a surgery area in a veterinary facility.

1. Cleaning is performed on a regular basis to reduce the amount of dust, organic material, and microbial presence in the surgery room.
2. The surgery room should be cleaned before and after each surgical procedure.
3. All horizontal surfaces in the surgery room should be damp-dusted before the first surgery of the day. In "damp dusting," a lint-free cloth dampened with water is used to wipe down the horizontal surfaces.
   Rationale: Proper cleaning of horizontal surfaces helps reduce airborne contaminants that may travel on dust and lint.
4. Surgical room equipment and furniture that are visibly soiled should be cleaned at the end of each procedure.
   Rationale: Items used for surgery are considered contaminated through contact with the patient's blood, tissue, and body fluids and should be cleaned before admittance of the next patient to the surgery room.
5. Surgery rooms should be "terminally cleaned" daily. *Terminal cleaning* is cleaning that is performed at the completion of the daily surgery schedule. It includes all the equipment in the surgery and prep areas and all the permanent and movable equipment.
6. Surgery rooms should be cleaned daily whether they are used or not.
   Rationale: A clean surgical environment reduces the number of microbial flora present.
7. Mechanical friction (a scrubbing motion) should be used to clean all surfaces, including (but not limited to) the following:
   - Surgical lights
   - Any fixed equipment
   - All furniture and equipment, including wheels, casters, step stools, foot pedals, telephones, and light switches
   - Handles of cabinets
   - Ventilation faceplates
   - Horizontal surfaces (doorway ledges)
   - Areas adjacent to surgery room
   - Scrub sinks
8. Refillable soap dispensers are not recommended because they can harbor bacterial growth.

BOX 9-1 Disinfectant Terms

Anionic detergent: Soap that has free, negatively charged ions that precipitate when combined with calcium and magnesium in hard water.
Antiseptic: Chemical that inhibits or prevents the growth of microbes on living tissue; compare with *disinfectant*.
Bactericide: Agent that destroys (kills) bacteria.
Bacteriostat: Agent that inhibits the growth of bacteria.
Biocide: Agent that kills living organisms.
Cationic detergent: Contains positively charged ions that remain suspended in solution (e.g., quaternary ammonium).
Detergent: Chemical that contains free ions and leaves a film on surfaces.
Disinfectant: Chemical used to inhibit or prevent the growth of microbes on inanimate objects; compare with *antiseptic*.
Fungicide: Agent that kills fungi.
Sanitize: To reduce the number of microbes to a safe level.
Sporicide: Agent that kills spores.
Sterilize: To eliminate all microbes by killing or inactivation.
Virucide: Agent that kills viruses.

9. Surgery rooms should be wet-vacuumed at the end of the day.
   Rationale: Terminal cleaning in the surgery room reduces the number of microorganisms, dust, and organic debris from the environment.
10. Cleaning equipment (mops, wet vacuums) should be disassembled, cleaned, and dried before storage.
    Rationale: This practice prevents growth of microorganisms during storage and subsequent contamination of the surgery room.

Disinfectants
Definitions

The basic definitions in Box 9-1 help in understanding how the different disinfectants work and interact with bacteria, viruses, spores, and even one another. The ideal disinfectant should have the following characteristics:

- Broad spectrum
- Nonirritating
- Nontoxic
- Noncorrosive
- Inexpensive

Effectiveness

The effectiveness of any disinfectant depends on the following factors:

Type of microorganism: Some microorganisms are more resistant to certain types of disinfectants.
Degree of contamination: This may affect the length of time and the amount of chemical disinfectant necessary to disinfect effectively.

Amount of protein in area: Proteins may absorb or inactivate the disinfectant.

Organic matter: Hair, feces, litter, and other organic matter decrease the effectiveness or render the disinfectant ineffective. Therefore, all organic matter should be removed from the area, and the area should be sanitized before the disinfectant is applied.

Additional sanitizing compounds: Other compounds used to sanitize the area may inactivate or react with the disinfectant. Therefore, thorough rinsing and drying after sanitizing should be attempted before a disinfectant is applied.

Concentration and quantity of chemical: Improper dilution or inadequate amount of the correct dilution may result in ineffective disinfection.

Contact time and temperature: Incorrect contact time or the temperature of the surface may result in ineffective disinfection.

Types of Disinfectants

Many types of disinfectants are available for use in a veterinary facility. Each facility should research the product information and determine the best policy for the facility. Most disinfectants require some form of dilution. The manufacturer's recommendations should be followed so that each disinfectant is used at its maximum effectiveness against bacteria, viruses, and other infective agents. Table 9-1 compares types of various disinfectants.

An example of a *chlorine-based* disinfectant is bleach (Figure 9-1). It can be used for cleaning as well as disinfecting. Bleach does corrode metals and causes fabrics to deteriorate. It can be irritating to eyes, mucous membranes, and skin. Bleach can be deactivated by fecal matter.

Decreased temperature and the pH of the water in which the bleach is diluted may alter its efficacy.

Phenol-based disinfectants include common household disinfectants (e.g., Lysol, Pine-Sol). Phenols are able to work in the presence of organic material. These disinfectants are relatively safe but can cause skin irritation. They are infrequently used in veterinary medicine.

An example of *quaternary amine–based* disinfectant is Roccal-D Plus (Pfizer, Inc., New York) (Figure 9-2). These disinfectants bind to and are inactivated by organic material, so the area must be cleaned before disinfection. They also react with soaps, so the area must be well rinsed. Hard water may also deactivate quaternary amine disinfectants.

Iodine disinfectants such as povidone-iodine are not generally used as disinfectants, but in veterinary medicine they are frequently used as antiseptics (Figure 9-3). The iodines can stain fabric and floors and can irritate tissue. They are also corrosive. Iodines are inactivated by organic material.

Chlorhexidine disinfectants are widely used in veterinary medicine as disinfectants for examination tables and for the disinfection of instruments for minor procedures (Figure 9-4). Chlorhexidine maintains its effectiveness in the presence of organic material but is not as effective against some bacteria and viruses as other disinfectants. It also has residual activity, which can be important. One drawback is that chlorhexidine must have sufficient contact time to be effective.

Technician Notes
- Disinfectants should be used according to the manufacturer's instructions.

FIGURE 9-1 Chlorine-based disinfectant.

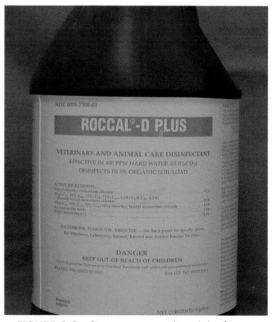
FIGURE 9-2 Quaternary amine–based disinfectant.

TABLE 9-1   Comparison of Different Types of Disinfectants

Disinfectant	Effectiveness	Advantages	Disadvantages
Chlorine based	Viruses: enveloped, nonenveloped Fungi Bacteria Algae *Not effective against:* Spores	Wide germicidal activity Relatively nontoxic Effective at low concentrations Low cost	Corrodes metal Deteriorates fabric Irritates mucous membrane, eyes, and skin Inactivated by organic material Area must be cleaned before use

Phenol based	Bacteria
	Viruses, enveloped
	Not effective against:
	  Viruses, nonenveloped
	  Spores
		Maintains effectiveness with organic matter
		Wide germicidal activity
		Relatively noncorrosive
		Limited toxicity
		Low to moderate cost
			Poor or limited residual activity
			Not sporicidal

Quaternary amine based	Bacteria: gram positive, gram negative
	Viruses: enveloped
	Not effective against:
	  Viruses, nonenveloped
	  Spores
	  Fungi
		Low toxicity
		Wide germicidal activity
		Noncorrosive
		Good for use on cleaned surfaces
		Low cost
			Binds to organic material and soaps
			Deactivated by hard water
			Areas must be cleaned and rinsed free of soap

Iodine (iodophor)	Bacteria Spores (some) Viruses Fungus	Wide germicidal activity Relatively nontoxic Better as sporicidal than chlorine Low cost	Inactivated by organic material Must be applied multiple times Stains fabric Poor residual activity Corrosive
Chlorhexidine	Bacteria Viruses, enveloped Fungus (some) Spores	Nonirritating to tissue Maintains effectiveness with organic matter Wide germicidal activity, but ineffective against some important species Nontoxic Effective at low concentrations Low cost	Less effective than other agents Must be in contact for 5 minutes Hard or alkaline water causes precipitation of active ingredients

Alcohols	Bacteria, gram-positive and gram-negative
	Viruses, enveloped
	Not effective against:
	  Viruses, nonenveloped
	  Spores
		Wide germicidal activity
		Noncorrosive
		Excellent instrument, disinfecting at 70%-95% concentration
			Requires time to work
			Does not penetrate organic material
			Irritates tissue
			Denatures protein, which may promote bacterial growth in open wounds
			Too expensive for general use

- There is no "ideal disinfectant," but many good disinfectants meet most of the criteria of an ideal disinfectant.
- The effectiveness of a disinfectant depends on many factors (e.g., microorganisms, contamination, organic matter).

Instrument Cleaning

Cleaning, decontaminating (or sanitizing), and sterilizing are the three cornerstones to providing sterile instruments in the surgery room. Each of these processes contributes to the overall destruction of microorganisms that could cause serious postoperative complications, including the death of the patient.

Basic cleaning procedures for instruments include presoaking, decontaminating, and ultrasonic cleaning. In the cleaning and sterilization of instruments, it is imperative to begin the process of presoaking immediately after a surgery.

Presoaking of Instruments

Presoaking or precleaning can make the cleaning process more efficient. *Presoaking* involves placing the soiled instruments in distilled water or water mixed with a detergent solution that is specifically approved for use with surgical instruments (e.g., HAEMO-SOL, HAEMO-SOL, Baltimore; Figure 9-5), without using mechanical agitation. The purpose of presoaking is to prevent blood and other surgical debris from drying on the instruments or to soften dried blood and debris on the instruments.

Precleaning involves rinsing the instruments in distilled water to rid them of tissue and blood. If this is not done, processing the instruments may take longer. Allowing tissue and blood to dry on the instruments makes

FIGURE 9-3 Povidone-iodine disinfectant.

FIGURE 9-5 Example of product approved for use as a cleaning solution for surgical instruments.

FIGURE 9-4 Chlorhexidine diacetate disinfectant.

cleaning much more difficult, especially in hinged areas and box locks. Debris can build up and harden in crevices, making decontamination more difficult as well.

Decontamination of Instruments

The *decontamination* process is the manual cleaning of an instrument in a detergent solution to assist in the

breakdown of biologic debris. Because this may be the only cleaning before sterilization, the instrument must be cleaned thoroughly. When cleaning instruments by hand, the technician must take care not to damage the more delicate items and must pay special attention to cleaning areas that have box locks or joints. Instruments should be decontaminated using the following procedural steps:

1. Prepare a basin with warm water and a detergent approved for use on surgical instruments.
2. Open all box locks and unlock ratchets as each instrument is gently placed in the basin.
3. Wash all surfaces of each instrument with a soft bristle brush. Pay special attention to box locks, joints, and serrations because biologic debris builds up in these areas. Use a brushing motion, directed away from you, to scrub the instruments; this method prevents biologic debris from splashing back toward you.
   - Never use a wire brush on instruments because it will damage instruments' surfaces and cause crevices that can harbor pathogens (microorganisms).
   - Instruments have a protective coating of chromium oxide to extend their usefulness as properly functioning devices. If the coating is removed, the instrument will be compromised, and then its surface can harbor pathogens that adversely affect the patient's health.
4. Rinse each instrument thoroughly with distilled water. This will prevent the buildup of "scale" on the instruments. If tap water is used, scale will eventually build up on instruments, and they will not work properly.
5. With locks and ratchets opened, place the instruments flat on an absorbent surface to drain and dry.
6. Cover the draining instruments with another layer of lint-free absorbent material.
7. When the instruments are clean and dry, check each for its general condition and its ability to function properly. Box locks should open and close smoothly;

FIGURE 9-6 Ultrasonic cleaning unit.

FIGURE 9-7 Example of enzymatic cleaning solution used in ultrasonic cleaning unit.

ratchets should engage and disengage easily; scissors should cut easily and smoothly; and the jaws and teeth should mesh as designed. One way to check the integrity of ratchets is to close them and firmly tap the ringed end of the instrument against a firm, smooth surface. If the ratchets pop open when tested, they cannot be trusted to hold the target tissue in surgery and should not be included in the surgery pack.

Instruments with broken or missing parts, malfunctioning parts, pitted or discolored parts, or rusted surfaces should be set aside for repair or replacement. It is best to buy high-quality instruments that will withstand repeated and excessive use.

Ultrasonic Cleaning of Instruments

After the decontamination process has been completed, the next step is ultrasonic cleaning with a solution of distilled water and chemicals (enzymes) (Figure 9-6). Several brands of enzymatic solutions are available, and the solution chosen should contain a *surfactant*, a product that reduces surface tension. An example of a surfactant solution is MetriClean 2 (Metrex, Orange, CA) (Figure 9-7). *Enzymes* are organic substances that cause a particular chemical reaction. Enzymes assist in the breakdown of soils and are generally formulated with a surfactant to improve their penetration into dried soil. Enzymes work most effectively when kept in water at a temperature recommended by the manufacturer. If the temperature is too high or too low, the enzymes may be inactivated. Enzymes can clean without mechanical action and are therefore used to clean instruments with lumens, such as endoscopes.

The benefit of ultrasonic cleaning is best demonstrated with hinged instruments or those with inaccessible areas (e.g., box lock), including hinged retractors and bone-cutting instruments. These devices should be in the open position for cleaning. An ultrasonic cleaner uses sound waves higher than those heard by the human ear, which create tiny bubbles. These bubbles form and collapse thousands of times each second, producing a scrubbing effect, known as *cavitation*, on the surface of items immersed in the liquid. Particles that have been agitated from instruments are suspended in solution and are subjected to negative pressure or suction. As a result, proteins are coagulated, the cell walls are disrupted, and microorganisms are destroyed.

The typical processing time of instruments in the ultrasonic machine is 3 to 6 minutes. Based on the manufacturer's recommendation, the temperature of the solution should be maintained in the range of 110° to 130° F. The temperature at which the chemical has greatest effect varies with the enzyme used. The instrument may be damaged if the enzyme is kept at too high a temperature. Additionally, if the solution is not maintained at the correct temperature, soil may be "heat set" on the instrument, making it more difficult to clean.

After the ultrasonic cleaning is complete, the instruments are rinsed with distilled water to remove mineral deposits left behind. At this point, application of a lubricant to prolong the life of the instruments and help prevent rust and corrosion is appropriate. Many different types of instrument lubricants are available. Some are used as a bath for soaking the instruments; other lubricants are sprayed on opened instruments spread out on a lint-free towel, then left to air-dry. Regardless of the type used, it is important to use only fresh, clean lubricant and to follow the manufacturer's directions. Lubricants can penetrate into difficult-to-reach areas such as box locks and leave a lubricating, microscopic film on the instrument. Most lubricants are steam permeable and do not interfere with the sterilization process. The instruments are now ready for wrapping.

Pack Wrapping

Recipes

Typically, each instrument pack has a "recipe" detailing pertinent information that is kept in a procedures manual. The recipe should include the names of all the instruments contained in each pack and the quantity of each type of instrument required to complete the pack. Additionally, the recipe should include the types and quantity of supplies that are necessary for pack completion, such as the number of gauze squares to include. It should contain a photo or illustration of each instrument and should specify whether linen or paper material should be used to wrap the pack. The procedures manual should also include the manufacturer's guidelines for any instrument in the pack that requires special handling and maintenance, any warranty that may be appropriate for items in the pack, and the manufacturer's telephone number.

Wrapping Material

Wraps used for sterilizing instruments are usually made of cotton or linen textiles and paper. These materials are able to sustain the heat and moisture of steam sterilization. For technicians working in a small animal facility that relies on steam sterilization for in-house procedures, the choice is usually linen or paper. The ideal wrap should have the following qualities:

Selective permeability: Steam or gas must be able to penetrate the wrapping for sterilization to occur and must be easily "exhausted" from the pack once the sterilization process is completed. Microbes and dust particles must not be able to penetrate from the outer surface of the wrap to the inner surface.
Resistance: The material should be resistant to damage when handled. Rips, punctures, or worn areas should be readily visible, to help ensure that contaminated packs will not be used.
Flexibility: The material should be able to conform to the shape of the pack.
Memory: After the pack has been opened, the wrapping material should return to the original flat position. This feature helps prevent accidental contamination of the pack contents.

Textile wraps traditionally are cotton textiles with a thread count of 140 to 288 threads per square inch. Textile wraps must be laundered, dried, and inspected for any damage before reuse as instrument pack wraps. The advantage of using textile wraps is that they are more resistant to rips and punctures than paper and generally have a higher degree of flexibility and memory. Cotton is the best option for textile wrappers. Synthetic wrap may contribute to static electricity in the operating room. Gray, light tones of green, and medium tones of blue are often preferred because they result in less eyestrain over

FIGURE 9-8 Sterilized pack with labeling information. Black strips along the indicator tape show that this pack has been autoclaved.

time than white. Fabric should be selected by thread count, not by its weight or texture.

Disadvantages of textile wraps are that they must be laundered after each use, and personnel may be reluctant to discard textile wraps that have become torn or ripped and may attempt to mend them. Continued use of damaged textile wrap is not recommended because each stitch in the wrap creates a passage for microbes. If heat-sealed patches are used, steam cannot penetrate the patches during sterilization as easily as it penetrates the body of the wrap.

There are many types of paper wraps, but crepe paper is preferred over the noncrepe papers. Crepe paper should not be reused because continuous autoclaving can destroy the integrity of the paper fiber.

Sealing of the Pack

Steam indicator tape is recommended when securing the wrapping material in place. Pretreated strips on the steam indicator tape change color from a pale yellow to black when the pack has been autoclaved. This indicates that conditions were met for sterilization. The name of the pack, the date the pack was sterilized, and the initials of the person who wrapped the pack should be written on the tape (Figure 9-8).

Packs can be wrapped with one wrap (single-wrapped) or with two wraps (double-wrapped). If a pack is double-wrapped, only the outer layer is sealed with steam indicator tape. Generally, when a pack is double-wrapped, the circulating nurse unwraps the outer layer, and the scrubbed-in assistant unwraps the inner layer. If inadvertent contamination occurs when the outer layer (circulating nurse accidentally touches outer surface of inner wrap) is unwrapped, a double-wrapped pack has the advantage of an additional layer of material protecting the instruments. The circulating nurse may then open the interior layer, and as long as contamination does not occur, the surgeon can use the pack. The disadvantage of double wrapping is the additional cost of the material used to wrap the pack.

When securing a wrapped package, personnel may attempt to use ordinary masking tape instead of indicator

FIGURE 9-9 Steps in accordion pleat folding of a hand or field towel. **A,** Spread towel flat on table. **B,** Fold towel in half lengthwise. **C,** Make first fold of accordion. **D,** Lateral view of first accordion fold. **E,** Completed accordion folding.

tape. This is not advisable because the adhesive on masking tape will not adhere adequately during steam sterilization.

The following guidelines should be followed in the preparation of packs:

1. All items to be sterilized must be clean and in good condition.
2. The wrap material used must be durable for the sterilization process.
3. Contents of frequently used packs should be standardized so that the same pack can be used for the same surgical procedure from session to session.
4. Pack size must be compatible for the size of the autoclave chamber.
5. Soft items such as towels and drapes should be folded using the accordion pleat technique (Figure 9-9). Items that have been folded in this manner can be lifted by one corner and allowed to fall open. No elaborate unfolding or shaking is necessary, reducing the potential for air currents that may circulate microbes.
6. All packs should be wrapped using the same method so that they can be unwrapped in the same way. One common method uses angled wrapping (Figure 9-10).

7. A sterilization indicator strip should be placed in the middle of the pack to verify that conditions were met for sterilization.
8. The outer wrap should be sealed with indicator tape to indicate the pack has been autoclaved and to keep the pack from opening (Figure 9-11).

Each step of this process is critical in providing sterile instruments; that is, each method used in these steps fulfills a particular function that cannot be omitted. Box 9-2 provides directions on how to wrap a surgical gown and towel pack.

Expiration Dating

Debate surrounds the issue of how long an item can be stored and still can be considered sterile. Shelf-life expiration and event-related expiration are the two types of dating for sterilized items. *Shelf-life expiration* includes a predetermined date that identifies how long an item should be considered sterile. For items wrapped in woven (linen) or nonwoven (crepe paper) materials, a shelf life of 2 weeks is an acceptable time to expiration. Items placed in peel-away pouches have an expiration date of 7 weeks.

FIGURE 9-10 Five steps in angle wrapping of a pack for sterilization. **A,** Spread wrap on a clean table with tray centered in middle of wrap. **B,** Bring bottom flap on top of tray, and fold back the corner to create a tab. **C,** Bring first side flap to center, and fold back the corner to create another tab. **D,** Bring second side flap to center, and fold back the corner to create another tab. **E,** Make final fold of pack wrap, and tuck under other flaps, leaving a short tab untucked to allow for easier unwrapping of the pack when opened for surgery.

In contrast, *event-related expiration* is determined from an environmental perspective. If damaged in any way, the pack would be considered nonsterile. Excessive handling of the pack, causing it to fall onto the floor, or accumulation of dust on the pack would lead personnel to question whether the pack is still sterile. Even under these conditions, packs have been found to be sterile after 50 weeks. However, whenever a pack's sterility is in question, it must be assumed that the pack is contaminated. Products that break down or alter over time, such as latex tubing, require expiration dating.

Sterilization

The last step in the cleaning process after presoaking/precleaning and decontamination is sterilization. *Sterilization* is defined as the use of a process to rid an object of all living microbes. Two types of sterilizers (autoclaves) are typically used in small animal practices: gravity air-displacement autoclaves and high-vacuum sterilizers (also known as prevacuum sterilizers). Both types use steam under pressure to kill microorganisms. Some autoclaves are capable of performing both methods of

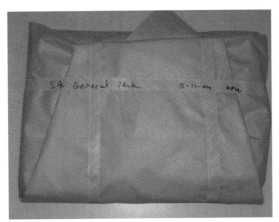

FIGURE 9-11 Wrapped and taped pack, ready for sterilization. Yellow strips on the indicator tape used to seal this pack have not yet changed to black, indicating that this pack has not yet been autoclaved.

BOX 9-2	**Wrapping Gowns and Hand Towels**

Gowns
1. Place a clean gown flat on a surface with the outer surface facing up.
2. Straighten out the sleeves and cuffs.
3. Fold the near edge of the gown to the center.
4. Fold the far edge of the gown toward the center to meet the near edge.
5. Fold the gown in half lengthwise.
6. Fold the gown lengthwise in accordion fashion into thirds.
7. Ensure that neck ties are easily accessible on the uppermost surface of the gown.

Hand Towels
1. Place a clean hand towel flat on a clean surface.
2. Use the accordion pleat technique to fold the towel on its long axis.
3. Fold the towel in accordion fashion into thirds or quarters.
4. Fold back a corner tab.

Gowns and Towels Together
1. Flatten out a clean outer wrap on a clean surface (single-layer wrap).
2. Place the folded gown in the center.
3. Place the folded hand towel on top of the gown.
4. Place an indicator strip inside the towel.
5. Wrap in same fashion as an instrument pack.*
6. Seal with tape, label "gown pack," note gown's size and the date, and initial.

*Most instrument packs are wrapped in two layers (double-wrapped). Gown packs typically are wrapped with one layer (single-wrapped).

sterilization. With both types of sterilizers, proper sterilization depends on the following three factors:
- Proper operation of the sterilizer.
- Proper preparation of the packs.
- Proper loading of the sterilizer.

Gravity Air-Displacement Sterilizer

The gravity air-displacement sterilizer found in most small animal hospitals is typically a tabletop-sized autoclave (Figure 9-12). Distilled water is placed in the bottom of the sterilizer and then heated electrically. As the water turns to steam, the steam forces air out of the sterilizer through a port. Once the air is out of the sterilizer, the steam pressure builds up until the operating temperature is reached. Once the cycle has been completed, the steam is removed and condenses back to water.

Several settings can be used in gravity air-displacement sterilization. The typical temperature is 250° to 270° F, and typical pressure is 15 to 27 pounds per square inch (psi). The cycle runs approximately 15 minutes to achieve the proper temperature and sterilizes in 3 to 15 minutes depending on the item. At the completion of the cycle, the door should be cracked open for approximately 15 minutes to allow any moisture to evaporate and prevent condensation on the pack.

High-Vacuum Sterilizer

High-vacuum sterilizers are most commonly found in teaching hospitals. They require additional plumbing and specialized installation. Proper operation of a high-vacuum gravity displacement sterilizer includes setting the sterilizer between 250° and 272° F for 4 minutes at 32 psi (Figure 9-13). The sterilizer should run through (1) a conditioning phase for about 17 minutes, (2) a sterilization phase for 4 minutes, (3) a high-vacuum exhaust for about 4 minutes, and (4) a drying cycle for about 20 minutes. The total sterilization process should take about 45 minutes. To ensure proper settings for specific types of packs (e.g., instruments, soft items), the user should consult the manufacturer's operating manual.

The main difference between gravity air-displacement and high-vacuum sterilizers is that the high-vacuum sterilizer forces steam into the sterilizing chamber, which causes steam to penetrate the pack more quickly. Additionally, after the sterilization cycle has been completed, the steam is vacuumed out of the chamber. This pulls the steam out of the pack to prevent condensation in or on the pack. This avoids a wet pack, which could compromise the pack's sterility.

Preparation and Loading

Proper pack preparation should be done in an area reserved for this purpose. For many small animal practices, however, this is not always possible. An acceptable alternative is to combine both the pack preparation area and the area used for preparation of operating room personnel. Traffic to and from this area should be minimized, and routine cleaning procedures should be in place to reduce the microbial load in the area as much as possible.

Proper loading of the sterilizer is a critical step in the sterilization process. The chamber of the sterilizer must

FIGURE 9-12   A, Tabletop gravity air-displacement sterilizer, with door closed. B, Same autoclave, with door opened.

FIGURE 9-13   High-vacuum sterilizer.

not be overloaded. The outer wraps of the packs should not touch the inner surface of the chamber. Steam will not be able to penetrate the packs effectively if they are crammed too tightly into the chamber.

Flash Sterilization

Flash sterilization is an abbreviated version of a regular sterilization cycle. Instruments sterilized by this method are not wrapped and are usually sterilized one or two instruments at a time. Special flash sterilization autoclaves are available, or the autoclaves just discussed can also be used to flash-sterilize individual, unwrapped instruments.

The autoclave settings should be 272° F, 32 psi, and 4 minutes. The conditioning phase is approximately 10 minutes, with a 4-minute sterilization phase. This is followed by a gravity exhaust of approximately 1 minute, then a 1-minute dry cycle. The dry cycle is shortened because no linen or paper was present for the steam to penetrate.

Typically, this process is used for individual instruments that have been dropped during surgery. Flash sterilization should not take the place of regular steam sterilization.

Ethylene Oxide (Gas) Sterilization

Another form of sterilization uses ethylene oxide (EtO), a colorless gas at room temperature. EtO is a toxin that can cause skin and mucous membrane irritation, however, and it is therefore considered a health hazard and has decreased in use.

EtO penetrates paper and plastic film packaging without melting these materials. EtO destroys metabolic pathways in the cells and is capable of killing all microorganisms. Effective sterilization with EtO depends on the concentration of gas, exposure time, temperature, and relative humidity. Moisture is necessary for the lethal action of EtO, and optimal relative humidity for this type of sterilization is 40%. Exposure time varies from 48 minutes to several hours, but 3 to 4 hours of exposure is typically used for sterilizing at room temperature. After EtO sterilization, materials should be quarantined in a well-ventilated area for a minimum of 24 hours. The aeration time can be reduced to 4 hours with the use of aerators that vent the gas outside the work environment (Figure 9-14).

Plasma Sterilization

The three most common states of matter are solid, liquid, and gas. The fourth, plasma, often occurs in nature, as

FIGURE 9-14 Ethylene oxide sterilizer.

FIGURE 9-15 Plasma sterilizer.

lightning and the aurora borealis (northern lights). The plasma state of matter is produced through the action of a strong electric or magnetic field.

Low-temperature *plasma sterilization* with hydrogen peroxide (H_2O_2) gas is produced when the gas is stimulated under a deep vacuum with radiofrequency (RF) or microwave energy. The plasma system uses H_2O_2 to form the reactive components to kill microorganisms. After a liquid solution of H_2O_2 is vaporized in a chamber, RF energy is applied to create an electric field that then creates low-temperature gas plasma (Figure 9-15). Within the plasma, H_2O_2 is broken into reactive components, including hydroperoxy-free and hydroxyl-free radicals. These radicals interact with cell membranes, killing the microorganisms in the process. After the components lose their energy, they recombine to form harmless by-products of oxygen and water.

One limitation to gas plasma sterilization is that it cannot penetrate the walls of an instrument with a lumen, and thus the area within the lumen is not sterilized.

Sterilization Indicators

Chemical and biologic indicators help determine whether items have been properly sterilized. *Chemical indicators* come in the form of strips or tape. Strips are placed inside the pack next to the instruments, whereas the tape is placed on the outside of the pack. The strips and tape change color if the conditions for sterilization have been met. This does not mean that the instruments are sterile, but only that the conditions were met for sterilization to have occurred.

Biologic indicators, on the other hand, demonstrate that the sterilizer has met all the sterilization parameters. A vial of *Bacillus stearothermophilus* is typically placed in the sterilizer with the first load to be sterilized for the day. At the end of the sterilization cycle, the vial is removed and placed in an incubator for 24 hours and checked for microbial colony growth. The vial should demonstrate that all the microorganisms have been killed, providing reassurance that the sterilizer worked appropriately at that time.

Specialty Instrument Cleaning
High-Level Disinfection

Cold sterilization is more of a high-level disinfection (see later) process than a true sterilization process. *Cold sterilization* is defined as the practice of immersing items in a disinfectant solution to reduce the level of contamination. Some instruments are cold-sterilized because they will not withstand repeated exposure to high-temperature steam sterilization.

Alcohol, used properly, exhibits strong bactericidal properties because of its ability to coagulate protein. Ethanol and isopropanol can be effective in a wide variety of applications. If used properly, alcohol solutions are effective against vegetative bacterial cells, including the bacterium that causes tuberculosis. However, alcohol cannot be relied on to kill bacterial spores or viruses and therefore should be used with caution.

Glutaraldehyde solution is considered a high-level disinfectant but not a sterilizing agent (Figure 9-16). Glutaraldehyde is bactericidal, tuberculocidal, and

FIGURE 9-16 A, Example of glutaraldehyde solution used for high-level disinfection. B, Instruments soaking in high-level disinfectant.

virucidal with an exposure time as short as 10 minutes. If exposure time is increased to several hours, the action is considered sporicidal. Prolonged exposure may adversely affect items made of rubber and plastic.

Drill Cleaning

Power drills are used in orthopedic surgery. Drills are not to be submerged in water or ultrasonically cleaned. They should be disassembled and inspected for any tissue or blood debris. If there is dried debris on the instrument, a foam disinfectant cleaner (e.g., Precise Hospital Foam Cleaner, Caltech Industries, Midland, MI is used on the drill) (Figure 9-17). The foam is allowed to loosen the debris so that it can be removed with a clean, lint-free towel. The drill should then be wiped with a clean, lint-free cloth moistened with isopropyl alcohol. Generally, power drills are wrapped and autoclaved according to the manufacturer's instructions in preparation for their use in orthopedic surgery. Frequently, this involves doubling the standard sterilization time used for soft tissue instrument packs.

Laparoscopic Instrument Cleaning

Laparoscopic equipment is expensive and should be handled gently. The scopes and fiberoptic light cables can be easily damaged. These items can be cleaned with gauze and alcohol after each procedure and stored in their cases. The scopes and light cable can then be gas sterilized (ethylene oxide) or cold sterilized (also known as high-level disinfection) before the procedure. Acceptable cold sterilization consists of the use of 2% glutaraldehyde (Cidex, CIVCO Medical Solutions, Kalona, IA).

A common alkylating agent approved by the U.S. Food and Drug administration (FDA) is 0.55% ortho-phthalaldehyde (Cidex OPA, CIVCO). It has a strong mycobactericidal activity level and a strong stability over a wide pH range of 3 to 9 and requires no activation.

FIGURE 9-17 Example of foaming disinfectant used to disinfect power drills.

Pentax and Olympus (two companies that manufacture laparoscopes) list OPA as a disinfectant compatible with flexible and rigid endoscopes for manual cleaning. Cindex states that 12-minute soaks are required to destroy all pathogenic organisms, but guidelines change and the manufacturer's instructions should be checked periodically. Gloves and eye protection should be worn to handle Cidex-OPA because it is a potential respiratory and dermal irritant. Cidex-OPA should be used in a well-ventilated area. The technician should refer to the manufacturer's detailed warnings and recommendations in the packet insert for further information. Once the instruments have been sterilized in Cidex, they should be rinsed thoroughly with sterile saline before entering the abdominal cavity. Laparoscopes and light cables should never be autoclaved unless the manufacturer states that they are "autoclave safe."

Endoscope Instrument Cleaning

Properly maintaining endoscopes and their accessory instruments is extremely important. Failure to adequately clean and disinfect endoscopes and their accessory instruments could lead to iatrogenic transmission of infection between patients. There are a variety of methods for cleaning and disinfecting endoscopes and instruments. Referring to the manufacturer's recommendations helps establish the cleaning protocol. This section covers the authors' preferred method for cleaning and disinfecting endoscopic equipment.

Endoscopes should be cleaned and disinfected immediately after the completion of any procedure. If this is not possible, abundant amounts of clean tap water should be suctioned to remove as much gross debris as possible. This practice prevents the adherence of large pieces of organic material to the channels and allows for easier cleaning once time permits.

To maximize the effect of the water moving through the suction channel, (1) the insertion tube is placed in a bowl of water, (2) the suction button is depressed for approximately 5 seconds while aspirating up the water, and (3) the suction button is released, breaking the suction and causing the water to "jump" or swish back and forth in the channel (like water being agitated in a washing machine). Afterward, the outer sheath should be gently wiped down with wet gauze sponges to remove gross debris.

Endoscopes should be inspected for damage before being submerged in solutions that may damage parts not designed for exposure. A leak test should be performed to ensure that the internal and external parts of the endoscope did not incur damage during a procedure.

Because of the gastrointestinal endoscope's delicate design, holes and tears of the inner lumen of the scope make it possible for water and other debris to contact otherwise impermeable areas of the scope. If the endoscope fails the leak test, it should not be submerged or used, and the manufacturer should be contacted immediately for inspection and repair. To perform a leak-test, the technician places the appropriate soaking caps and then attaches the leak tester and uses it according to the manufacturer's instructions (Figure 9-18). The cleaning and disinfecting protocol then can be completed.

The most important step in prevention of infection during endoscopy is manual cleaning. Organic soil (blood, feces) may contribute to the failure of disinfection by harboring embedded microbes and preventing the penetration of germicides. Also, some disinfectants are inactivated by organic material. After the endoscope has been disassembled and passed the leak test, the following channels should be cleaned with a cleaning brush: suction, air/

FIGURE 9-18   Leak testers are manufacturer specific. This Pentax leak tester is compatible with all Pentax endoscopes. (Courtesy MJR-VHUP, Philadelphia.)

water and biopsy, including the detachable suction and air/water valves; the biopsy channel cover; and the whole exterior of the endoscope. This cleaning process should take place in an enzymatic cleaner designed to clean organic material by breaking down proteins and enhancing the efficacy of brushing and flushing. Endozime (Ruhof Corporation, Mineola, NY), a bacteriostatic enzymatic cleaner, is a unique formulation of protease and amylase enzymes, digesters, and buffers that can clean in 2 to 3 minutes. Allowing the endoscope to be submerged in Endozime for at least 10 minutes after precleaning is sufficient. Endozime needs to be diluted, and as with any enzymatic solution, dilution protocols specified by the manufacturer should be followed.

After the appropriate time has elapsed with the endoscope submerged in the enzymatic cleaner, the exterior should be rinsed off with water, including the appropriate channels that do not need soaking caps, and then purged with air before being exposed to the disinfectant. The endoscope should be purged with water, followed by air, before disinfection. This helps prevent contamination of the disinfectant with the enzymatic solution and dilution of the disinfectant itself.

High-level disinfection (HLD) is recommended for endoscopes because they cannot withstand available sterilization methods. HLD is a cleaning process that kills all microorganisms except large numbers of bacterial spores. Because they are not rendered sterile, endoscopes cleaned using HLD are considered semicritical items. These endoscopes may contact broken skin or mucous membranes, which are usually resistant to common spores, but they should not contact vascular or other sterile body tissue. The FDA-approved alkylating agent Cidex-OPA is often used, as discussed earlier for laparoscopes. Submerging an endoscope in Cidex-OPA for 40 minutes is sufficient, and it should not be submerged for longer than 60 minutes. After it is removed from Cidex-OPA, the interior and exterior portions of the endoscope should be thoroughly rinsed and flushed with sterile or filtered water. If tap water is used for rinsing, 70% alcohol should be the final rinse, because tap water may contain microbes (e.g., *Pseudomonas, Mycobacterium*). The endoscope can then be purged with air and allowed to hang to dry either on a wall mount or in a well-ventilated storage cabinet.

As with the endoscope, failure to adequately clean the biopsy and retrieval instruments can spread disease. With inadequate cleaning, instruments also may not open or may break when opened. Not only should instruments be precleaned with water, followed by an enzymatic cleaner with a brush; detachable parts (e.g., valves, biopsy channel covers) should be cleaned as well. The same cleaning protocol used on the endoscope can be used on the biopsy instruments. Cleaning brushes are usually disposable, but if they are thoroughly cleaned by HLD, they can be reused. Water bottles and tubes used for endoscopic irrigation are difficult to clean and disinfect, so sterile water should be used rather than tap water.

NOTE: Reported iatrogenic infections from endoscopes not thoroughly disinfected include *Escherichia coli, Pseudomonas, Klebsiella, Serratia,* and *Salmonella.* Other organisms of concern in gastroenterology settings include *Campylobacter, Clostridium difficile,* and *Helicobacter pylori,* as well as many viral pathogens.

Biopsy forceps cups tend to lock in the position in which they dry after cleaning, which will require releasing any tension before use. If locked in a closed position, cups can be soaked in warm water or mineral oil for several seconds, then gently separated with a small-gauge needle. Once the biopsy forceps cup is open, the finger control at the top of the instrument is used to open and close the cup several times to ensure free movement. If locked in an open position, cups can be soaked for several seconds in warm water, and then gentle digital pressure can be applied to the cups to work them closed. The finger control is used to ensure that the cups are moving freely.

Rotating and Restocking Supplies

Supplies in the surgery room should be limited to an amount that would be used over a short time. Necessary supplies in the surgery room vary greatly among veterinary facilities, depending on the number and types of procedures performed and what is needed for each one. Supplies should not be excessive because increased inventory can tie up the facility's money unnecessarily. The veterinary technician plays a vital role in communicating with the veterinarians on staff about their needs for the surgery area. The veterinary technician is often the person who restocks and organizes the room. It is important to keep lines of communication open and to closely monitor the supplies used in the room. Supplies can be broken down into two categories: disposable and reusable.

Disposable Supplies

Disposable supplies consist of the supplies purchased for single-time use, such as scalpel blades, suture, and surgical gloves. These items are purchased as sterile items and usually are labeled with a date specifying when they should be "used by" or when they are considered "outdated." These items need to be checked and rotated each time the surgery area is stocked. Items with expiration dates that are shortest (or closest) should be rotated so that they are used before items with longer (further) dates. If too much stock of one item is kept in the area, the potential for outdating increases. For this reason, keep only a minimum of what is needed in a day. This practice keeps the stock rotated, and the potential for outdated items decreases.

Reusable Supplies

Reusable supplies are the items that the veterinary facility uses and resterilizes between patients. These items consist of surgery packs, clean and laundered reusable cloth drapes, hand towels, and separate instruments. These items are often cleaned after surgery, repackaged, sterilized, and placed back in the storage cabinets of the surgery room. For reusable supplies, as with disposable items, the oldest packs should be placed so that they are used first and the stock is continually rotated. If the veterinary facility has more than one spay pack, it is important to rotate the packs so that they do not fall out of the rotation.

Current practice in human medicine is that packs do not automatically become outdated after a certain number of days. An event must occur to cause the item to become nonsterile. An "event" is something that occurs to cause a breach of the item's sterility. Examples of events are opening of the pack, the pack's coming in contact with moisture, and the pack's being dropped on the floor.

Many veterinary facilities still operate on the assumption that an item is outdated after a certain arbitrary period, such as 30 days. For items sterilized in a veterinary facility, is it necessary to keep everything wrapped and sterilized, just in case it might be needed? It would be a better practice for the facility to sterilize only the items that will be needed in the next few days or weeks. Although the veterinary profession is not always predictable and emergencies do occur, not all the spay packs need to be sterile unless multiple spays are scheduled for the next day. This practice would save on storage of sterile items in the surgery room and facilitate a more organized rotation of supplies.

The veterinary profession has few legal guidelines in surgery room cleanliness and supply rotation in comparison with the human medical profession, but this does not mean these areas can be ignored. For the well-being of the patients and the financial well-being of the veterinary facility, it is important that veterinary technicians take a proactive role in establishing protocols for cleanliness, stock rotation, and sterilization of surgical items. A breakdown in any of these areas can be costly for the veterinary facility. By being organized, efficient, and detail oriented, the veterinary technician can serve the best interests of the patient, the client, and the veterinary facility.

KEY POINTS

1. Surgery rooms should be spot-cleaned after each procedure.
2. Surgery rooms should be terminally cleaned at the end of each day.
3. Mechanical friction should be applied during cleaning.
4. Disinfectants should be used according to the manufacturer's instructions.
5. There is no "ideal disinfectant," but there are many good disinfectants that meet most of the criteria of an ideal disinfectant.
6. The effectiveness of a disinfectant depends on many factors (e.g., microorganisms, contamination, organic matter).
7. The stock of disposable surgical supplies should be limited so that expiration does not occur.
8. Reusable supplies are items that are cleaned and resterilized.
9. All surgical supplies should be rotated so that the items are used in a rotating order (oldest first).
10. In event-related contamination, an event must occur to cause an item to become nonsterile (contaminated).
11. Appropriate cleaning procedures begin with a thorough presoaking of instruments to rid the items of any blood or tissue.
12. Decontamination of instruments is vital in removing debris from the instrument's box locks and hinges.
13. Lubricants make instruments easier to open and close and help prevent the buildup of protein on the instruments.
14. Ultrasonic cleaning is a critical step in removing microbes from instruments.
15. Enzymes are used to assist in the breakdown of debris to allow more thorough ultrasonic cleaning of instruments.
16. Each instrument pack should contain a "recipe" that specifies the types of instruments, quantity of each, type of wrapping material, manufacturers' guidelines, and any warranty.
17. Pack wraps are made of linen or paper and should have selective permeability, flexibility, memory, and resistance to damage.
18. Textile wraps are selected based on thread count (140-288 threads/square inch), not weight or texture.
19. Torn wraps repaired by stitching can allow an avenue for microbes to penetrate the pack, and patches can hamper steam penetration during sterilization; torn wraps should be discarded and replaced.

20. Steam indicator tape is used in securing wraps; a black stripping effect indicates that conditions were met for sterilization.
21. Guidelines for preparing a pack for sterilization address the items' condition, wrap material, standardization of contents, compatibility with autoclave, folding of soft items, use of similar wrapping methods, placement of indicator strips, and sealing of the outer pack.
22. Expiration dating may be used for packs with items that degrade over time (e.g., latex tubing).
23. Sterilization takes place after presoaking, decontaminating, and ultrasonic cleaning. The sterilization process rids the instruments of any living microbes.
24. Sterilization depends on three factors: proper sterilizer operation, proper pack preparation, and proper loading.
25. Gravity air-displacement sterilization is typically done on a tabletop. Steam enters the chamber by gravity and is set at a lower pressure.
26. High-vacuum sterilizers force steam into the sterilizer chamber for quicker penetration.
27. If a separate area is unavailable for proper pack preparation, it can be done in the preparation area for surgical personnel.
28. Flash sterilization is used for items dropped in the surgery suite.
29. Use of ethylene oxide is an excellent means to sterilize instruments and supplies wrapped in paper and plastic, but health and environmental risk factors have decreased its use over the years.
30. Plasma sterilization offers a safe technique for sterilization, but it is not an effective means of sterilizing items with lumens.
31. Chemical and biologic indicators determine whether items have been properly sterilized. Biologic indicators show that the sterilizer has met all the sterilization parameters.
32. Alcohol exhibits strong bactericidal properties but may not kill spores or viruses. Glutaraldehyde is considered a high-level disinfectant and is bactericidal, tuberculocidal, and virucidal.
33. Orthopedic drills should not be immersed in liquid and should be cleaned with a foaming disinfectant and alcohol before sterilization.
34. Maintaining endoscopes involves proper cleaning and disinfection, leak testing and inspection, microbial monitoring, and storage.

REVIEW QUESTIONS

1. In what room should anal sac surgeries and abscessed wounds be lanced and flushed?
   a. In the surgery room.
   b. In the preparation room.
   c. In the scrub room.
   d. In the examination room.

2. What items should be located in the scrub area/room?
   a. Hair clippers.
   b. Scrub sink.
   c. Autoclave.
   d. Table/counter to hold open gown packs.
   e. Answers b, c, and d.

3. *True or False:* All procedures should be performed in the surgery room, whether they are considered "clean" or "dirty."

4. *True or False:* The surgery room needs to have easy access, so doors should not be placed between surgery rooms and scrub or prep areas.

5. *True or False:* The air pressure in the surgery room should be greater than that in the rest of the hospital to reduce the influx of bacteria into the surgery room.

6. *True or False:* Movable equipment (i.e., equipment that is not permanently affixed) in the surgery room should not leave the surgery room.

7. When movable equipment is removed from the surgery room:
   a. It should not be brought back into the surgery room.
   b. It should be thoroughly cleaned and disinfected before being returned to the surgery room.
   c. It is considered contaminated and must be sterilized before being returned to the surgery room.
   d. It can be returned directly to the surgery room when it is no longer needed outside the surgery room.

8. In the absence of cleaning instructions from the manufacturer, stethoscopes, blood pressure cuffs, and other noncritical items can be cleaned in what manner for use in the surgery room?
   a. Autoclaved.
   b. Immersed in high-level disinfectants.
   c. Cleaned and then disinfected with alcohol.
   d. Put through a cycle in a washing machine or dishwasher.
   e. None of the above.

9. How often should the surgery room floor be cleaned?
   a. Only as needed.
   b. Daily.
   c. Morning and evening.
   d. Weekly.
   e. It does not matter.

10. *True or False:* Surgery rooms should be cleaned daily whether they are used or not.

11. Why are refillable soap dispensers not recommended for use in the surgery prep or scrub area?
    a. They always run out just when they are needed.
    b. They take too long to refill if they run out of soap during the hand prep process.
    c. They can harbor bacterial growth.
    d. All of the above.
    e. None of the above.

12. What is the difference between antiseptics and disinfectants?
    a. Antiseptics are intended for use on living tissues, and disinfectants are intended for inanimate objects.
    b. Antiseptics are intended for use on inanimate objects, and disinfectants are intended for living tissues.
    c. There is no difference, and they are used interchangeably.
    d. Antiseptics are used daily, and disinfectants are only used weekly.
    e. Disinfectants are sporicidal, bactericidal, and virucidal, whereas antiseptics are only bactericidal and virucidal.

13. Regarding disinfectants, what does "contact time" refer to?
    a. The time required for the disinfectant to be in contact with the microorganisms to achieve its intended effect (i.e., significantly reduce the number of microorganisms).
    b. The time of day when the manufacturer can be contacted for assistance.
    c. The time required for a microorganism to develop resistance to the disinfectant.
    d. The latent phase of microorganisms, giving the disinfectant a "window of opportunity" to kill the microorganisms.

14. Which of the following affect a disinfectant's effectiveness?
    a. Amount of protein present in the area.
    b. Type of microorganisms present.
    c. Concentration of the disinfectant.
    d. Both b and c.
    e. All of the above.

15. What is the correct order of events used to achieve the level of disinfection required for surgical supplies and instruments?
    a. Decontaminate→sanitize→sterilize.
    b. Clean→sanitize→sterilize.
    c. Sterilize→sanitize→decontaminate.
    d. Sterilize→ sanitize→clean.
    e. None of the above.

16. Basic cleaning of surgical instruments involves which order of the following steps?
    a. Presoaking→decontaminating→ultrasonic cleaning.
    b. Ultrasonic cleaning→rinsing→lubricating.
    c. Decontaminating→ultrasonic cleaning→presoaking.
    d. None of the above.

17. What is the purpose of presoaking?
    a. To scrub the instruments with mechanical cleaning.
    b. To prevent blood and other surgical debris from drying on the instruments.
    c. To soften blood and other surgical debris already dried on the instruments.
    d. Both b and c.
    e. All of the above.

18. What process involves manually cleaning surgical instruments in a detergent?
    a. Presoaking.
    b. Decontaminating.
    c. Sterilizing.
    d. All of the above.
    e. None of the above.

19. After ultrasonic cleaning, instruments:
    a. Are ready for sterilizing.
    b. Should be rinsed with distilled water.
    c. Should be individually inspected and towel-dried.
    d. Should be rinsed in tap water and air-dried.

20. *True or False:* Steam indicator tape is recommended for securing the wrapping material of an instrument pack.

21. *True or False:* Both the inner and the outer wraps of a surgical pack should be closed with steam indicator tape.

22. What are two methods used to identify how long a previously sterilized item is considered sterile?
    a. Expiration dating and event-related expiration of sterility.
    b. Double wrapping or single wrapping.
    c. Autoclaving or ethylene oxide sterilizing.
    d. Paper- or linen-wrapped packs.
    e. High-level disinfecting or gas plasma disinfecting.

23. Which of the following are acceptable ways to sterilize items for use in surgery?
    a. Gravity air-displacement autoclave.
    b. High-vacuum autoclave.
    c. Ethylene oxide unit.
    d. All of the above.
    e. None of the above.

24. What is an example of a chemical sterilization indicator?
    a. Steam indicator tape.
    b. Vial of *Bacillus stearothermophilus*.
    c. Both a and b.
    d. None of the above.

25. *True or False:* Power drills used in orthopedic surgery should not be submerged in liquids (high-level disinfectants) or cleaned in ultrasonic units.

26. *True or False:* Endoscopes are routinely submerged in high-level disinfectants rather than steam-sterilized.

ANSWERS

1. b	8. c	15. b	22. a
2. e	9. b	16. a	23. d
3. False	10. True	17. d	24. a
4. False	11. c	18. b	25. True
5. True	12. a	19. b	26. True
6. True	13. a	20. True	
7. b	14. e	21. False	

BIBLIOGRAPHY

Adler S, Scherrer M, Daschner FD: Cost of low temperature plasma sterilization compared with other sterilization methods. J Hosp Infect 40:125, 1998.

Association of periOperative Registered Nurses: Recommended practices for environmental cleaning in the surgical practice setting. AORN J 76:1071, 2002.

Blankenau R: Shedding light on flash sterilization. Mater Manag Health Care 3:32, 1994.

Carlile F: Sterilization or disinfection: that is the question. Surg Technologist 27:8, 1995.

Catanzaro T: Veterinary Practice Building Design Starter Kit, ed 2, Denver, 1990, American Animal Hospital Association.

Centers for Disease Control and Prevention (CDC), Healthcare Infection Control Practices Advisory Committee (HICPAC): Draft Guidelines for Environmental Infection Control in Healthcare Facilities, Atlanta, 2001, CDC.

Copich W: Avoiding the common errors made in the designing of animal hospitals. Vet Clin North Am 2:537, 1972.

Crawford L, et al: A comparison of commonly used surface disinfectants. Infect Control Today Nov, 2000. Available at http://www.infectioncontroltoday.com/articles/0b1feat2.html.

Detwiler MS: Ultrasonic cleaning in the hospital. J Healthc Mater Manage 7:46, 1989.

Frey KB: The new alternative: plasma sterilization. Surg Technologist 26:8, 1994.

Harrison SK, Evans WJ Jr, LeBlanc DA, et al: Cleaning and decontaminating medical instruments. J Healthc Mater Manage 8:36, 1990.

Kennedy J, Bek J, Griffin D: Selection and use of disinfectants, Lincoln, NB, 2000, Institute of Agriculture and Natural Resources, University of Nebraska, Available at http://ianrpubs.unl.edu/animaldisease/g1410.htm.

Klapes NA, Greene VW, Langholz AC, et al: Effects of long term storage on sterile status of devices in surgical packs. Infect Control 8:289, 1987.

Lind D: Steam sterilization. J Healthc Mater Manage 12:56, 1994.

Lind N: Cleaning in decontamination. J Healthc Mater Manage 12:48, 1994.

Magne ML, Tams TR: Laparoscopy: instrumentation and technique. In Tams TR, editor: Small animal endoscopy, ed 2, St Louis, 1999, Mosby.

Mathias JM: Draft guideline on processing practices. OR Manager 18:7, 2002.

O'Connor LM: Event-related sterility assurance. Surg Technologist 26:8, 1994.

Recommended practices for environmental cleaning in the surgical practice setting. Association of Operating Room Nurses. AORN J 67:448, 1998.

Reichert M, Schultz JK: Coping with drills and other powered equipment, OR Manager 18:21, 2002.

Reichert M, Schultz JK: When and how to use ultrasonic cleaning, OR Manager 14:20, 1998.

Sacred cow survey. OR Manager 14:1, 1998.

Schumway R, Broussard J: Maintenance of gastrointestinal endoscopes. Clin Tech Small Anim Pract 18:254, 2003.

Simmons BL: Fundamentals of cleaning: the effects of water and detergents. J Sterile Serv Manage 5:16, 1987.

Thro E: Surgical instruments: their care and characteristics. J OR Res Inst 3:3, 1983.

Client Education for Postoperative Care

Marianne Tear

10

LEARNING OBJECTIVES

After completion of this chapter, the reader will be able to:
- Provide instructions to the owner describing the proper care of a patient after general anesthesia.
- Provide instructions to the client describing proper care of a patient with postoperative drains.
- Describe client education for postoperative care of a patient with a bandage, splint, or cast.
- Provide instructions to the owner describing proper care of a patient after the following surgical procedures:
  - *Tooth extraction*
  - *Gastrointestinal surgery*
  - *Feeding tube placement*
  - *Cystotomy*
  - *Declaw*
  - *Aural hematoma*
  - *Ear canal resection or ablation*
  - *Orthopedic surgery*
  - *Cesarean section*

Discharge Instructions

The role of the veterinary technician does not end when the patient is ready to go home; the owner (client) must be taught how to care for the animal properly. The responsibility for explaining the patient's aftercare to the owner is typically assigned to the veterinary technician. This is a logical policy because the technician has been the postoperative caregiver and understands the patient's needs and reactions. Every patient cannot be treated in the same manner. The approach to providing the prescribed treatments is dictated by the patient's reaction and willingness to cooperate. The veterinary technician assigned to care for the patient has determined which restraint techniques work, what method to use to administer oral medication, and how effective the analgesic drugs have been for the patient. Areas to discuss with the client include timing of drug administration, wound care, and daily walks. For example, antibiotics and analgesics may be administered with a meal. The wound care should be delayed for about an hour after the analgesic is given. This technician knows the patient, can advocate for the patient, and can best educate the owner on how to care for the patient.

Postoperative education can begin before the actual procedure is started. Providing the client with a generalized handout on the procedure (Figure 10-1) can give him/her the opportunity to become familiar with the condition. By having information on the causes, signs, and follow-up care, the client will feel more actively involved. Many clients then come to the discharge with questions of their own.

In addition to the verbal discussion, written instructions explaining how to care for the postoperative patient should be sent home with the client. The hospital often has generic instructions that are prepared for all routine postoperative patients. Special instructions are added for certain nonroutine surgical procedures or medical conditions. However, each patient is an individual, and each client appreciates and deserves an explanation of the specific observations of the pet's reactions and the specific care techniques used. The veterinary technician personally discharging the pet to its owner can provide this communication. It is best to explain the discharge instructions in a quiet area of the clinic. The client's full attention needs to be directed to the technician's instructions, so the animal should not be brought to the client until all the information has been provided. Alternatively, the veterinary technician can write out special instructions and add these to the generic instructions (Figure 10-2).

Regardless of the type of procedure that was performed, the technician must be certain that all the client's questions have been answered. In a busy hospital a technician may discharge ten animals who have undergone spay procedures in a single day. It is easy to talk at the client rather than with them. The technician should include the owner in the discussion by asking non-leading questions to make sure the information has been understood. "What time will you be feeding Fluffy tonight?" allows for more interaction than "You understand what time to feed Fluffy, right?" The client's response to the first question allows the technician to gauge the client's understanding of postoperative feeding.

General Postanesthesia Instructions

All patients that have been under sedation or general anesthesia should go home with instructions regarding their care for at least the first 24 hours. The instruction sheet should address (1) confinement, (2) feeding, (3) medications, (4) signs of possible adverse reactions, and (5) how to reach the hospital or 24-hour emergency

clinic. If possible, a contact person, such as the technician, should also be listed. This helps personalize the treatment and makes the client feel more comfortable contacting the clinic with questions or concerns.

The client may need to confine the pet to a recovery crate or room. The pet may still be sedated and unable to walk normally. The pet may need to be accompanied or carried up and down stairs. Other pets in the household may disturb the patient, and it may be preferable to have the patient isolated from other animal housemates for a specified time. Over the long term it may be necessary to keep cats inside and to walk dogs only with a leash.

The owner needs instructions regarding when and how much to feed the animal after returning home. The time to resume the normal feeding schedule should also be addressed. The technician should take the time to discuss the possibility of nausea after anesthesia. The owner should be instructed to start with water first and then offer smaller meals more frequently to the patient. Special diets may be prescribed and may be introduced gradually. The technician should give detailed examples of how to mix the new food in with the old to prevent gastrointestinal (GI) upset. Also, the owner should be given some helpful suggestions on how to make the new food more palatable—heating, adding water, and so on. Specific instructions regarding the special diet should be written in the space provided on the postoperative form.

Medications may be sent home with the patient. Specific instructions regarding their administration are written on the label of the medication bottle. The instructions are repeated on the discharge instructions with more details, including whether the medication should be administered with food or on an empty stomach. In addition, the necessity of giving one medication at a separate time from other medications can be explained to the owner at discharge. Colored labels can be preprinted and placed on the medication bottles to help the owner remember specific requirements. Also, possible side effects of the medication should be addressed.

Animals under anesthesia or sedation may experience undesirable side effects. GI motility may be slowed down (ileus), which may cause inappetence, vomiting, constipation, or bloating. Lethargy, ataxia, and/or depression may be a symptom of prolonged recovery from anesthesia. These symptoms should be discussed with the client or listed on the instruction sheet. The informed owner will be an observant advocate for the patient.

Finally, instructions should be clearly provided regarding how to reach the hospital or a referral emergency center 24 hours a day.

General Postsurgical Instructions

In addition to the postoperative instructions already mentioned, the client is instructed on the need to observe the patient's surgical site. The integrity of the surgical site

Dystocia in Dogs and Cats

Ronald M. Bright, DVM, MS, DACVS

BASIC INFORMATION

Description

Dystocia is the inability to initiate the act of labor or the delivery of pups or kittens at the end of a pregnancy. Dog breeds at increased risk for dystocia include the Yorkshire terrier, miniature poodle, Pomeranian, English bulldog, dachshund, Chihuahua, and Scottish terrier.

Causes

The causes of dystocia can generally be classified into those caused by the mother and those caused by the fetus.

Uterine inertia is a condition in which the uterine muscles either do not contract (primary uterine inertia) or become fatigued during labor (secondary uterine inertia) from persistent straining against an obstruction within the birth canal. Secondary uterine inertia is almost never the sole cause of dystocia.

A narrow birth canal caused by a previous fracture of the pelvis can prevent passage of the fetus. The head of the fetus may be too large to pass through the birth canal, or the fetus may be oversized or malformed. Sometimes an improper position of the fetus as it approaches the birth canal makes passage difficult.

Psychological stress can delay the onset of labor. A rare cause of dystocia is twisting of the uterus on itself (uterine torsion).

Clinical Signs

The following are signs of dystocia:

- Active straining has occurred for more than 30-60 minutes without the birth of a fetus.
- Straining for 2 or more hours has not resulted in delivery of a fetus.
- The resting stage between expulsion of fetuses is greater than 4 hours and there is no sign of straining even though it is known that more fetuses remain in the uterus.
- Signs of systemic illness, such as vomiting, weakness, or fever, are present.
- Abnormal vaginal discharge, such as frank blood or pus, is present.
- The pregnancy is known to be a high risk (predisposed breed); only one, large fetus is present; or narrowing of the birth canal has occurred from a prior pelvic fracture.
- Attempts to expel a fetus are painful.
- Obvious signs of distress are present.

Diagnostic Tests

The diagnosis of dystocia is often derived from the clinical signs and a thorough physical examination. Other tests that may be recommended include x-rays, an abdominal ultrasound, and laboratory tests, such as measurement of blood calcium levels. Low blood calcium may be associated with uterine inertia. Commercially available external whelping monitors can be used to detect diminished fetal viability (fetal stress) and abnormal patterns in the uterine contractions.

TREATMENT AND FOLLOW-UP

Treatment Options

The treatment of dystocia varies, depending on the underlying cause. If a fetus has passed part of the way through the birth canal but is now caught, it may be possible to dislodge the fetus through cautious use of fingers or instruments. Administering a tranquilizer to relieve stress in an apprehensive bitch or queen may be helpful.

If uterine inertia is diagnosed, medical therapy may be attempted, provided that the birth canal is a normal size, the cervix is open, the fetus is not too large to pass through the canal, and no other obstruction is identified. Medical therapy involves administration of the hormone, oxytocin, to stimulate uterine contractions. If calcium levels are low, supplementation of calcium is indicated, because it enhances uterine contractions and increases the effects of oxytocin.

If medical therapy fails, surgery to perform a cesarean section (C-section) is indicated. Your veterinarian may discuss the option of spaying the mother at the time of the cesarean section. If there are no further plans for breeding the mother or if a uterine rupture is present, ovariohysterectomy (spaying) may be recommended.

Follow-up Care and Prognosis

Following resolution of the current dystocia, emphasis must be placed on preventing dystocia during future pregnancies. Such measures include providing consistent and adequate amounts of exercise during the pregnancy and making sure the mother is fed a well-balanced diet.

To increase the chances of an optimal litter size, it is often recommended that bitches be bred 2 days after ovulation. All queens and bitches should be provided a quiet, dark, stress-free, and sanitary birthing environment.

FIGURE 10-1 Example of a client handout explaining dystocia in dogs and cats. (From Morgan R: Small animal practice: client handouts. St Louis, 2010, Saunders/Elsevier.)

DISCHARGE INSTRUCTIONS
Elsewhere Veterinary Clinic
123 Street Road
Somewhere, USA
123-555-1234

Client name:_____ Patient's name: _____

Date admitted: _____ Date discharged: _____

Procedure or diagnosis: _____

Medications:
- ☐ None dispensed
- ☐ Dispensed—directions on medication bottle
- ☐ Start medication _____

Food and water:
- ☐ Only offer ___ cup water and _____ food today
- ☐ Offer normal meal tonight
- ☐ Normal feeding may resume _____

         Special diet _____

Exercise:
- ☐ Restrict running, jumping, playing until _____
- ☐ If cat, confine indoors for _____ days
- ☐ If dog, leash walk only for _____ days

Sutures:
- ☐ Discourage your pet from licking or chewing at incision site.

    If excessive licking or chewing occurs, please call the clinic for a collar to prevent this.

- ☐ Check the incision daily for swelling, redness, or discharge.

    If it appears irritated, swollen, or bleeding please notify us.

- ☐ **Please make an appointment for suture removal in _____ days.**
- ☐ Sutures are absorbable and do not need to be removed.
- ☐ No sutures.

Please notify the clinic if any of the following occur:

- ☐ Loss of appetite for more than _____ days
- ☐ Pain
- ☐ Straining to urinate/defecate

- ☐ Excess drainage from incision
- ☐ Excessive vomiting/diarrhea
- ☐ Depression

*Special instructions: _____
_____
_____
_____
_____
_____

Emergency clinic numbers:_____

Veterinarian's signature: _____

FIGURE 10-2 Example of general postoperative instructions for clients (owners) after a veterinary patient's discharge.

should be monitored at least twice daily. The number of sutures should be counted. The client should observe for swelling, redness, and discharge. If sutures are missing or if excessive swelling, discharge, or redness is noted, the owner should be instructed to call the veterinary hospital.

The owner is encouraged to call for advice regarding the management of the patient and any changes involving the surgical site. If possible, the owner should be shown pictures of a normally healing incision and then pictures of seromas, hematomas, and inflamed incisions. This knowledge will allow the owner to better understand the terms and conditions being described.

Specific instructions on confining the pet should be discussed with the owner. Each situation is unique, and residences vary, for example, in the presence and number of stairs to the outside. Other pets in the household may necessitate new routines regarding feeding, litter boxes, and walks outside. Children may need to be restricted from handling the pet until the patient is fully recovered. During the pet's recuperative phase at home, the family's routines and lifestyle will be disrupted, which can be stressful. The technicians should remind the client that the pet cannot articulate their pain or discomfort; it becomes vitally important for the client to track changes, improvements, or declines in behavior. These small clues can help the veterinary staff determine whether the animal is progressing as anticipated or there might be underlying complications.

If the animal is sent home with an Elizabethan collar (E-collar) or a BiteNot Collar (BiteNot Products, Inc., San Francisco), the technician needs to stress the importance of leaving the collar in place. Removing the collar for even a short period of time can lead to disaster; it only takes a matter of seconds for the animal to remove the skin sutures or completely open the incision. The owner should also be advised that the collar will not prevent the other animals in the household from licking the site and causing damage. An E-collar can also impede the animal's ability to eat or drink. Even properly fitted collars can touch the floor around the food bowl before the animal can reach the food with its mouth or can hit the bowl itself and prevent eating. If this occurs, the animal should be provided with elevated bowls and/or bowls with a smaller diameter.

If possible, before leaving the hospital, appointments are scheduled for rechecks, suture removal, and drain removal. The hospital should also have a policy on calling the client to check on the animal's progress. Many clients assume that abnormal behavior is common after surgery. Having the technician call 24 hours after discharge and then at a preset time (times) after that can put clients at ease; they will also be more likely to voice what they may feel are minor concerns.

Postoperative Care of Patients with Drains

Many surgical procedures involve the implanting of drains. These devices are temporarily placed to channel unwanted fluid or gas from a wound or body cavity. Often the patient is sent home with a passive drain. The owner is required to clean the discharge from the drain site and ensure that the drain is not disturbed by the patient. Clear and detailed instructions regarding drain care are important. Owners should also be informed that the discharge from an unbandaged drain can get on to furniture, carpet, and clothing. In multi-pet households the owner should also be reminded that the E-collar will not prevent the other animals from licking at the site or removing the drain.

FIGURE 10-3 Care of postoperative drains. Clean the area where the drain exits the wound with a warm compress of gauze. Apply warm soaks to the area to soften the discharge. Once the discharge is soft and loose, wipe the area clean.

The owner needs a demonstration of as well as written instructions regarding the care of the surgical site with the drain. Warm soaks to loosen and remove dried serous discharge will be necessary (Figure 10-3). The skin may need to be protected from the development of a moist dermatitis caused by contact with the discharge. A thin film of petroleum jelly can be spread over the area where the discharge tends to dry to the skin. The petrolatum serves as a protective barrier and facilitates skin cleaning.

Inadequate cleaning of discharge can prevent the drain from functioning and block further discharge. Fluid then becomes trapped under the wound or in the body cavity. This will slow the healing process or compromise a successful outcome in other ways. The veterinary technician must emphasize to the client the importance of proper and thorough cleaning of the drain site.

The client also needs instructions about effective restraint of the pet while the drain is being cleaned. The technician who has been caring for the patient knows the most effective means to restrain the patient safely and effectively. If possible, this technician should be present when the patient is discharged. These "customized" instructions can be written on the discharge information form in the area for special instructions.

If the pet pulls out the drain, the owner should report this to the clinic. The owner should search for any parts or pieces of the drain. These pieces can help the veterinary technician determine whether a portion of the drain is still in the patient. If a piece of the drain remains deep in the wound or body cavity, it will need to be surgically retrieved.

Postoperative Care of Patients with a Bandage, Splint, or Cast

When a bandage, splint, or cast has been applied to a limb, the pet should be kept quiet. Cats are confined indoors and restricted from jumping. Dogs may need to be

FIGURE 10-4 *Patient relaxing at home with an unbandaged feeding tube.*

confined in a recovery crate. Play with other dogs and humans in the household must be suspended. Dogs are walked only by leash.

Weekly in-hospital rechecks should be scheduled. The owner is instructed to examine the pet carefully each day and note the condition of the bandage and the extremity (Box 10-1). Toes should be checked for smell, warmth, and color. Foul odor can indicate tissue damage under the bandage; if swelling is occurring the toes will move apart, or if the bandage is too tight, the toes may become cyanotic or extremely pale. In the event that any abnormalities are noted, the owner should be instructed to contact the hospital for bandage removal and or replacement. The client should be made aware of the serious complications that can arise from a damaged bandage.

The owner is given instructions regarding how to protect the cast, bandage, or splint from wet grass, snow, puddles, and other sources of moisture. A plastic bag taped to the limb can effectively cover and protect the bandage (cast, splint) while the pet is outside. Empty fluid bags are made of heavy plastic that holds up well to repeated use. The bag should be removed as soon as the pet is back inside because the animal's body heat can create condensation within the bag, leading to a moist bandage.

Postoperative Instructions for Common Procedures
Dental Extraction

While the mouth is healing after a tooth extraction, the pet will have a soft-food diet, such as canned, semi-moist

pet food or dry food soaked in water until mushy. The socket will heal in 1 to 2 weeks. During the healing phase the pet may be gradually returned to his/her usual dry-food diet.

The client should watch for a number of specific signs. For the first day the owner may see the water in the bowl tinged red after the pet drinks. If this does not subside, the veterinarian should be notified. Long-term bleeding from the mouth indicates delayed healing, infection, or a coagulation problem. The pet rubbing or pawing at its face is an indication of pain, and the veterinarian should be notified. Crying out while eating or refusing to eat any hard food after several days to weeks have passed indicates an ongoing problem. The patient that refuses to eat will not heal promptly or properly.

Feeding Tube Placement

An enteral feeding tube may be placed for many reasons to aid in the patient's nutritional support (see Chapter 8). This tube may stay in place for many weeks. Because of the critical support the feeding tube provides and the possible long-term need for it, the client caring for the patient at home requires detailed instructions on the tube's use and care (Box 10-2; Figure 10-4).

Commercially prepared liquid diets (e.g., CliniCare, Jevity) are mandated when the tube has a very small diameter. Gastric and esophageal tubes are often large enough in diameter that pureed canned pet foods can be used in larger patients. It is important that large chunks of food be eliminated during preparation and not be forced down the tube.

Gastrointestinal Enterotomy or Anastomosis

Surgery of the GI tract is indicated to remove foreign body obstructions, collect tissue biopsy samples, remove growths, and resect diseased areas of intestine (e.g., cancer,

BOX 10-2 Client Instructions for Care and Use of a Feeding Tube

1. When cleaning the area where the tube exits the skin, warm water soaks may be needed to soften any dried discharge. The discharge may be clear or slightly red tinged. Thick, cloudy, or foul-smelling discharge may indicate an infection at the site. Adding an antiseptic cleanser, such as chlorhexidine at a 1:40 dilution, helps kill microbial invaders. (However, this may not be necessary for a normally healing site.) An antiseptic ointment or plain petroleum jelly can be applied to help with the removal of dried discharge, and the site is covered with a light bandage or stockinette if the veterinarian chooses. The end of the feeding tube should be incorporated in the bandage. The skin site should be inspected and cleaned one or two times daily, or with each feeding.

2. During inspection of the tube, a measurement should be taken to ensure that the tube is the same length; using a permanent marker a line can be drawn on the tube at skin level to help ensure that the tube does not migrate. If the tube length has changed, the tube has migrated. An Elizabethan collar helps prevent the patient from pulling out the tube with its teeth.

3. Before and after each feeding, the tube is flushed with 10-15 mL of warm water. The end of the tube is securely plugged with a Luer-Slip catheter plug between feedings.

4. If the tube becomes clogged, instilling carbonated water (soft drinks, soda) repeatedly into the tube will eventually dislodge most obstructions. If the owner is unable to open the tube in this way, the veterinarian must be notified.

5. In regard to feeding, the technician or veterinarian will have calculated the exact dietary amount that will be administered at each feeding based on the patient's weight, body condition, and disease state.

6. Liquid medications may be administered through the feeding tube. Flushing with warm water is necessary before and after medication administration as well as after feeding.

7. The patient should also have food available to eat during the day. Using measured feedings will allow the owner to monitor the amount being consumed. As soon as the patient is eating on his/her own and able to maintain his/her caloric needs, the feeding tube can be pulled. Ideally the animal will be completely self-feeding for 2 weeks prior to tube removal without any weight loss occurring.

---

necrosis, intussusception). Fluid therapy is continued until the animal is drinking and not vomiting. Feeding is resumed after the animal is able to consume water without vomiting. Prophylactic antibiotic therapy is typically discontinued within hours postoperatively.

Animals recovering from GI surgery need to be observed with great care. If the intestinal surgical site does not hold and intestinal contents leak into the abdominal cavity, a serious infection will ensue. This complication, peritonitis, can occur within hours or days after surgery. Peritonitis is an extremely painful condition that responds only slightly to analgesics. The patient will also have a fever, so postoperative monitoring of body temperature is important. If the patient spikes a fever, laboratory procedures (e.g., complete blood count) may be ordered. As peritonitis progresses, fluid accumulates in the abdominal cavity, and the patient appears bloated. An abdominocentesis procedure may be performed to obtain a culture sample, and abdominal ultrasound may be helpful in diagnosing peritonitis.

The owner should be instructed to monitor the patient closely at home immediately following and for several weeks postoperatively for signs of peritonitis (Box 10-3)

Two other postoperative concerns may not appear for weeks or months. First, the intestinal lumen may narrow because of scar formation. Second, a small, slow leak from the enterotomy site can lead to an abdominal abscess. Both complications may cause clinical signs associated with an obstruction. If an abdominal abscess has formed, vomiting, anorexia, lack of bowel movements, and abdominal pain may occur.

BOX 10-3 Client Postoperative Instructions Following Gastrointestinal or Anastomosis Surgery

1. Check the abdominal incision daily for redness, swelling, discharge, and tenderness.
2. Monitor the pet's temperature twice daily, if possible. If a fever is detected, the hospital should be notified.
3. Alert the hospital if vomiting, diarrhea, constipation, or inappetence occurs.
4. Alert the hospital if the patient appears unusually lethargic or in excessive pain.
5. Alert the hospital if the patient appears bloated.

Perianal Surgery

Surgery around and involving the anus is indicated for removal of tumors, débridement and drainage of fistulas and anal sacs, and removal of anal sacs. In addition to the general postsurgical instructions, special instructions should be given to the client (Box 10-4).

Cystotomy

One major concern following bladder surgery is bladder distension. To prevent the bladder from becoming overly distended, the patient needs to be able to and allowed to empty his/her bladder frequently. See Box 10-5 for postoperative instructions for the owner of a pet with a procedure involving surgical incision of the bladder (cystotomy).

BOX 10-4 Client Postoperative Instructions Following Perianal Surgery

1. A special diet high in fiber may be prescribed to keep the stools soft. The diet may or may not be a permanent change.
2. Stool softeners such as lactulose may be prescribed for short-term therapy.
3. If diarrhea occurs, the veterinary hospital should be notified. Discontinue the stool softener, and clean the surgical site by flushing thoroughly with warm tap water. Do not scrub the site.
4. Observe the pet while it passes a bowel movement. If the pet is straining or crying in pain, the veterinary hospital should be notified. Fecal incontinence, inability to stop or leakage of feces, also warrants hospital contact.

BOX 10-5 Client Postoperative Instructions Following a Cystotomy

1. Expect bloody urine (hematuria) for 12 to 36 hours. The amount of blood in the urine should diminish as time passes. The owner can monitor the color of the urine by lining the litter box with a white paper towel or placing a white paper towel under the pet when it urinates. Blood in the urine is more easily observed when soaked into a white paper towel.
2. A special diet may be prescribed. Instructions may recommend a gradual change to the new diet by mixing the previous and new diets together for several days.
3. Antibiotic therapy may be prescribed. The choice of antibiotic may change when the results of the urine culture and sensitivity test are known.
4. The dog should be walked outside frequently, and the amount and color of the urine should be monitored. Having the dog urinate on a white paper towel is helpful.
5. If the pet is straining to urinate or exhibiting pain when urinating, the hospital should be notified.
6. If the pet is not passing urine, it should be immediately examined. This is an emergency. Stones remaining in the bladder or blood clots in the bladder can cause obstructions.

BOX 10-6 Client Postoperative Instructions Following an Onychectomy

1. Shredded paper, dried beans, or a pelleted paper product replaces clay or clumping litter. The paper litter is less likely to leave foreign material in the surgical sites. If the paper sticks to the surgical wounds, it is easily seen and removed.
2. The cat should be restricted from jumping and running. This may mean "crating" the cat during the recuperative period.
3. If swelling of a toe is noted or the cat is non-weight bearing on one paw, the hospital should be notified.
4. Bleeding from the toes is not expected postoperatively. The hospital should be notified if bleeding from the toes occurs.
5. The cat should be kept inside for the remainder of its life because it will not be able to protect itself.

BOX 10-7 Client Postoperative Instructions Following an Aural Hematoma

1. The area where the drain exits the pinna needs to be cleaned of discharge. Warm water and a clean face towel or gauze work well. The drains usually stay in for 2 to 3 weeks (Figure 10-5).
2. Some animals may also need to have an infected ear canal treated with topical drops and ear cleansers. The pinna may be sore to the touch, so take extra care when instilling medication into the ear canal.
3. Some patients may have their head wrapped in a bandage. The same observations outlined earlier for extremity bandages apply to head bandages. Watch for soiling, slipping, moisture, foul odor, and skin irritation along the edges of the bandage.

Feline Declaw (Onychectomy)

An onychectomy is a painful procedure regardless of the method used. Pain management preoperatively, perioperatively, and postoperatively will ensure that the patient recovers quickly and with few complications. Owners need to understand that jumping must be forbidden, because the force of even the smallest jump could damage the paws. This may mean confining the cat to a small bathroom or even a kennel during the healing processes. Even though the site of the phalange removal is covered or closed, it still needs to be treated like any other surgical incision. The paws should be checked daily for swelling, redness, discharge, and odor. Clay or clumping litter should be replaced as it can leave material in the surgical site (Box 10-6).

Aural Hematoma

Aural hematomas are typically messy, and the bandaging can be quite distressing to the owner. The technician needs to stress the importance of treating the underlying cause of the hematoma as well as keeping the pinna clean (Box 10-7).

Lateral Ear Canal Resection or Ablation

The ear canal is ablated, or surgically removed, when it is so chronically diseased that medical treatment is unable to establish a healthy canal. This surgery is a last resort. The theory is that if the diseased part is removed, the pain and discomfort will disappear. Part or all of the ear canal can be removed. If the entire ear canal is removed, the pet may be rendered deaf in that ear.

FIGURE 10-5 Aural hematoma repair using soft Penrose drain.

The pet is usually not released to the owner's care until the need for daily bandage changes has passed and all drains have been removed. Postoperative infection may be caused by preexisting disease or contamination during surgery. Facial nerve paralysis is a well-recognized complication that usually resolves within 2 weeks. In some patients the vestibular system can be adversely affected when the entire ear canal is ablated. In these cases the pet exhibits a head tilt, nystagmus, and difficulty walking. Overall, many complications may occur, and intensive nursing care in the hospital setting is needed for a variable time after ear canal resection or ablation surgery.

The patient typically tries to scratch at the surgical site. An Elizabethan collar is an important piece of equipment used to help protect the integrity of the surgical site. Postoperative pain often drives the pet to self-trauma. Lateral ear canal resection or ear canal ablation tends to be very painful. Administration of analgesic medication and close observation of the surgical site are the owner's primary directives.

Orthopedic Procedures

The client with a pet that underwent orthopedic surgery should receive postoperative instructions specific to that procedure. The animal may need additional support such as a bandage, cast, or non–weight-bearing sling. Exercise and even moderate activity may be severely restricted for weeks or months. Extensive pain management may also be indicated. See Box 10-8 for general home care instructions following orthopedic procedures.

Cesarean Section

After a cesarean section, the mother and newborns are kept apart until all have completely recovered from anesthesia. The neonates are at risk of being crushed if introduced to a mother that is still heavily sedated or ataxic. Even when fully recovered, the mother may reject the newborns. The staff must watch the mother carefully for any sign of aggression toward the neonates.

BOX 10-8 Client Postoperative Instructions Following an Orthopedic Procedure

1. The pet will need to be confined. Dogs are walked only by leash. Cats must stay indoors during the recuperative period. Excessive activity and exercise can slow the healing process by allowing weight bearing too early or causing excessive movement of the affected joint or fracture site.
2. Dogs especially may need help standing and walking. A bath towel can be placed under the abdomen or chest to act as a sling (Figure 10-6).
3. If a bandage or cast has been applied, the owner receives specific instructions regarding its care (see Box 10-1).
4. If the patient has an external fixation device, the stainless steel pins and connecting pieces need particular attention, as follows:
   - The site where the pin exits the skin will not heal while the pin is in place. Dried discharge is cleaned from the area once or twice daily as needed. An antimicrobial ointment can be applied to the skin around the exit site.
   - The connecting pieces are covered with tape to prevent sharp edges from catching on furniture or the opposite limb.

FIGURE 10-6 Towel sling. Place a towel under the dog's abdomen. Pull up with one or both arms. The towel sling takes some of the weight off the dog's hind end, allowing the animal to walk more easily.

The newborns should be weighed at least once daily. Each one should be steadily gaining weight every day. If any newborn is not gaining weight, it should have extra time by itself on the mammary glands. If the newborn is not nursing, the owner should be shown how to supplement the neonate's feeding with milk replacer (e.g., KMR, Esbilac).

The mother's surgical incision is at risk of irritation and injury from her licking or the newborns' suckling. The owner should inspect the incision daily. A bloody, mucous discharge is expected from the vulva for several days postsurgically. The color of the discharge may change from red to brown as the days pass. A foul odor to the discharge is not normal, and the hospital should be notified.

It is common for the new mother to have loose stools after giving birth. The mother's appetite should be good. It is important that the new mother have plenty of high-calorie food because she must eat enough for herself and all her offspring. The new mother that is not eating will not heal promptly and cannot produce enough milk to feed the newborns.

The owner should be shown how to express milk from each mammary gland to check it for milk production and color and consistency. Colostrum (the first milk, generally rich in antibodies) is usually slightly yellow and sticky. After the newborns have nursed for approximately 24 hours, the milk becomes thinner and whiter. If the mammary glands stop releasing milk or become painful

or red, or if the milk is thick or discolored (any color other than white), the owner must contact the veterinarian. The mother will need to be treated, and the newborns will need to be fed milk replacer. The veterinary technician often must instruct clients on how to bottle-feed or tube-feed the newborns.

Pet supply stores carry milk replacers for puppies and kittens. Bottles with nipples of appropriate size for the newborn should be purchased at the same time. Milk replacers come in canned as well as powdered forms. The process of tube or bottle feeding neonates can be very labor intensive. The technician should discuss the pros and cons of both options with the owner. Detailed description and hands-on demonstrations will be necessary to ensure that the young animals get the proper nutrition with minimal complications.

There are several veterinary textbooks dedicated to the pediatric patient; *Small Animal Pediatrics: The First 12 Months of Life* is one example.

KEY POINTS

1. As the primary caregiver in the hospital setting, the veterinary technician is the best team member to discharge the patient to the owner's care.
2. Instructions for all postanesthesia patients address confinement, feeding, medication, possible adverse reactions, and hospital contact information.
3. The client should receive written instructions as well as a demonstration of cleaning steps for passive drains.
4. To prevent distraction, all discharge instructions should be given in a quiet area where there will be minimal distractions. The pet and owner should not be reunited until after all home care has been thoroughly discussed.
5. It is important to ask non-leading questions to assess the client's understanding of home care.
6. The client should be given a point of contact person, typically that of the technician, so that he/she feels more comfortable calling with questions.
7. The technician or other staff member should call the owner 24 hours after discharge to see how the patient is doing and then again at set intervals during the recovery.
8. Patients with a bandage, cast, or splint need to be strictly confined. The owner must understand the importance of this measure.
9. The owner needs to report any change in the appearance or position of the bandage, splint, or cast to the veterinary hospital.
10. Within a week, the patient that has undergone one to several tooth extractions should be pain free, and the tooth sockets should be almost healed.
11. If a patient is sent home with an E-collar, the owner must make sure that the animal is able to eat and drink normally.
12. Owners in multi-pet households should be reminded that the E-collar will not prevent the other animals from licking the patient's incision and causing damage.
13. A feeding tube may be needed for several weeks, so the owner must care for the tube properly.
14. To assess the necessity of maintaining the feeding tube, the patient must have food available when it is ready to eat.
15. The patient exhibiting signs of unrelenting pain hours to days after gastrointestinal surgery most likely has peritonitis.
16. The heavier and older the cat, the longer it will take for the cat to recover from declaw surgery. Confining the cat to an indoor lifestyle is ideal after onychectomy because the animal no longer has the ability to defend itself.
17. Insufficient confinement of the patient after an orthopedic procedure is the most common reason for delayed healing.
18. The bladder of the patient recovering from a cystotomy should be kept small by allowing the patient to void every few hours.
19. After aural hematoma surgery, passive drains usually remain in place for several weeks. The pinna may heal with scar tissue and significant wrinkling.
20. The patient recovering from a cesarean section must heal and also raise a litter. The newborns' feeding may have to be supplemented with milk replacer.

REVIEW QUESTIONS

1. Which of the following statements is true regarding postoperative at-home nursing care?
   a. The general principles are the same regardless of what specific surgery was performed, such that every patient can be treated exactly the same when he/she leaves the hospital.
   b. Only the veterinarian who performed the procedure should explain postoperative nursing care to the owners at discharge.
   c. The veterinary technician knows the patient, can advocate for the patient, and can educate the owner regarding what postoperative techniques work the best for that specific animal.
   d. Well-written instructions make verbal discharge instructions unnecessary.
   e. It is best to have the patient in the examination room when discharge instructions are given to the owner.

2. Which of the following may be clinical signs of prolonged recovery from anesthesia?
   a. Lethargy.
   b. Ataxia.
   c. Depression.
   d. All of the above.

3. How often should the surgical site be observed once the patient is discharged to the owners?
   a. Once daily.
   b. Twice daily, as a minimum.
   c. Twice daily, as a maximum.
   d. Continuously.
   e. The surgical site does not need to be observed after the patient leaves the hospital, because the patient would not be released if this were necessary.

4. When checking the surgical site, which of the following should be noted?
   a. The number of sutures.
   b. Any swelling.
   c. Any redness or discharge from the incision.
   d. All of the above.

5. Serous discharge tends to accumulate where a surgical drain exits the skin. What can be done to prevent this accumulation from occluding the drainage site and thereby preserve the intended function of the drain?
   a. Application of warm soaks around the exit site.
   b. Application of a thin film of petroleum jelly.
   c. Suturing the drain exit site closed.
   d. Both a and b.

6. *True or False*: When a dog has a bandage, splint, or cast on a limb, it should be walked only by leash.

7. *True or False:* A plastic bag may be continuously kept over a bandage, splint or cast to prevent it from getting dirty or damaged.

8. If a feeding tube becomes clogged, which of the following techniques usually resolves most occlusions?
   a. Instilling carbonated water into the tube.
   b. Instilling cold water.
   c. Instilling distilled water.
   d. Instilling coffee.
   e. Instilling IV fluids through the tube.

9. *True or False:* If a large enough feeding tube is placed, chunks of kibble can be administered.

10. Which of the following may occur after an intestinal resection and anastomosis?
    a. Peritonitis.
    b. Narrowing of the intestinal lumen at the anastomosis site.
    c. Slow leak from the anastomosis site leading to an abdominal abscess.
    d. All of the above.
    e. Both b and c.

11. All of the following are indications of post–tooth extraction complications except:
    a. Pawing at the mouth.
    b. Refusal to eat.
    c. Red-tinged water in the bowl for the first day postoperatively.
    d. All of the above are indications of complications.

12. How long should hematuria be expected following a cystotomy?
    a. No longer than 12 hours.
    b. No longer than 24 hours.
    c. Up to 36 hours.
    d. Weeks after surgery.
    e. Any hematuria following a cystotomy is abnormal, and the veterinarian should be alerted immediately.

13. Why should the typical clay, clumping cat litter be avoided for the first few weeks after a declaw procedure?
    a. Most cats refuse to use clumping litter after a declaw.
    b. Most cats are so clean that they refuse to use clay litter after a declaw.
    c. The clay granules tend to stick to the surgical site and can become embedded in the healing wound, leading to pain and infection.
    d. This litter is too expensive.
    e. None of the above.

14. What is another name for a declaw procedure?
    a. Orchidectomy.
    b. Onychectomy.
    c. Osteotomy.
    d. Oclawotomy.

15. Which of the following statements regarding ear canal ablations is true?
    a. Postoperative infection may occur.
    b. Facial nerve paralysis is a common complication that usually resolves within 2 weeks.
    c. Head tilt, nystagmus, and difficulty walking are signs of a compromised vestibular system.
    d. All of the above.

16. Which of the following statements regarding postoperative care of cesarean section patients is true?
    a. The veterinary technician should show the owner how to express milk from each mammary gland.
    b. It is important that the mother eat a high-calorie diet while nursing the newborns.
    c. A bloody, mucous vaginal discharge is to be expected for several days.
    d. All of the above.

ANSWERS

1. c
2. d
3. b
4. d

5. d
6. True
7. False
8. a

9. False
10. d
11. c
12. c

13. c
14. b
15. d
16. d

BIBLIOGRAPHY

Bassert JM, McCurnin DM, editors: McCurinin's clinical textbook for veterinary technicians, ed 7, St Louis, 2010, Elsevier.

Peterson ME, Kutzler M: Small animal pediatrics: the first 12 months of life, St Louis, 2011, Saunders.

Piermattei DL, Flo GL, DeCam CE: Brinker: Piermattei and Flo's handbook of small animal orthopedics and fracture repair, ed 4, St Louis, 2006, Elsevier.

Sirois M: Principles and practice of veterinary technology, ed 3, St Louis, 2011, Mosby.

Wortinger A. Nutrition for the veterinary technician and nurse, Ames, Iowa, 2007, Wiley-Blackwell.

The Technician's Role in Pain Management

Marianne Tear

11

OUTLINE

LEARNING OBJECTIVES

After completion of this chapter, the reader will be able to:
- Define pain.
- Discuss the importance of pain management.
- Discuss the physiologic effects of pain.
- Understand key terms associated with pain and pain management.
- Discuss the importance of preoperative, intraoperative, and postoperative pain management.
- Identify painful procedures.
- Distinguish the difference between dysphoria and pain.
- Describe behavioral changes associated with pain.

This chapter is not meant to be a stand-alone text on pain management. There are many excellent books whose entire content is devoted to the subject of analgesia. One such text is the *Handbook of Veterinary Pain Management* by Gaynor and Muir. Several dedicated veterinarians and technicians have spent almost their entire careers advocating for the recognition, prevention, and treatment of animal pain. One has only to Google the name Nancy Shaffran to receive multiple references on pain management. The purpose of this chapter is to discuss the technician's role in recognizing and helping to prevent pain in our animal patients. It is meant to complement Chapter 2's discussion on the general mechanism of pain transmission and general classes of drugs used to prevent pain.

As advances in veterinary medicine continue, the role and responsibility of the veterinary technician will increase. Technicians will be expected to know more, do more, and be more in almost every hospital setting. Although this addition of duties will be gratifying, it is imperative that the primary role of the technician not be lost or pushed to the side. Regardless of the clinical setting, the technician is first and foremost the patient advocate. No single person in the hospital spends more time with the patients than the technician. Nowhere is this strong, compassionate, knowledgeable advocacy more necessary than in the realm of pain management. As the primary caregiver, it is the technician who needs to communicate the animal's needs to the veterinarian. The doctor is ultimately responsible, but it is the technician's job to ensure that the doctor has the most current information to facilitate the best medical care.

Gone are the days when pain was considered necessary to keep the animal from further injuring itself. The perception that pain is not felt or processed by animal patients is also being disproved. Pain is now considered one of the five parameters that should be monitored. Animals should no longer have to prove that they have pain to receive analgesia.

Understanding Pain

What is pain and how can it be quantified? The International Association for the Study of Pain classifies it as "an unpleasant sensory and emotional experience associated with actual or potential tissue damage or described in terms of such damage." The inability to communicate this discomfort in no way negates the experience, nor should it exclude the patient from receiving pain-relieving treatment. It has been argued by some that animals do not feel pain the same way as humans. On a physiologic level, pain is processed in a similar fashion in all mammals.

"It is possible that animal pain is worse than human pain because lacking the language and sophisticated reasoning skills and temporal concepts, animals cannot understand the reasons for and causes of pain, and thus lack the ability to hope for and anticipate its cessation," says Bernard Rollin, in *Handbook of Veterinary Pain Management.*

Pain creates adverse physiologic changes that can delay healing and even lead to a patient's decline or demise. With this realization, more and more concerned professionals are advocating the concept of preemptive analgesia—to prevent as much of the pain as possible rather than trying to alleviate it once it has already occurred. The American Animal Hospital Association (AAHA) encourages veterinary professionals to consider pain a vital sign, requiring that all hospitals seeking its accreditation have a comprehensive pain management protocol in place (Box 11-1).

Communication, whether it be among the health care team or with clients, is the best way to ensure that pain management is initiated. Having a standardized vocabulary will help ensure that the team is "on the same page" and working together toward the common goal (Box 11-2).

BOX 11-1 AAHA Pain Standards

- Pain assessment for every patient regardless of presenting complaint.
- Assessment recorded in the patient's record.
- Utilization of preemptive pain management.
- Appropriate pain management for the anticipated level and duration of pain.
- Pain management with all surgical procedures.
- Reassessment throughout the procedure.
- Written protocols.
- Teaching clients to recognize pain in their pets.

The Technician's Role in Pain Management

The role of the technician in pain management encompasses everything from assessing the patient to providing the veterinarian with information, to administering and logging the drugs prescribed, to educating the owner on proper home analgesia. Box 11-3 gives a brief overview of some of the pain management tasks technicians perform on a daily basis. It is by no means an exhaustive list.

Communicating with Clients

Pain management should begin before the animal enters the clinic. Elective procedures are planned painful events and should be prepared for as such. Communicating the need for analgesia with the client *before* the animal comes in or at the time of admission helps lay the foundation for quality care. Analgesia should not be considered optional treatment. This gives the client a mixed message, that "pain management is important only if you can afford it." Educating the client on the process of pain and the importance of preventing it should be standard operating procedure. Most owners want to do what is best for their pets; they just lack an understanding of why something is being recommended. Many have had pets that have undergone surgery without the benefit of analgesia and are legitimately concerned about why protocols have changed.

Many animals mask signs of pain in the hospital, so owners need to be advised as to what to watch for once the patient is discharged. Client education should include verbal and written orders along with hospital contact information in case additional questions arise. At-home pain management should be tailored to the animal and the home situation; this includes the type of medication, and the route, and frequency of administration.

Anticipating Painful Procedures

All tissue damage, including that caused by surgery, has the potential to cause pain. Therefore it is in the best interest of the pet to start analgesics before, rather than after, the painful event. Preemptive therapy can reduce the likelihood of wind-up: progressive stimulation of pain receptors leads to hyperexcitability, hyperalgesia, and allodynia. Once wind-up has occurred, treatment becomes exponentially more difficult and in some cases impossible.

When considering the amount of postoperative pain a patient may experience, several factors should be considered: the expectation of pain associated with the procedure to be performed, the individual animal's response to the procedure, and its response to the analgesic protocol. Although two of the three factors cannot be assessed until the animal awakens, the expectation of pain can be anticipated. Table 11-1 lists the estimation of pain associated with common procedures. It should be stressed that this is just estimation and should not be used as a reason to deny pain medications.

BOX 11-2 Definitions of Pain-Related Terms

Acute pain: pain that follows some bodily injury, disappears with healing, and tends to be self-limiting.

Adaptive pain: normal response to tissue damage; includes inflammatory pain.

Allodynia: pain caused by a stimulus that does not normally cause pain.

Analgesia: the loss of sensitivity to pain.

Anesthesia: total or partial loss of sensation.

Breakthrough pain: a transient flare-up of pain in the chronic pain setting, which can occur even when chronic pain is under control.

Central sensitization: an increase in the excitability and responsiveness of nerves in the spinal cord.

Chronic pain: pain that lasts several weeks to months and persists beyond the expected healing time, when nonmalignant in origin.

Hyperalgesia: an increased response to a stimulation that is normally painful either at the site of injury or in surrounding undamaged tissue.

Hyperesthesia: increased sensitivity to sensation.

Hypoalgesia: decreased sensitivity to pain.

Hypoesthesia: decreased sensitivity to stimulation.

Maladaptive pain: hypersensitivity to pain resulting from abnormal processing of normal input; can also occur if adaptive pain is left untreated.

Multimodal analgesia: the use of multiple drugs with different actions to produce optimal analgesia.

Neuroplasticity: the idea that the nervous system can be changed by the effect of the environment, external stimuli, and the effects of physiologic stimuli, e.g., pain.

Nociception: the transaction, conduction, and CNS processing of nerve signals generated by the stimulation of certain receptors.

Pain threshold: the minimal amount of pain that a patient can recognize.

Pain tolerance level: the greatest level of pain that a patient can tolerate.

Pathologic pain: pain that has an exaggerated response beyond its protective usefulness. It is often associated with tissue injury incurred at the time of surgery or trauma.

Physiologic pain: pain that acts as a protective mechanism that incites individuals to move away from the cause of potential tissue damage or to avoid movement or contact with external stimuli during a reparative phase.

Preemptive analgesia: the administration of an analgesic drug before painful stimulation to prevent sensitization of neurons, or wind-up, thus improving postoperative analgesia.

Regional anesthesia: the loss of sensation in part of the body caused by interruption of the sensory nerves that conduct impulses from that region of the body.

Somatic pain: pain that originates from damage to bone, joints, muscle, or skin and is described by humans as localized, constant, sharp, aching, and throbbing.

Visceral pain: pain that arises from stretching, distention, or inflammation of the viscera and described by humans as deep, cramping, aching, or gnawing without good localization.

Wind-up: temporal summation of painful stimuli in the spinal cord. Mediated by C fibers and responsible for "second" pain.

Adapted from Gaynor J, Muir W: Handbook of veterinary pain management, St Louis, 2002, Mosby.

BOX 11-3 Technician's Role in Pain Management*

Administer medications and perform analgesic techniques.
Anticipate painful procedures.
Assess the patient postoperatively.
Communicate with clients.
Log controlled substances.
Monitor and treat drug effects.
Recognize signs of pain.
Request appropriate analgesia.

*Not listed in order or according to frequency that tasks are performed.

Pain is often increased in anxious or stressed animals, so tranquilizers or sedatives should be included in the premedication process. See Chapter 2 for premedication discussion.

Administering Intraoperative Pain Management

Good preemptive pain management protocols are designed to transition the patient through the surgical period and into the recovery phase (see the Appendix for suggested pain management protocols). However, patients undergoing surgical procedures of more than several hours' duration often require additional analgesia intraoperatively. In addition, patients undergoing procedures necessitating major tissue or nerve damage (e.g., back, knee, or hip procedures, amputation, multiple anastomoses, and ear or rectal procedures) will benefit from intraoperative analgesia and analgesic techniques. Finally, patients with poor tolerance for gaseous anesthesia can be effectively managed with constant-rate infusions (CRIs) of opioids, which can greatly decrease the inhalant requirements.

In any of these cases, increased duration or intensity of surgical pain, often evidenced by sudden elevation in heart or respiratory rate, should not be addressed by merely increasing the concentration of inhaled anesthesia. Although "turning up the gas" will keep the patient immobile on the table, it will not manage acute pain, which will become evident as soon as the patient returns to consciousness.

Administration of additional bolus doses of opioids is determined by the patient's response to surgical stimulation. Such responses include movement, audible sounds

TABLE 11-1   Estimates of Pain Associated with Various Types of Surgery*

Most Painful	Moderately to Severely Painful	Mildly to Moderately Painful
Thoracotomies (particularly median sternotomies), amputations, ear resections, pelvic fracture repair, nephrectomy, cervical disk surgery	Mastectomy, mandibulectomy, thoracic or lumbar disk surgery, stabilization of a fractured femur or humerus, cranial abdominal procedures	Tracheotomy; aural hematoma; stabilization of a fractured radius, ulna, tibia, or fibula; castration; caudal abdominal procedures; dental cleaning; tooth extraction

*The practitioner's expectations of the level of pain should not be grounds for denying a patient analgesic relief.
Modified from Carroll GL: Small animal pain management, Lakewood, CO, 1998, American Animal Hospital Association Press.

BOX 11-4   Morphine CRI

Avoids the peaks and valleys typically seen with opioid bolus dosing.

Allows a reduction in inhalant anesthesia, which can be advantageous in patients with adverse reaction to gaseous agents.

Allows for a lower dose of morphine to be used in CRI than in bolus dosing, which can reduce the unwanted side effects of morphine (e.g., dysphoria, panting).

Useful to manage any severe surgical pain and can be safely combined with ketamine or lidocaine.

Dosage
- Dogs: 0.2-0.5 mg/kg slow IV loading bolus, followed by 0.1-0.3 mg/kg/hr CRI.
- Cats: 0.05-0.1 mg/kg IV loading bolus, followed by 0.025-0.2 mg/kg/hr CRI.

BOX 11-5   Fentanyl CRI

The main advantages of fentanyl over morphine are rapid onset of action and short half-life, which allow for rapid cessation of unwanted side effects.

The major disadvantage is that fentanyl is considerably more expensive than morphine.

Dosage
- Dogs: 2-5 μg/kg IV loading dose, followed by 1-6 μg/kg/hr CRI intraoperatively.
- Cats: 1-2 μg/kg IV loading dose, followed by 1-4 μ mg/kg/hr CRI.

BOX 11-6   Lidocaine CRI

Provides excellent systemic analgesia when delivered intravenously.

Safe for use in patients with gastrointestinal disturbances.

Provides benefit for patients undergoing procedures with excessive nerve trauma, such as complicated back procedures or limb amputations.

Extremely short-acting and can be discontinued without residual effect almost immediately.

Should be discontinued if the patient shows signs of toxicity (e.g., muscle tremors, seizures, nausea or vomiting).

Dosage
- Dogs: 2 mg/kg IV followed by 0.025-0.08 mg/kg/min.
- Cats: Not recommended.*

*There are reported lidocaine CRI dosages for cats, but lidocaine usually is not recommended for use in cats because of the potential for severe cardiotoxic effects.

BOX 11-7   Ketamine CRI

As an NMDA receptor antagonist, ketamine given as an intraoperative CRI binds at central nervous system (CNS) receptors and prevents wind-up.

Best used to manage neuropathic pain, particularly when the pain has been longstanding and the patient has not shown good response to other analgesics.

Should always be given in combination with an opioid, and both can be delivered in the same infusion.

Dosage
- Dogs and cats: 0.5 mg/kg IV loading bolus, followed by 0.3-0.6 mg/kg/hr CRI during surgery and 0.1-0.3 mg/kg/hr for 24 hours after surgery.

such as growling or crying (if patient is not intubated), and increases in heart rate, blood pressure, or respiratory rate. Intraoperative boluses should be delivered intravenously for fastest onset of action. The full opioid agonists, morphine, hydromorphone, and oxymorphone, are optimum choices. Fentanyl is not recommended for one-time bolus use because of its short half-life, and it is best administered as a constant-rate infusion.

Intraoperative analgesia is best administered by CRI. Many agents can be delivered by this method, but the drug groups most often given by CRI are local anesthetics (lidocaine), opioids (morphine or fentanyl), and *N*-methyl-s-aspartate (NMDA) antagonists (ketamine). Regardless of the drug, a loading dose is typically given immediately before CRI is begun. These drugs can be used as single agents or in combination with one another. See Boxes 11-4 through 11-7 for information on specific analgesics.

For other procedures, regional local anesthesia, or nerve blocks, can aid in pain management. Ring blocks can be utilized to add additional analgesia during declaw procedures by blocking nerve impulses before they enter the CNS. Subcutaneous injections of bupivacaine or bupivacaine/lidocaine can be used to block the three major nerves in the forelimb (Figure 11-1). Blocking the infraobrital and mandibular foremen enables the animal's entire muzzle to be anesthetized; this approach greatly

FIGURE 11-1 Nerve block for onychectomy. The median and palmar branches of the ulnar nerve are blocked medial to the accessory carpal pad; the dorsal branch of the ulnar nerve is blocked lateral and proximal to the accessory carpal pad. The superficial radial nerve branches are blocked at the dorsomedial aspect of the proximal carpus. (From Fossum TW, Hedlund CS, Hulse DA, et al: Small animal surgery, ed 3, St Louis, 2007, Mosby.)

reduces the pain association with dental extractions (Figures 11-2 and 11-3). Each of these blocks can be successfully administered by the technician.

Assessing the Postoperative Patient

The ease and success of managing postoperative pain are directly related to preoperative analgesia. That is, the more successful the attempts to preempt surgical pain, the easier it is to control postoperative pain with minimal additional analgesics. Assuming adequate preemptive analgesia, the overall goal of postoperative pain management should be to maintain the analgesic plane achieved throughout surgery.

The patient should recover quietly and calmly without displays of overt signs of pain (e.g., vocalization, excessive movement, abnormal body posturing). At no time should the patient be required to return to a painful state and "request" additional analgesics during the immediate

FIGURE 11-2 Infraorbital blocks in a dog and a cat. (From Fossum TW, Hedlund CS, Hulse DA, et al: Small animal surgery, ed 3, St Louis, 2007, Mosby.)

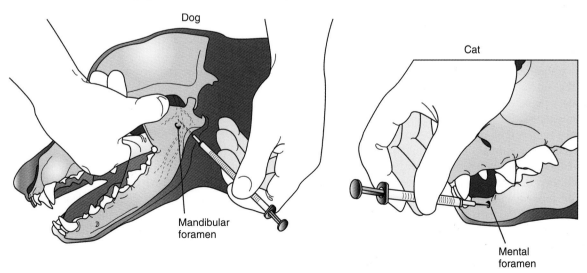

FIGURE 11-3 **A,** A mandibular block in a dog. **B,** A mental block in a cat. (From Fossum TW, Hedlund CS, Hulse DA, et al: Small animal surgery, ed 3, St Louis, 2007, Mosby.)

TABLE 11-2   Behavioral and Physiologic Responses to Pain

Response	Signs of Pain
Behavioral responses	Vocalization: Groaning, whining, growling, purring. Facial expression: Fixed stare, glazed or squinted eyes, dilated pupils, furrowed brow. Body posture: Hunched, rigid, prayer position or other abnormal position. Activity: Restless or restricted movement, trembling. Attitude: Aggression, fearfulness, timidity, comfort-seeking. Appetite: Decreased. Urinary and bowel habits: Increased urination, failure in house training or failure to use litter box. Grooming: Loss of hair coat sheen, unkempt appearance. Guarding and self-mutilation: Protects wound or limb; fails to bear weight; may lick, chew, or rub surgical area.
Physiologic responses	Cardiovascular system: Increased heart rate and blood pressure, vasoconstriction. Pulmonary system: Increased respiratory rate, shallow breathing, splinting. Digestive system: Inappetence, salivation; possibly vomiting, diarrhea or constipation, evacuation of anal glands. Musculoskeletal system: Tense muscles, muscle tremors. Immune system: Diminished resistance, stress leukogram; increased metastasis. Neuroendocrine system: Increased catabolism, decreased anabolism.

Modified from Carroll GL: Small animal pain management, Lakewood, CO, 1998, American Animal Hospital Association Press.

postoperative period. Some patients experience pain that persists or that develops despite adequate doses of analgesics and must be treated with additional analgesia or analgesic techniques. This type of pain is termed *breakthrough pain* because it has "broken through" the usual analgesic barriers.

Postoperatively, pain and dysphoria, a state of restlessness with or without vocalization, can occur at the same time. It is important to differentiate between the two. An animal that is experiencing pain can be temporarily quieted with a calm voice and reassuring petting. Painful behavior resumes when the human interaction stops. On the other hand, an animal experiencing dysphoria or emergence delirium cannot be quieted by interaction.

Once the animal is completely recovered from the effects of anesthesia, change in behavior is often the most common sign of pain (Table 11-2). Every animal that is admitted to the hospital for a surgical procedure should undergo a complete physical examination. That examination should include an assessment of the animal's behavior: Is it outgoing and inquisitive or hesitant and shy? Having the "normals" on behavior can help in monitoring the animal's pain response postoperatively.

Physiologic signs, such as increased heart rate and respiratory rate, can be good indicators of pain or stress in the recovering animal. They should not be the sole indicator of whether pain medication should be administered. Rather, these changes and the behavioral changes should be looked at in combination in an attempt to objectively determine pain.

There are many different types of pain scoring systems, each with advantages and disadvantages (Box 11-8). It is important that the clinic have a standard method to assess all patients that is comprehensive but easy to use (Figure 11-4).

BOX 11-8   Components of a Comprehensive Pain Scoring System

- Physiologic parameters
- Anticipated pain associated with the procedure
- Behavior
- Patient's response to current therapy

Each animal should be treated as an individual, regardless of the scoring scale used. Animals undergoing the same procedure with the same preemptive analgesia protocol may exhibit different levels of pain. This variation can reflect differences in genetics or other underlying conditions. For example, a geriatric dog may experience more pain during a routine spay than a younger dog, because of the onset of arthritis and positioning during the procedure. Some animals are also naturally more stoic than others; reluctance to show pain should not penalize the animal.

Pain should be assessed at least every 2 hours postoperatively, and treatment should be adjusted according to the patient's response.

Requesting Appropriate Analgesia

While technicians are the primary care-givers, they lack the authority to initiate therapy without the veterinarian's approval. This can prove to be daunting and frustrating. Technicians can leverage their knowledge and skill set to advocate for their patients. Giving the veterinarian objective details about the patient's conditions, including heart rate, respiratory rate, and food intake, balanced with a detailed summary of what has already been implemented allows the technician to more effectively argue the case for (increased) analgesia.

Colorado State University

Date _____

Time _____

**Colorado State University
Veterinary Medical Center
Canine Acute Pain Scale**

Rescore when awake	☐ Animal is sleeping, but can be aroused - Not evaluated for pain ☐ Animal can't be aroused, check vital signs, assess therapy

Pain Score	Example	Psychological & Behavioral	Response to Palpation	Body Tension
0		☐ **Comfortable** when resting ☐ **Happy, content** ☐ Not bothering wound or surgery site ☐ Interested in or curious about surroundings	☐ **Nontender** to palpation of wound or surgery site, or to palpation elsewhere	Minimal
1		☐ **Content to slightly unsettled** or restless ☐ **Distracted easily** by surroundings	☐ **Reacts to palpation** of wound, surgery site, or other body part by **looking around, flinching, or whimpering**	Mild
2		☐ Looks **uncomfortable** when resting ☐ May **whimper** or cry and may **lick or rub wound** or surgery site when unattended ☐ Droopy ears, **worried facial expression** (arched eye brows, darting eyes) ☐ **Reluctant to respond** when beckoned ☐ **Not eager to interact** with people or surroundings but will look around to see what is going on	☐ Flinches, whimpers cries, or guards/pulls away	Mild to Moderate **Reassess analgesic plan**
3		☐ **Unsettled, crying, groaning, biting or chewing** wound when unattended ☐ **Guards or protects** wound or surgery site by altering weight distribution (i.e., limping, shifting body position) ☐ **May be unwilling to move** all or part of body	☐ May be **subtle** (shifting eyes or increased respiratory rate) if dog is too painful to move or is stoic ☐ May be **dramatic**, such as a sharp cry, growl, bite or bite threat, and/or pulling away	Moderate **Reassess analgesic plan**
4		☐ Constantly groaning or screaming when unattended ☐ May bite or chew at wound, but unlikely to move ☐ **Potentially unresponsive** to surroundings ☐ **Difficult to distract** from pain	☐ Cries at non-painful palpation (may be experiencing allodynia, wind-up, or fearful that pain could be made worse) ☐ May react aggressively to palpation	Moderate to Severe **May be rigid to avoid painful movement** **Reassess analgesic plan**

O Tender to palpation
X Warm
■ Tense

RIGHT   LEFT

Comments _____

A © 2006/PW Hellyer, SR Uhrig, NG Robinson

FIGURE 11-4 Colorado State University (CSU) pain scales for dogs (**A**) and cats (**B**). Acute animal pain scales developed by P. Hellyer and colleagues at CSU for assessing pain in dogs and cats. Available at www.IVAPM.org. (From Bassert JM, McCurnin DM, editors: Mccurnin's clinical textbook for veterinary technicians, ed 7, St Louis, 2010, Saunders.)

Understanding the pharmacology of different pain medications is also an advantage for a skilled technician. Explaining to the veterinarian how monitoring and assessment of the patient will change with the addition of or a change in pain management protocol will increase the likelihood of cooperation. In the end, pain management is the responsibility of the team. The veterinarian relies on the technician's keen observation and nursing skills to ensure that adequate analgesia is on board. By working together the animal is the ultimate winner.

Colorado State University

Date _____

Time _____

**Colorado State University
Veterinary Medical Center
Feline Acute Pain Scale**

Rescore when awake	☐ Animal is sleeping, but can be aroused - Not evaluated for pain ☐ Animal can't be aroused, check vital signs, assess therapy

Pain Score	Example	Psychological & Behavioral	Response to Palpation	Body Tension
0		☐ **Content and quiet** when unattended ☐ **Comfortable** when resting ☐ Interested in or **curious** about surroundings	☐ **Not bothered** by palpation of wound or surgery site, or to palpation elsewhere	Minimal
1		☐ **Signs are often subtle and not easily detected in the hospital setting**; more likely to be detected by the owner(s) at home ☐ Earliest signs at home may be **withdrawal from surroundings or change in normal routine** ☐ In the hospital, may be content or slightly unsettled ☐ **Less interested** in surroundings but will look around to see what is going on	☐ May or may not react to palpation of wound or surgery site	Mild
2		☐ Decreased responsiveness, **seeks solitude** ☐ **Quiet**, loss of brightness in eyes ☐ **Lays curled up or sits tucked up** (all four feet under body, shoulders hunched, head held slightly lower than shoulders, tail curled tightly around body) with eyes partially or mostly closed ☐ **Hair coat appears rough** or fluffed up ☐ May intensively groom an area that is painful or irritating ☐ Decreased appetite, **not interested in food**	☐ **Responds aggressively or tries to escape** if painful area is palpated or approached ☐ Tolerates attention, may even perk up when petted as long as painful area is avoided	Mild to Moderate **Reassess analgesic plan**
3		☐ Constantly **yowling, growling, or hissing** when unattended ☐ May bite or chew at wound, but **unlikely to move** if left alone	☐ **Growls or hisses at non-painful palpation** (may be experiencing allodynia, wind-up, or fearful that pain could be made worse) ☐ **Reacts aggressively to palpation**, adamantly pulls away to avoid any contact	Moderate **Reassess analgesic plan**
4		☐ Prostrate ☐ Potentially **unresponsive** to or unaware of surroundings, difficult to distract from pain ☐ Receptive to care (even mean or wild cats will be more tolerant of contact)	☐ **May not respond to palpation** ☐ **May be rigid to avoid painful movement**	Moderate to Severe **May be rigid to avoid painful movement** **Reassess analgesic plan**

RIGHT   LEFT

○ Tender to palpation
✕ Warm
■ Tense

Comments _____

B © 2006/PW Hellyer, SR Uhrig, NG Robinson

FIGURE 11-4, Cont'd

KEY POINTS

1. The technician is first and foremost the patient advocate.
2. It is the technician's job to ensure that the doctor has the most current information to facilitate the best medical care.
3. Pain is considered one of the five parameters that should be monitored.
4. Animals should not have to prove that they are in pain to receive analgesia.
5. On a physiologic level, pain is processed in a similar fashion in all mammals.
6. Pain can delay healing and even lead to a patient's decline.

7. Communication is the best way to ensure that pain management is initiated.
8. The role of the technician encompasses everything including assessing the patient, providing the veterinarian with information to administer and log the drugs prescribed, and educating the owner on proper home analgesia.
9. Pain management should begin before the animal enters the clinic.
10. Analgesia should not be considered optional.
11. Many animals mask the signs of pain in the hospital.
12. All tissue damage has the potential to cause pain.
13. Pain is often increased in anxious or stressed animals.
14. Increased duration or intensity of surgical pain should not be addressed by increasing the concentration in inhaled anesthesia.
15. Postoperatively pain and dysphoria can occur at the same time; care must be taken to differentiate between the two.

REVIEW QUESTIONS

1. *True or False:* Pain creates adverse physiologic changes.

2. *True or False:* A constant-rate infusion of an intraoperative opioid can greatly reduce the gas anesthetic requirements of the anesthetized patient.

3. *True or False:* Increasing the amount of gas anesthesia will decrease the amount of pain felt by the animal.

4. *True or False:* It is possible to anticipate the amount of postoperative pain on the basis of the procedure performed.

5. *True or False:* Because each animal is an individual, it is in the best interest of the pet to wait until it shows signs of pain before administering analgesia.

6. *True or False:* Dysphoria can be quieted with calm interaction.

7. *True or False:* Fentanyl is recommended for one-time bolus use.

8. *True or False:* The overall goal of postoperative pain management should be to maintain the analgesic plane achieved throughout surgery.

9. When might a patient need an IV bolus of an analgesic drug?
   a. If the patient moves during surgical stimulation.
   b. If the heart rate rapidly increase.
   c. If the blood pressure markedly rises.
   d. All of the above.
   e. None of the above.

10. The drug group(s) most often given by CRI is/are:
   a. Local anesthetics.
   b. Opioids.
   c. *N*-methyl-D-aspartate (NMDA) antagonists.
   d. All of the above.
   e. None of the above.

ANSWERS

1. True
2. True
3. False
4. True
5. False; the animal should not have to "request" pain medication.
6. False
7. False; its half life is too short.
8. True
9. d
10. d

BIBLIOGRAPHY

Allen DG, Dowling PM, Smith DA, et al: Handbook of veterinary drugs, ed 3, Baltimore, 2005 Lippincott Williams & Wilkins.

American Animal Hospital Association, American Association of Feline Practitioners, AAHA/AAFP Pain Management Guidelines Task Force Members; Hellyer P, Rodan I, Brunt J, et al: AAHA/AAFP pain management guidelines for dogs & cats. J Am Anim Hosp Assoc 43:235-248, 2007.

Anderson C: Introduction to pain management. In Michigan Veterinary Conference Proceedings, Lansing, 2010.

Bassert JM, McCurnin DM, editors: McCurnin's clinical textbook for veterinary technicians, ed 7, St Louis, 2010, Saunders.

Dyson DH: Perioperative pain management in veterinary patients. Vet Clin North Am Small Anim Pract 38:1309-1327, 2008.

Fossum TW, Hedlund CS, Hulse DA, et al: Small animal surgery, ed 3, St Louis, 2007, Mosby.

Gaynor JS, Muir WW: Handbook of veterinary pain management, St Louis, 2002, Mosby.

Merskey H, Bogduk N: Part III: "Pain Terms, A Current List with Definitions and Notes on Usage" pp 209-2214) Classifiication of Chronic Pain, Second Edition, ISAP Task Force of Taxonomy, edited by H, IASP Press, Seattle, 1994.

Plumb DC: Plumbs' veterinary drug handbook, ed 5, Ames, 2005, Blackwell.

Shaffran N: Pain management: the veterinary technician's perspective. Vet Clin North Am Small Anim Pract 38:1415-1428, 2008.

Shaffran N: The psychology of animal pain management. In Proceedings of the International Veterinary Emergency and Critical Care Symposium, September 11-15, 2010, San Antonio, TX.

Thomas JA, Lerche P: Anesthesia and analgesia for veterinary technicians, ed 4, St Louis, 2011, Mosby.

APPENDIX

Quick Reference for Common Intravenous Infusions and Analgesic Protocols

Intravenous Fluid Flow Rate

Occasionally, it is necessary to administer intravenous (IV) fluids without an infusion pump. The following table is a quick reference that allows the veterinary technician to count the number of seconds between drops of fluid (not the number of drops per second) into the drip chamber of the administration set to estimate the hourly infusion rate, as long as the type of fluid administration set is known.

15 drops/mL	60 drops/mL
1 drop/sec = 240 mL/hr	1 drop/sec = 60 mL/hr
1 drop/2 sec = 120 mL/hr	1 drop/2 sec = 30 mL/hr
1 drop/3 sec = 80 mL/hr	1 drop/3 sec = 20 mL/hr
1 drop/4 sec = 60 mL/hr	1 drop/4 sec = 15 mL/hr
1 drop/5 sec = 48 mL/hr	1 drop/5 sec = 12 mL/hr
1 drop/6 sec = 40 mL/hr	1 drop/6 sec = 10 mL/hr
1 drop/7 sec = 35 mL/hr	1 drop/7 sec = 8.8 mL/hr
1 drop/8 sec = 30 mL/hr	1 drop/8 sec = 7.5 mL/hr
1 drop/9 sec = 27 mL/hr	1 drop/9 sec = 6.7 mL/hr
1 drop/10 sec = 24 mL/hr	1 drop/10 sec = 6 mL/hr

mL/hr, Milliliters per hour; *sec*, second(s).

Maintenance Fluid Flow Rate

Determining a patient's fluid flow rate is achieved with the following formula:

Total fluids = Maintenance fluids +

Replacement fluids + Ongoing losses

Many formulas are available for calculating a patient's maintenance fluid requirements. However, a simple, easy-to-remember formula for estimating an animal's hourly maintenance fluid requirements is 1 mL per pound of body weight (lb BW); two times (or twice) the maintenance requirement is 2 mL/lb BW.

Body Weight (lb)	Maintenance Fluids	Twice Maintenance Fluids
1	1 mL/hr	2 mL/hr
10	10 mL/hr	20 mL/hr
20	20 mL/hr	40 mL/hr
40	40 mL/hr	80 mL/hr
80	80 mL/hr	160 mL/hr

"Spiking the Bag" with Potassium Chloride

- Patients undergoing fluid diuresis are prone to hypokalemia.
- To prevent hypokalemia, the IV fluids can be "spiked," or supplemented, with potassium chloride (KCl).
- To figure out how much KCl supplementation is needed, it is necessary to know the patient's serum potassium level.
- Normal serum potassium level = 3.5 to 5.5 mEq/L.
- Failure to correct hypokalemia can result in muscle weakness, lethargy, and vomiting.
- KCl must be given in a slow drip, diluted in another fluid.

Serum Potassium Level (mEq/L)	Supplemental Potassium Chloride (Per 250 mL Fluid)*
3.5-5.5 (normal)	5 mEq (20 mEq/L)
3.0-3.4	7 mEq (28 mEq/L)
2.5-2.9	10 mEq (40 mEq/L)
2.0-2.4	15 mEq (60 mEq/L)
<2.0	20 mEq (80 mEq/L)

*Never administer fluids supplemented with potassium chloride faster than twice the maintenance rate; with more potassium, adjust the rate even slower.
mEq/L, Milliequivalents per liter.

"Spiking the Bag" with Dextrose

- If a patient is prone to hypoglycemia, debilitated, septic, or anorectic, a dextrose supplement may be required.
- If the blood glucose (BG) is less than 40 mg/dL, dextrose should be added to fluids to make a 2.5% dextrose solution.
- If BG continues to remain at or below 40 mg/dl, the solution should be increased to a 5% dextrose solution.

Size of Fluid Bag*	To Make 2.5% Dextrose Solution	To Make 5% Dextrose Solution
250 mL	Add 12.5 mL of 50% dextrose	Add 25 mL of 50% dextrose
500 mL	Add 25 mL of 50% dextrose	Add 50 mL of 50% dextrose
1000 mL	Add 50 mL of 50% dextrose	Add 100 mL of 50% dextrose

*Before adding dextrose to fluid bag, withdraw an amount of fluid from bag equal to the amount of dextrose to be added.

Heparinized Saline ("Hep-Saline," "Flush")

Size of Fluid Bag of 0.9% Sodium Chloride (NaCl)	Amount of Heparin [1000 Units/mL] to Add
250 mL	1.25 mL (1250 units)
500 mL	2.5 mL (2500 units)
1 liter	5 mL (5000 units)

Drug Doses Used to Treat Surgical Pain in Animals*

Drug Name	Indication(s)	Dose	Onset of Action	Duration of Action	Precautions
NONSTEROIDAL ANTI-INFLAMMATORY DRUGS (NSAIDS)					
Carprofen *Oral:* 25-, 75-, and 100-mg tablets or chewables	Pain and inflammation associated with arthritis and soft tissue and orthopedic surgery in dogs **FDA-approved for use in dogs**	Dog: 2.2 mg/kg PO bid *or* 4.4 mg/kg PO sid	1 hr 1 hr	12 hr 24 hr	Do not use in patients with GI or renal disease Discontinue use if vomiting or diarrhea develops NSAIDs are not recommended in hypovolemic or dehydrated patients or patients with bleeding disorders Do not use concurrently with corticosteroids
Injectable: 50 mg/mL		*Dog:* 4.4 mg/kg SC *Cat:* 1-2 mg/kg SC			
Deracoxib *Oral:* 25- and 100-mg tablets	Control of pain and inflammation associated with orthopedic surgery and chronic pain (osteoarthritis) **FDA-approved for use in dogs**	Postoperative pain: 3-4 mg/kg PO sid for 7 days Chronic pain: 1-2 mg/kg PO sid	1 hr	24 hr	As for carprofen Do not use in patients less than 4 pounds or 16 weeks of age (see listing on label) Contraindicated in patients receiving any corticosteroids
Etodolac *Oral:* 150- and 300-mg tablets	Control of pain and inflammation associated with osteoarthritis **FDA-approved for use in dogs**	*Dog:* 10-15 mg/kg PO sid	1 hr	24 hr	As for carprofen Not recommended for dogs weighing less than 5 kg

Drug Name	Indication(s)	Dose	Onset of Action	Duration of Action	Precautions
Meloxicam *Oral solution: 1.5 mg/mL* *Injectable: 5 mg/mL*	Postoperative and chronic pain (not labeled for postoperative use, only for osteoarthritis) **FDA-approved for use in dogs**	*Dog:* 0.2-0.3 mg/kg PO sid for 1 day, then 0.1 mg/kg PO sid *Cat:* 0.2 mg/kg PO on day 1, followed by 0.1 mg/kg PO sid for 2-4 days, then 0.1 kg/cat PO sid *Dog:* 0.2 mg/kg IM sid	1 hr	18-24 hr	As for carprofen Loading dose can be by injection or oral administration Do not administer drug concurrently or within 24 hours of other steroidal or nonsteroidal anti-inflammatory drugs, aminoglycoside antibiotics, or anticoagulation products
Tepoxalin *Oral: 30-, 50-, 100-, and 200-mg disintegrating tablets*	Control of pain associated with osteoarthritis in dogs weighing more than 3 kg **FDA-approved for use in dogs**	*Dog:* 10 mg/kg PO sid; 20 mg/kg once on initial dose	1 hr	18-24 hr	Tablets in foil blister packs Administer with food or water; place in mouth for a minimum of 4 seconds to allow tablet to dissolve
ALPHA2-ADRENERGIC AGONISTS					
Medetomidine*† *Injectable: 1 mg/mL*	Sedative, analgesic **FDA-approved for use in dogs**	*Dog:* 10-60 µg/kg IM *Cat:* 10-20 µg/kg IM, IV 5.0-10 µg/kg IV	20 min 20 min 3 min	1.0-3.0 hr 1.0-3.0 hr 0.5-1.5 hr	Do not use in patients with underlying cardiopulmonary or renal disease The lower IV dose is to be used as adjunct to opioid analgesia or as premedication before anesthesia Even lower doses may be used for anxiety and dysphoria (see Sedatives below)
Xylazine*† *Injectable: 20 and 100 mg/mL*	Sedative, analgesic **FDA-approved for use in dogs and cats**	*Dog:* 0.1-0.5 mg/kg IM, SC 0.05-0.1 mg/kg IV *Cat:* 0.1-0.5 mg/kg IM, SC 0.05-0.1 mg/kg IV	20 min 1 min 20 min 1 min	0.5 hr 20 min 0.5 hr 20 min	Do not use in patients with underlying cardiopulmonary or renal disease The lower IV dose is to be used as an adjunct to opioid analgesia, not by itself
OPIOIDS					
Morphine	Acute and cancer- related pain				
Oral: 10-, 15-, and 30-mg tablets		*Dog:* 0.5-4 mg/kg PO tid or qid *Cat:* 0.25-1.0 mg/kg PO tid or qid	1 hr 1 hr	3-4 hr 8-12 hr	Higher doses may induce sedation or dysphoria
Oral sustained-release: 15-, 30-, 60-, 100-, and 200-mg tablets		*Dog:* 0.5-4.0 mg/kg PO bid or qid	15 min	3-6 hr	Increase frequency of administration before increasing dose if duration is insufficient

Continued

Drug Name	Indication(s)	Dose	Onset of Action	Duration of Action	Precautions
		Cat: Not recommended because of size of tablets, which should not be scored	1 min	1 hr	
Injectable: preservative free: 1 mg/mL		*Dog:* 0.5-2.2 mg/kg SC, IM 0.1-0.5 mg/kg IV (slowly)	15 min	3-6 hr	IV administration should be avoided in dogs that are not normovolemic and normotensive because morphine may induce histamine release and vasodilation
		Cat: 0.1-0.5 mg/kg SC, IM 0.05-0.1 mg/kg IV (slowly)	1 min	1 hr	
Hydromorphone *Injectable:* 2 mg/mL	Perioperative and acute pain	*Dog:* 0.22 mg/kg SC, IM	20 min	4-6 hr	Hydromorphone is less likely to induce vomiting or hypotension than morphine
		0.1-0.2 mg/kg IV	1 min	30-45 min	
		Cat: 0.05-0.1 mg/kg IV	20 min	3-4 hr	
		0.1-.02 mg/kg sc, IM	1 min	30-45 min	
Fentanyl *Injectable:* 50 µg/mL	Perioperative and acute pain	*Dog:* 10 µg/kg SC	20 min	40-60 min	Duration may be variable from individual to individual because of variations in liver metabolism
		2-5 µg/kg IV loading dose, followed by	1 min	15-30 min	
		5-20 µg/kg/hr CRI intraoperatively	Continuous	Continuous	
		2-5 µg/kg/hr CRI perioperatively	1 min	15-30 min	
		Cat: usually no SC or IM administration			
		1-2 µg/kg IV loading dose followed by 5-20 µg/kg/hr CRI	Continuous	Continuous	
Fentanyl *Transdermal:* 25-, 50-, 75-, and 100-µg/hr patches	Acute and chronic pain	Dog and cat: 3-5 µg/kg/hr	12-24 hr	72 hr	Most cats can tolerate a 25-µg/hr patch Fentanyl patches alone should not be relied on for relief of acute postoperative pain
Butorphanol *Oral:* 1-, 5-, and 10-mg tablets	Pain associated with surgical procedures **FDA-approved for use in dogs as antitussive**	*Dog:* 1.0-4.0 mg/kg PO *Cat:* 0.5-2.0 mg/kg PO	0.5 hr	1-4 hr	Oral butorphanol usually will not achieve the same degree of analgesia as morphine, hydromorphone, or fentanyl

Drug Name	Indication(s)	Dose	Onset of Action	Duration of Action	Precautions
Butorphanol *Injectable:* 2 and 10 mg/mL	Pain associated with trauma and surgical procedures **FDA-approved for use in cats**	*Dog:* 0.2-0.4 mg/kg SC, IM 0.1-0.4 mg/kg IV *Cat:* 0.1-0.4 mg/kg SC, IM 0.05-0.2 mg/kg IV	20 min 1 min 20 min 1 min	1-2 hr 45 min 4 hr 45-60 min	Injectable butorphanol usually will not achieve the same degree of analgesia as morphine, hydromorphone, or fentanyl
Buprenorphine *Injectable:* 0.3 mg/mL	Acute and perioperative pain	*Dog:* 0.01-0.03 mg/kg SC, IM, IV *Cat:* 0.005-0.01 mg/kg SC, IM, IV *or* 0.01-0.02 mg/kg buccal/sublingual	45-60 min	6-12 hr 6-12 hr 6-8 hr	Cats tolerate buccal administration well. Owing to its high affinity for the μ receptor, buprenorphine is virtually impossible to reverse. Injectable buprenorphine usually will not achieve the same degree of analgesia as morphine, hydromorphone, or fentanyl
LOCAL ANESTHETICS Lidocaine *Injectable:* 20 mg/mL	Acute pain	Dog: 1-2 mg/kg infiltration or epidurally 2 mg/kg IV, followed by 20-50 μg/kg/min for continuous systemic analgesia	2 min 2 min	60 min Continuous	Epidural administration will result in hindlimb motor paralysis
Bupivacaine *Injectable:* 5 and 7.5 mg/mL (Marcaine)	Acute pain	Dog and cat: 1-2 mg/kg infiltration 0.1-0.75 mg/kg epidurally	10-20 min 10-20 min	6-8 hr 6-8 hr	Inadvertent IV injection can result in cardiac arrest. Low concentrations or doses administered epidurally can potentially block sensory nerves without resulting in hindlimb motor paralysis
OTHER DRUGS Tramadol *Oral:* 50-mg tablets	Acute and cancer-related pain	*Dog:* 8-10 mg/kg PO sid 2-5 mg/kg PO bid or tid 0.2-0.4 mg/kg IV *Cat:* 0.1-0.2 mg/kg IV; oral dose unknown	1 hr 1 hr 1 min 1 min	24 hr 8-12 hr 4-6 hr 4-6 hr	Tramadol has opioid-like effects without being a controlled substance
Ketamine *Microdose:* 100 mg/mL	Prevention and treatment of "wind-up" (central hypersensitization)	*Dog and cat:* (CRI) 0.5 mg/kg IV, followed by 10 μg/kg/min during surgery and 2 μg/kg/min for 24 hr after surgery	1 min	Continuous	Does not provide analgesia directly but helps prevent and treat wind-up caused by NMDA receptor antagonist activity. Potential for CNS excitation when ketamine is given alone

Continued

Drug Name	Indication(s)	Dose	Onset of Action	Duration of Action	Precautions
Amantidine Oral: 100-mg capsule; 10-mg/mL liquid	Prevention and treatment of "wind-up"	Dog and cat: 3 mg/kg PO sid	1 hr	24 hr	Does not provide analgesia directly but helps prevent and treat wind-up caused by NMDA receptor antagonist activity
Gabapentin Oral: 100-, 300-, and 400-mg tablets	Neuropathic pain	Dog and cat: 5-10 mg/kg PO sid	1 hr	24 hr	Does not provide analgesia directly but may help control abnormal neural processing in patients with peripheral and central neuropathic pain and chronic pain
SEDATIVES AND ANXIETY-DYSPHORIA–RELIEVING DRUGS					
Acepromazine Injectable: 10 mg/mL	Provides sedation **FDA-approved for use in dogs**	Dog and cat: 0.01-0.2 mg/kg SC, IM, IV	10-20 min	4-6 hr	May last considerably longer in geriatric patients and patients with liver disease Should be avoided in patients that have a history of seizures or are currently hypotensive or dehydrated
Acepromazine Oral: 10- and 25-mg tablets	Provides sedation **FDA-approved for use in dogs**	Dog and cat: 0.5 mg/kg PO	30-60 min	As above. 6-12 hr	
Diazepam or midazolam Injectable: 5 mg/mL	Relieves anxiety	Dog and cat: 0.1-0.2 mg/kg IV	1 min	20-60 min	May cause excitement instead of sedation in younger animals
		0.1-0.2 mg/kg/hr CRI	Continuous	Continuous	
Medetomidine Injectable: 1 mg/mL	Provides sedation **FDA-approved for use in dogs**	Dog and cat: 0.5-3.0 µg/kg IV	3 min	20-60 min	To be avoided in patients with cardiopulmonary or renal disease Lower IV dose is to be used as an adjunct to opioid analgesia and to help relieve anxiety; not intended for use alone
Xylazine Injectable: 20 and 100 mg/mL	Provides sedation **FDA-approved for use in dogs and cats**	Dog and cat: 0.05-0.1 mg/kg IV	1 min	20 min	As for medetomidine

Data from Dr. James S. Gaynor, DVM, MS, DACVA, and other members of the Companion Animal Pain Management Consortium.

bid, Twice daily; *CNS*, central nervous system; *CRI*, constant-rate infusion; *CVM*, Center for Veterinary Medicine; *FDA*, U.S. Food and Drug Administration; *GI*, gastrointestinal; *IM*, intramuscularly; *IV*, intravenously; *µg*, micrograms; *NSAID*, nonsteroidal anti-inflammatory drug; *PO*, orally; *SC*, subcutaneously; *sid*, once daily; *tid*, three times daily.

NOTE: Some of the dosages in this table are based on the previous authors' personal experiences and observations. Dosages were also checked in Saunders Handbook of veterinary drugs, ed 3. Veterinarians should ensure that their actions in administering drugs are in accordance with the latest legislation and standards of good practice.

All dosages listed in this table are referenced in the veterinary literature. However, unless otherwise stated, not all the drugs or dosages are approved by the FDA for use in dogs and cats.

*α_2-agonists have significant sedative effects. Sedation lasts longer than analgesia and frequently may be two to five times longer. The combination of α_2-agonists with opioids or anesthetics greatly enhances the levels of CNS depression and level of analgesia unless dosages are adjusted. There is an effective ceiling effect of α_2-agonists. Dosages above the effective level result in increased duration of effect.

†Duration of analgesic varies with dosage and route of administration. IV administration generally results in a more rapid onset and shorter duration, whereas SC administration usually results in a slower onset and longer duration than listed for IM administration. The CVM-approved dosage of medetomidine in dogs as a sole agent is 750 µg/body surface area (m²) IV or 1000 µg/m² IM. For convenience, this relates to a dosage range of 30 to 80 µg/kg for most dogs, with smaller dogs requiring the higher dosage. Medetomidine at 5 and 10 µg/kg IM has been evaluated as a preanesthetic to propofol anesthesia. Alpha₂-agonists may be reversed with atipamezole, 25 to 300 µg/kg IM.

Sample Surgical Analgesia Protocols

The following protocols are taken from the Pfizer Animal Health Pain Management Toolkit. These protocols were created by the Companion Animal Pain Management Consortium (CAPMC) and include drugs and dosages that may or may not be approved by the FDA for use in animals. However, all drugs and dosages are referenced in the veterinary literature and have been used by one or more members of the CAPMC for treatment of acute or chronic pain in animals. Two protocols are offered for each procedure, without preference for protocol A or B. These protocols are meant to serve as examples of good surgical analgesia practice.

Surgical Procedure	Anticipated Degree of Pain	Protocol A	Protocol B
Canine OHE	Moderate	*Premedication:* Acepromazine, 0.02 mg/kg SC Buprenorphine, 0.01 mg/kg SC ± Atropine, 0.01-0.04 mg/kg SC Carprofen, 4 mg/kg SC *Postoperative analgesia:* Incisional block: bupivacaine, 1.5 mg/kg (with 1:200,000 epinephrine) Carprofen, 4 mg/kg PO sid for 3 or 4 days, starting day after surgery	*Premedication:* Medetomidine, 0.005-0.010 mg/kg IM Morphine, 0.5-1.0 mg/kg IM *or* Hydromorphone, 0.2 mg/kg IM ± Atropine 0.01-0.04 mg/kg IM Carprofen, 4 mg/kg SC *Postoperative analgesia:* Repeat dose of opioid 4-6 hours after initial dose, or sooner if needed Carprofen, 4 mg/kg PO sid for 3-4 days, starting 24 hours after initial dose
Canine castration	Mild to moderate	As for OHE	As for OHE
Feline OHE	Moderate	*Premedication:* Medetomidine, 0.02 mg/kg IM Hydromorphone, 0.05 mg/kg IM ± atropine 0.01-0.04 mg/kg IM *Postoperative analgesia:* Incisional block: bupivacaine, 1.5 mg/kg (with 1:200,000 epinephrine) NSAID (see previous table on drug doses for recommendations)	*Premedication:* Medetomidine, 0.02 mg/kg IM Buprenorphine, 0.02 mg/kg IM Ketamine, 2 mg/kg IM ± carprofen, 1-2 mg/kg SC *Postoperative analgesia:* Repeat buprenorphine 6-8 hours (IM or buccal) after initial dose On discharge (postop day 1): buprenorphine, 0.02 mg/kg (buccal) q8-12h for 1 day, followed by 0.01 mg/kg q8-12h for 2-3 days
Feline castration	Mild to moderate	*Premedication:* Medetomidine, 0.02 mg/kg IM Buprenorphine, 0.02 mg/kg IM Ketamine, 2 mg/kg IM ± carprofen, 1-2 mg/kg SC	As for OHE, but may omit the postoperative opioid.
Feline onychectomy	Moderate to severe	*Premedication:* Medetomidine, 0.02 mg/kg IM Hydromorphone, 0.05 mg/kg IM ± atropine 0.01-0.04 mg/kg IM *Additional intraoperative analgesia:* Declaw block: lidocaine, 1.5 mg/kg; bupivacaine, 1.5 mg/kg	*Premedication:* Apply fentanyl patch, 25 μg/hr (may cover half the absorptive surface of patch in cats <10 kg) Medetomidine, 0.02 mg/kg IM Morphine, 0.2-0.5 mg/kg IM ± atropine 0.01-0.04 mg/kg IM *Additional intraoperative analgesia:* Declaw block: bupivacaine, 1-2 mg/kg

Continued

Surgical Procedure	Anticipated Degree of Pain	Protocol A	Protocol B
		Postoperative analgesia: Hydromorphone, 0.05 mg/kg SC q3h for duration of supervised hospitalization Carprofen, 1-2 mg/kg SC (once) Buprenorphine, 0.02 mg/kg (buccal) q8-12h starting 3 hours after last dose of hydromorphone	*Postoperative analgesia:* Morphine, 0.2-0.5 mg/kg IM q4h for up to two doses Remove fentanyl patch within 3-5 days
Canine abdominal exploratory (e.g., GDV repair, splenectomy)	Moderate to severe	*Premedication:* Morphine, 0.5-1.0 mg/kg or Hydromorphone, 0.2 mg/kg IM ± atropine, 0.01-0.04 mg/kg IM *Postoperative analgesia:* Incisional block: bupivacaine, 1.5 mg/kg (with 1:200,000 epinephrine Morphine, 0.05-0.2 mg/kg/hr (CRI) Oral morphine, 0.5-1.0 mg/kg after discontinuation of CRI	*Premedication:* Morphine, 0.5-1.0 mg/kg IM or Hydromorphone, 0.2 mg/kg IM Fentanyl patch (refer to drug dose table for dosing) ± atropine 0.01-0.04 mg/kg IM *Additional intraoperative analgesia:* Repeat preoperative opioid at half-dose to full dose as needed (IV or IM) *Postoperative analgesia:* Repeat morphine or hydromorphone q4h for 12-24 hours NSAID therapy for 7-10 days after discharge (if not a GI procedure)
Feline abdominal exploratory (e.g., cystotomy, linear foreign body removal)	Moderate to severe	*Premedication:* Hydromorphone, 0.05 mg/kg IM ± medetomidine, 0.02 mg/kg IM ± atropine 0.01-0.04 mg/kg IM *Postoperative analgesia:* Incisional block: bupivacaine, 1.5 mg/kg (with 1:200,000 epinephrine) Hydromorphone, 0.03-0.05 mg/kg/hr (CRI) Buprenorphine, 0.02 mg/kg (buccal) q8-12h starting immediately after discontinuation of hydromorphone CRI	*Premedication:* Morphine epidural (0.1 mg/kg) Morphine, 0.25 mg/kg IM ± medetomidine, 0.02 mg/kg IM ± atropine 0.01-0.04 mg/kg IM Apply fentanyl patch, 25 μg/hr *Postoperative analgesia:* Morphine IM may have to be repeated once or twice until fentanyl patch becomes effective
Canine repair of ruptured cranial cruciate ligament or other hindlimb orthopedic procedure (e.g., repair of femoral fracture)	Moderate to severe; can be severe to excruciating	*Premedication:* Acepromazine, 0.01-0.04 mg/kg SC Morphine, 1.0 mg/kg SC ± atropine 0.01-0.04 mg/kg SC Carprofen, 4 mg/kg SC *Additional intraoperative analgesia:* Epidural: morphine, 0.1 mg/kg; bupivacaine, 1.0 mg/kg Bupivacaine, 1.0-2.0 mg/kg intra-articularly	*Premedication:* Medetomidine, 0.005-0.010 mg/kg IM Hydromorphone, 0.2 mg/kg IM ± atropine 0.01-0.04 mg/kg IM Carprofen, 4 mg/kg SC Appropriate-size fentanyl patch applied 12 hours preoperatively *Additional intraoperative analgesia:* Bupivacaine, 1.0-2.0 mg/kg intra-articularly

Surgical Procedure	Anticipated Degree of Pain	Protocol A	Protocol B
		Postoperative analgesia: Morphine, 1.0 mg/kg SC, 4 hours after initial dose Carprofen, 4 mg/kg PO sid, starting day after surgery for 7-10 days	*Postoperative analgesia:* Hydromorphone, 0.2 mg/kg IM, 4 hours after initial dose Carprofen, 4 mg/kg PO sid, starting day after surgery for 7-10 days
Canine radius/ulna fracture repair or other forelimb orthopedic procedure	Moderate to severe; can be severe to excruciating	Same as hindlimb orthopedic procedure, but omit epidural and intra-articular block *Additional intraoperative analgesia:* Brachial plexus block: bupivacaine, 1.0-2.0 mg/kg (for procedures distal to elbow)	Same as hindlimb orthopedic procedure, but epidural is omitted *Additional intraoperative analgesia:* Lidocaine, 0.025-0.050 mg/kg/min (CRI) Repeat preoperative opioid at half-dose to full dose as needed (IV or IM)
Feline radius/ulna fracture repair or other forelimb orthopedic procedure	Moderate to severe; can be severe to excruciating	*Premedication:* Medetomidine, 0.02 mg/kg SC Hydromorphone, 0.05 mg/kg SC ± atropine 0.01-0.04 mg/kg IM *Additional intraoperative analgesia:* Brachial plexus block: bupivacaine, 1.0-2.0 mg/kg (for procedures distal to elbow) *Postoperative analgesia:* Carprofen, 1-2 mg/kg SC (once) Buprenorphine, 0.02 mg/kg (buccal) q8-12h starting 4-6 hours after initial dose of hydromorphone	*Premedication:* Acepromazine, 0.05-0.1 mg/kg IM Morphine, 0.25 mg/kg IM ± atropine, 0.01-0.04 mg/kg IM ± carprofen, 1-2 mg/kg SC (once) Fentanyl patch, 25 µg/hr *Additional intraoperative analgesia:* Consider ketamine CRI (0.002 mg/kg/min) *Postoperative analgesia:* Morphine IM nay have to be repeated once or twice until fentanyl patch becomes effective

Data from Dr. James S. Gaynor, DVM, MS, DACVA.

CNS, central nervous system; *CRI,* constant-rate infusion; *CVM,* Center for Veterinary Medicine; *FDA,* U.S. Food and Drug Administration; *GI,* gastrointestinal; *GDV,* gastric dilatation and volvulus; *h,* hours; *IM,* intramuscularly; *IV,* intravenously; *µg,* micrograms; *NSAID,* nonsteroidal anti-inflammatory drug; *OHE,* ovario-hysterectomy; *PO,* orally; *q,* every; *SC,* subcutaneously; *sid,* once daily.

Sample Calculations for Constant-Rate Infusion of Analgesics

Constant pain requires constant-rate infusion (CRI) of analgesics. The following sample calculations show how to determine the number of milliliters (mL) of the different analgesics to add to different sizes of fluid bags to deliver a CRI of analgesics through an IV drip.

Overview

1. Give an initial loading dose as a bolus to the desired effect.
2. Begin a CRI of one of the analgesics discussed below either in a syringe pump or as an IV drip.
3. Monitor for signs of inadequate pain control, and evaluate the following behavioral categories hourly while the patient is receiving CRI:

a. Posture:
   - Painful signs: hunched back, tense muscles, anxious facial expression, withdrawn, cowering.
   - Managed pain: grooming, sleeping in normal posture.
b. Vocalization:
   - Painful signs: whining, whimpering, growling, distressful yowling.
   - Managed pain: quiet, purring.
c. Mobility:
   - Painful signs: unable to lie quietly (restless) or unwilling/reluctant to get up or move.
   - Managed pain: gets up, sits, lies down, walks willingly.
d. Response to touch (specifically, palpation of wound if present):

- Painful signs: trembling, guarding wound, baring teeth.
- Managed pain: affectionate, relaxed.
4. Evaluate the following physiologic parameters hourly while the patient is receiving CRI:
   - Temperature, pulse, respiration.
   - Mucous membrane color and capillary refill time.
   - Blood pressure.
5. Titrate delivery rate accordingly (increase if painful).
   or

If pain is unrelenting, a combination CRI of morphine, lidocaine, and ketamine may be needed.
6. Monitor for signs of excessive dosing:
   - Dysphoria.
   - CNS depression.
7. Titrate delivery rate accordingly (decrease or discontinue).
   or
   Consider an opioid antagonist if an opioid was administered.

Fentanyl CRI

Loading Dose
- Canine: 2 to 5 µg per kilogram body weight (µg/kg) intravenously (IV)
- Feline: 1 to 2 µg/kg IV
- Give to effect.

Constant-Rate Infusion
For this example, the patient is a 10-pound (10-lb) domestic short-hair cat.
1. Determine the hourly flow rate of IV fluids for the patient:
   - For this example, maintenance fluid flow rate is used as the hourly rate, as calculated by the following formula: 1 mL/pound (lb)/hour (hr):

$$10\,lb \times (1\,mL/lb/hr) = 10\,mL/hr$$

Hourly IV fluid flow rate $= 10\,mL/hr$

2. Determine the hourly analgesic dose rate:
   - Fentanyl CRI dose range, the units are micrograms (µg) for cats: **5 to 20 µg/kg/hr.**
   - *NOTE:* The low end of the given dose range is appropriate for postoperative, awake analgesia. The high end of the given dose range is more appropriate for intraoperative analgesia when very little inhaled anesthesia is desired.
   - Convert lb to kg: 10 lb × (1 kg/2.2 lb) = 4.5 kg.
   - Calculate the lower and upper limits of the dose range:

$$4.5\,kg \times (5\,\mu g/kg) = 23\,\mu g$$
$$4.5\,kg \times (20\,\mu g/kg) = 90\,\mu g$$
$$Range = 23\ to\ 90\,\mu g/hr$$

   - Select a dose in the calculated range based on the patient's level of pain and purpose of analgesia

(awake vs. intraoperative). For this example, select **23 µg/hr.**
3. Determine how many units of analgesic per mL of IV fluids:
   - In this case, using fentanyl, µg.
   - Use the hourly IV fluid flow rate determined in step 1 in the following formula:

$$(23\,\mu g/hr) \times (1\,hr/10\,mL) = \textbf{2.3}\,\mu g/mL\ \textbf{of IV fluids}$$

4. Determine how many units of analgesic to add to a 1-liter (1-L) bag of fluids:
   - In this case, using fentanyl, the units are µg:

$$(2.3\,\mu g/mL) \times (1000\,mL/L) = \textbf{2300}\,\mu g/L$$

If using a 500-mL (half-liter; ½-L) bag of fluids, add 1150 µg of fentanyl to the bag.
If using a 250-mL bag of fluids, add 575 µg of fentanyl to the bag.

5. Determine how many mL of analgesic to add to the bag of fluids.
   NOTE: Before adding analgesic to the fluid bag, remove an equal volume of fluid from the bag.
   - Determine concentration of analgesic, which is stated on the vial; in this case, fentanyl concentration is [50 µg/mL]:

$$(2300\,\mu g) \times ([mL/50\,\mu g]) = \textbf{46 mL}$$

   - 46 mL of fentanyl should be added to a 1-L bag.

Or add 23 mL of fentanyl to a half-liter bag (500-mL).
Or add 11.5 mL of fentanyl to a 250-mL bag.
Or connect the patient to a syringe pump of fentanyl and deliver IV fluids separately.

Morphine CRI

- Monitor for signs of histamine release (pruritus, hypotension) whenever morphine IV is administered.
- Morphine analgesia continues for approximately 30 minutes after CRI has been discontinued.
- Dysphoria associated with morphine may be alleviated with a low dose of a sedative.

Loading Dose

- Canine: 0.2 to 0.5 mg/kg IV
- Feline: 0.05 to 0.1 mg/kg IV
- Give to effect.

Constant-Rate Infusion

For this example, the patient is a 50-lb dog.

1. Determine the hourly fluid flow rate of IV fluids for the patient:
   - For this example, maintenance fluid flow rate is used as the hourly rate, as calculated by the following formula: 1 mL/lb/hr:

   $$50\,lb \times (1\,mL/lb/hr) = 50\,mL/hr$$

   Hourly IV fluid flow rate = **50 mL/hr**

2. Determine the hourly analgesic dose rate:
   - Morphine CRI dose range, the units are milligrams (mg) for canines: **0.1 to 0.3 mg/kg/hr.**
   - Convert lb to kg:

   $$50\,lb \times (1\,kg/2.2\,lb) = 23\,kg$$

   - Calculate the lower and upper limits of the dose range:

   $$23\,kg \times (0.1\,mg/kg) = 2.3\,mg$$
   $$23\,kg \times (0.3\,mg/kg) = 6.9\,mg$$
   $$Range = 2.3\,to\,6.9\,mg/hr$$

   - Select a dose in the calculated range based on patient's level of pain. For this example, select **5 mg/hr.**

3. Determine how many units of analgesic per mL of IV fluids:
   - In this case, using morphine
   - Use the hourly IV fluid flow rate determined in step 1 in the following formula:

   $$(5\,mg/hr) \times (1\,hr/50\,mL) = \textbf{0.1 mg/mL of IV fluids}$$

4. Determine how many units of analgesic to add to liter (L) bag of fluids:
   - In this case, using morphine, the units are mg:

   $$(0.1\,mg/mL) \times (1000\,mL/L) = \textbf{100 mg/L}$$

   - If using a 500-mL bag of fluids, add 50 mg of morphine to the bag.
   - If using a 250-mL bag of fluids, add 25 mg of morphine to the bag.

5. Determine how many mL of analgesic to add to the bag of fluids.
   NOTE: Before adding analgesia to fluid bag, remove an equal volume of fluid from the bag.
   - Determine the concentration of analgesic, which is stated on the vial; in this case, morphine = [15 mg/mL]:

   $$(100\,mg) \times ([mL/15\,mg]) = \textbf{6.7 mL}$$

   - 6.7 mL of morphine should be added to a 1-L bag. *Or* add 3.4 mL of morphine to a half-liter bag (500-mL).

   Or add 1.7 mL of morphine to a 250-mL bag.
   Or connect the patient to a syringe pump of morphine and deliver IV fluids separately.

Lidocaine CRI

Loading Dose

- Canine: 2 mg/kg IV
- Give to desired effect.
- Feline: not recommended for use in cats.

Constant-Rate Infusion

For this example, the patient is a 50-lb dog.

1. Determine the hourly fluid flow rate:
   - For the following example, maintenance fluid flow rate is based on the formula 1 mL/lb/hr:

   $$50\,lb \times (1\,mL/lb/hr) = \textbf{50 mL/hr}$$

   Hourly IV fluid flow rate = 50 mL/hr

2. Determine the hourly analgesic dose rate:
   - Lidocaine CRI dose range for canines: **20-50 µg/kg/min.**
   - Convert lb to kg: 50 lb × (1 kg/2.2 lb) = 23 kg.

   - Calculate the lower and upper limits of the dose range:

   $$23\,kg \times (20\,µg/kg) = 460\,µg$$
   $$3\,kg \times (50\,µg/kg) = 1150\,µg$$
   $$Range = 460\,to\,1150\,µg/min$$

   - Select a dose in the calculated range based on patient's level of pain. For this example, select 600 µg/min.
   - Convert the minute rate to an hourly rate:

   $$(600\,µg/min) \times (60\,min/hr) = 36,000\,µg/hr$$
   $$36,000\,µg = 36\,mg.$$
   $$Hourly\,rate = \textbf{36 mg/hr}$$

3. Determine how many units of analgesic per mL of IV fluids:

- In this example, using lidocaine, the units are now in milligrams (mg).
- Use the hourly IV fluid flow rate determined in step 1 in the following formula:

$$(36\,mg/hr)\times(1\,hr/50\,mL)=0.72\,mg/mL$$

4. Determine how many units to add to a 1-liter (1-L) bag of fluids:
   - In this example, using lidocaine, the units are now in mg:

$$(0.72\,mg/mL)\times(1000\,mL/L)=720\,mg/L$$

   If using a 500-mL bag of fluids, add 360 mg of 2% lidocaine to the bag.
   If using a 250-mL bag of fluids, add 180 mg of 2% lidocaine to the bag.

5. Determine how many mL of analgesic to add to a bag of fluids:
   NOTE: Before adding analgesia to fluid bag, remove an equal volume of fluid from the bag.
   - Determine the concentration of analgesic, which is stated on the vial; in this case, 2% lidocaine = [20 mg/mL].

$$(720\,mg)\times([mL/20\,mg])=\textbf{36 mL}$$

   - 46 mL of lidocaine should be to a 1-L bag.

   Or add 18 mL to a half-liter bag.
   Or add 9 mL to a 250-mL bag.
   Or connect the patient to a syringe pump of lidocaine and deliver IV fluids separately.

Ketamine CRI

Loading Dose
- Canine and feline: 0.5 mg/kg IV
- Give to desired effect.

Intraoperative Dose
- Canine and feline: 10 μg/kg/min

Constant-Rate Infusion (up to 24 Hours Postoperatively)
In this example, the patient is a 10-lb cat.
1. Determine hourly fluid flow rate:
   - For the following example, maintenance fluid flow rate will be based on the following formula: 1 mL/lb/hr:

$$10\,lb\times(1\,mL/lb/hr)=10\,mL/hr$$
$$\text{Hourly IV fluid flow rate}=\textbf{10 mL/hr}$$

2. Determine the hourly analgesic dose rate:
   - Postoperative ketamine CRI dose for felines: **2 μg/kg/min**
   - Convert lb to kg: 10 lb × (1 kg/2.2 lb) = 4.5 kg
   - Calculate the minute rate of ketamine:

$$(4.5\,kg)\times(2\,\mu g/kg)=9\,\mu g/min$$

   - Convert the minute rate to an hourly rate:

$$(9\,\mu g/min)\times(60\,min/hr)=540\,\mu g/hr$$
$$\text{Hourly dose}=\textbf{540 μg/hr}$$

3. Determine how many units of analgesic per mL of IV fluids:

- In this example, using ketamine, the units are in micrograms (μg).
- Use the hourly IV fluid flow rate determined in step 1 to the following formula:

$$(540\,\mu g/hr)\times(1\,hr/10\,mL)=\textbf{54 μg/mL}$$

4. Determine how many units to add to a 1-liter (1-L) bag of IV fluids:
   - Note shift from μg to mg in this example:

$$(54\,\mu g/mL)\times(1000\,mL/L)=54{,}000\,\mu g/L$$
$$54{,}000\,\mu g=54\,mg$$

   - Add **54 mg** of ketamine to a 1-liter bag of fluids.

   Or add 27 mg to a half-liter bag.
   Or add 13.5 mg to a 250-mL bag.

5. Determine how many mL of ketamine to add to a bag of fluids:
   - Determine the concentration of analgesic, which is stated on the file; in this case, the ketamine concentration is [100 mg/mL].

$$(54\,mg)\times([mL/100\,mg])=0.54\,mL$$

   - **0.54 mL** of ketamine should be added to a 1-L bag of fluids.

   Or add 0.27 mL of ketamine to a half-liter bag.
   Or add 0.14 mL of ketamine to a 250-mL bag.
   Or connect the patient to a syringe pump of ketamine and deliver IV fluids separately.

GLOSSARY

Abdominocentesis: puncture and aspiration of the abdominal cavity.

Ablation: removal, especially by cutting.

Absorbable (suture): a strand of organic or synthetic material used for closing wounds that becomes dissolved in the body fluids and disappears.

ACL: anterior cruciate ligament.

Active drain: a surgically placed implant that creates negative-pressure gradients to facilitate the removal of unwanted fluid or gas.

Acute pain: pain that follows some bodily injury, disappears with healing, and tends to be self-limiting.

Adaptive pain: normal response to tissue damage; includes inflammatory pain.

Adrenergic: activated by or capable of releasing epinephrine or an epinephrine-like substance, or having physiologic effects similar to those of epinephrine.

Aerophagia: habitual swallowing of air.

Agonal breathing: the spasmodic opening of the mouth with contraction of the diaphragm usually associated with death; no respiration is taking place.

Agonist: a drug that can combine with a receptor on a cell to produce a physiologic reaction; a drug that binds to a receptor and causes it to express its function.

Allodynia: pain caused by a stimulus that does not normally cause pain.

Analgesia: the loss of sensitivity to pain.

Anastomosis: surgical, traumatic, or pathologic formation of a connection between two normally distinct structures.

Anesthesia: total or partial loss of sensation.

Anionic detergent: soap that has free, negatively charged ions that precipitate when combined with calcium and magnesium in hard water.

Anticholinergic: a drug that inhibits the action of acetylcholine by competing at the receptor sites; an agent that is antagonistic to the action of parasympathetic or other cholinergic nerve fibers.

Antiseptic: chemical that inhibits or prevents the growth of microbes on living tissue; compare with *disinfectant*.

Anuria: complete suppression of urine formation.

A-O: Arbeitsgemeinschaft für Osteosynthesefragen, Swiss for the Association for the Study of Internal Fixation (ASIF). These abbreviations are frequently seen together but separated by a slash: AO/ASIF. The AO is involved in research and development of medical devices used in orthopedic surgery. Their devices are available through a company called Synthes.

Articular: pertaining to a joint.

Asepsis: the absence of pathogenic microorganisms that cause infection.

Aseptic loosening: breakdown of bone and loosening of prosthesis in the absence of microorganisms.

ASIF: Association for the Study of Internal Fixation.

Assisted ventilation: the depth of spontaneous ventilation is augmented by the anesthetist.

Atraumatic: not producing injury or damage.

Auscultation: listening with a stethoscope.

Autotransfusion: re-infusion of the patient's own blood.

Bactericide: agent that destroys (kills) bacteria.

Bacteriostat: agent that inhibits the growth of bacteria.

Balanced anesthesia: anesthesia protocol that offsets the depressing effects of anesthetic agents on the motor, sensory, reflex, and mental aspects of nervous system function by combining different agents.

Biocide: agent that kills living organisms.

Biologic indicator: a vial containing the spore state of a specific bacteria is placed in a sterilizer to show that a sterilizer is functioning properly.

Blepharospasm: squinting, blinking.

Bone wax: a composition of beeswax and isopropyl palmitate used to seal the cut end of bone; also called *bone sealant*.

Box lock: hinged part of a needle holder, tissue forceps, or hemostatic forceps.

Brachycephalic: head shape that is shortened in the rostrocaudal dimension, as seen with breeds such as Pugs, Boston Terriers, and Boxers.

Breakthrough pain: a transient flare-up of pain in the chronic pain setting that can occur even when chronic pain is under control.

Callus: unorganized network of woven bone formed about ends of a broken bone that is reabsorbed as healing is completed.

Capillarity: the action by which the surface of a liquid where it is in contact with a solid is elevated or depressed.

Capnography: the measurement of carbon dioxide concentration in the exhaled air, especially of anesthetized animals.

Cationic detergent: cleaning agent that contains positively charged ions that remain suspended in solution (e.g., quaternary ammonium).

CCL: cranial cruciate ligament.

Celiotomy: surgical incision into the abdominal cavity.

Central sensitization: an increase in the excitability and responsiveness of nerves in the spinal cord.

Chemical indicator: an item in the form of a strip or tape that shows, by changing color, that conditions for sterilization were met.

Chief complaint: the most apparent clinical sign in a patient's illness.

Chronic pain: pain that lasts several weeks to months and persists beyond the expected healing time, when nonmalignant in origin.

Circulating nurse: a nonsterile person who opens items for the surgical team and helps maintain surgical conscience.

Closed reduction: nonsurgical realignment of fracture or joint.

Coaptation: application of external appliance, such as a splint or cast.

Conjunctivitis: inflammation of the conjunctiva.

Cryotherapy: therapeutic techniques to decrease tissue temperature.

Cryptorchid: animal with undescended testes.

Crystalluria: presence of crystals in the urine.

Cyanosis: a bluish discoloration of the skin and mucous membranes due to excessive concentration or reduced hemoglobin in the blood.

Cystectomy: excision or resection of the urinary bladder.

Cystostomy: surgical formation of an opening into the bladder.

Cystotomy: a surgical incision into the bladder to expose the lumen or interior of the urinary bladder.

Cystourethrogram: radiograph of the urinary bladder and urethra.

Débridement: the removal of all foreign material and all contaminated and devitalized tissues from or adjacent to a traumatic or infected lesion until surrounding healthy tissue is exposed.

Decontamination: the manual cleaning of an instrument in a detergent solution to assist in the breakdown of biologic debris.

Dehiscence: a splitting open; the breakdown of a surgical incision such that the tissue layers separate from each other.

Delayed union: prolonged renewal of continuity in a broken bone or between the edges of a wound.

Detergent: chemical that contains free ions and leaves a film on surfaces.

Disarticulation: amputation or separation at a joint.

Disinfectant: chemical used to inhibit or prevent the growth of microbes on inanimate objects; compare with *antiseptic*.

Dislocation: complete separation of the articular surfaces of a joint.

Dissociative anesthesia: loss of perception of certain stimuli while that of others remains intact.

Dissociative anesthetic: a class of anesthetic agent that cause a disruption of the nerve transmission in some parts of the brain and elective stimulation in others; this combination of actions causes the animal to appear awake but immobile and unaware of its surroundings.

Dysuria: difficulty urinating.

Elective: referring to surgical procedure that can wait for later scheduling.

Emergence delirium: delirious behavior resulting from incomplete recovery from gas anesthesia.

Endogenous contamination: contamination from the patient.

Endotoxemia: the presences of endotoxins in the blood.

Enophthalmos: pulling back of the eye and a secondary, raised third eyelid.

Enteral feeding: delivery of nutrients directly into the stomach, duodenum, or jejunum; also called *enteral nutrition.*

Enterotomy: incision of the intestine.

Entropion: inversion or turning inward of the margin of an eyelid.

Enzymes: organic substances that assist in the breakdown of soils and are generally formulated with a surfactant to improve their penetration into dried soil.

Ethylene oxide (gas) sterilization: a sterilization process used for items that cannot be steam sterilized because the heat would destroy the item.

Event-related expiration: a method that uses environmental causes to determine item sterility. If a sterile item is damaged in any way, it would be considered nonsterile.

Evisceration: extrusion of the viscera or internal organs.

Exogenous contamination: contamination that comes from the surgical team or the environment.

Fenestrated: to have one or more window-like openings.

Fenestration: an opening in a surface.

Flash sterilization: an abbreviated version of a regular sterilization cycle used for individual instruments that have been dropped during surgery.

Flexibility: the state of being unusually pliant.

Fungicide: agent that kills fungi.

Gastrectomy: excision of the stomach or a portion of the stomach.

Gastritis: inflammation of the lining of the stomach.

Gastropexy: surgical fixation of the stomach.

Gastrotomy: the creation of an opening into the stomach.

Gravity air-displacement: a method of steam sterilization that relies on gravity to assist steam in penetrating items within the chamber. It is the most common sterilization method in veterinary practices.

Hematuria: blood in urine.

Hemostasis: the arrest of bleeding by either natural (clot formation) or artificial (compression or ligation) means.

Herniation: abnormal protrusion of an organ or other body structure through a defect or natural opening.

High-level disinfection: immersing items in a disinfectant solution to reduce the level of contamination. Items are not sterile.

High-vacuum sterilizer: a steam sterilizer that forces steam into the sterilizing chamber, causing steam to penetrate the pack more quickly; after the sterilization cycle has been completed, the steam is vacuumed out of the chamber.

Hip dysplasia: abnormal development of coxofemoral joint characterized by subluxation or complete luxation of femoral head in younger patients and mild to severe degenerative joint disease in older patients.

HOD: Hypertrophic osteodystrophy; developmental disease that causes disruption of metaphyseal trabeculae in long bones of young, rapidly growing dogs.

Hyperalgesia: an increased response to a stimulation that is normally painful either at the site of injury or in surrounding undamaged tissue.

Hyperesthesia: increased sensitivity to sensation.

Hypoalgesia: decreased sensitivity to pain.

Hypoesthesia: decreased sensitivity to stimulation.

Hypoglycemia: lower than normal levels of blood glucose resulting in lack of fuel to the brain and other organ systems.

Hypotension: lowered blood pressure.

Hypothermia: abnormally low body temperature.

Iatrogenic: any adverse condition in a patient caused by the action of the doctor or medical staff.

Ileus: functional obstruction of the intestines or failure of peristalsis; partial or complete nonmechanical blockage of the small and/or large intestine.

Inappetence: partial lack of appetite; inferred in animals with depressed food intake.

Indicator tape: pretreated strips on the sterilization tape that change color when the pack has been through the sterilization process.

Insufflation: blowing or a powder, vapor, or gas into a body cavity.

Interfragmentary: bone fragments of a fracture that may or may not be able to be reconstructed and stabilized.

Intussusception: prolapse of one part of the intestine into the lumen of an immediately adjacent part, causing intestinal obstruction.

Ischemia: deficiency of blood in a part.

IVDD: intervertebral disc disease associated with disc degeneration and extrusion, causing spinal cord compression and nerve root entrapment.

Keratitis: inflammation of the cornea.

Lacrimation: tearing.

Laparotomy: flank incision into the abdominal cavity; sometimes used interchangeably with *celiotomy*.

Lavage: to wash out or irrigate.

Ligate: to tie off or constrict blood vessels or tissue.

Luxation: complete separation of a bone from its articulation.

Maladaptive pain: hypersensitivity to pain resulting from abnormal processing of normal input; can also occur if adaptive pain is left untreated.

Malunion: incorrect anatomical alignment of the fragments of a fractured bone; faulty union and alignment of the fractured bone.

Mechanical friction: a scrubbing motion used to clean all surfaces.

Memory (suture): a property of some synthetic fibers that encourages the spontaneous untying of knots.

Movable equipment: pieces of equipment that can be transported from the surgery room to other areas of the hospital.

MPL: medial patellar luxation.

Multimodal analgesia: the use of multiple drugs with different actions to produce optimal analgesia.

Neoplasia: the formation of abnormal growth.

Neuroplasticity: the idea that the nervous system can be changed by the effect of the environment, external stimuli, and the effects of physiologic stimuli, such as pain.

Nociception: the transaction, conduction and central nervous system processing of nerve signals generated by the stimulation of certain receptors; term used to describe three neuralgic phases of the pain pathway: transduction, transmission, and modulation.

Nonelective: surgical procedures that cannot wait for later scheduling.

Nonmovable (permanent) equipment: pieces of equipment that are attached to the floor, wall, or ceiling in the surgery room.

Nonreducible: unable to be restored to the normal place or position.

Non-union: failure of the ends of a fractured bone to unite.

Normothermic: normal body temperature.

Nosocomial infection: infection acquired during hospitalization or during attendance at any veterinary medical facility.

Occlusive wound dressing: a dressing used on the skin that retains moisture and heat while increasing the concentration and absorption of medication being applied; impermeable to air and fluid.

OCD: osteochondritis dissecans; inflammation of bone and cartilage that results in the splitting of cartilage pieces into the affected joint.

Onychectomy: declawing; the removal of the claw and its associated third phalanx.

Open reduction: surgical opening and exposure to realign a fracture or joint.

Orchiectomy: castration.

Osteomyelitis: bone infection.

Pain threshold: the least experience of pain that a patient can recognize.

Pain tolerance level: the greatest level of pain that a patient can tolerate.

Passive drain: a surgically placed implant that uses gravity and overflow to facilitate the removal of unwanted fluid or gas.

Pathologic pain: pain that has an exaggerated response beyond its protective usefulness. It is often associated with tissue injury incurred at the time of surgery or trauma.

Percutaneous: performed through the skin.

Peritonitis: an inflammatory process that involves the serous membrane of the abdominal cavity.

Pétrissage: a type of massage that consists of kneading, rhythmic lifting, squeezing, and releasing the tissue.

Photophobia: sensitivity to light.

Physiologic pain: pain that acts as a protective mechanism that incites individuals to move away from the cause of potential tissue damage or to avoid movement or contact with external stimuli during a reparative phase.

Plasma sterilization: low-temperature plasma sterilization with hydrogen peroxide (H_2O_2) gas used for items that cannot be steam sterilized.

Pollakiuria: abnormally frequent passage of urine.

Preemptive analgesia: the administration of an analgesic drug before painful stimulation to prevent sensitization of neurons, or *windup*, thus improving postoperative analgesia.

Premedication: preliminary medication, particularly internal medication, to produce sedation or narcosis prior to general anesthesia.

Preparation area: a room used for patient preparation and the storage of surgical supplies.

Presoaking: placing soiled instruments in distilled water or water mixed with a detergent solution without using mechanical agitation.

Pronate: to turn the palm downwards or from the body to face the ground.

Prophylaxis: use of an agent that tends to ward off disease.

Pulse deficit: the difference between the apical pulse (that heard over the heart with a stethoscope) and the arterial pulse.

Pulse oximetry: an instrument that measures pulse rate and the percentage of oxygenated and reduced hemoglobin.

Recipe: details pertinent information about surgery pack preparation and contents. It is often maintained in a procedures manual.

Reducible: able to be restored to the normal place or relation of parts, as in a reducible fracture.

Regional anesthesia: the loss of sensation in part of the body caused by interruption of the sensory nerves that conduct impulses from that region of the body.

Sanitize: to reduce the number of microbes to a safe level.

Scrub area: an area near the surgery room with the scrub sink, autoclave, and room to gown and glove.

Semiocclusive wound dressing: bandage that allows air to penetrate and exudates to escape from the wound surface.

Sepsis: the presence of pathogenic microorganisms or their toxins in blood or other tissue.

Septicemia: systemic disease associated with the presence of pathogenic microorganisms and their toxins.

Seroma: a serosanguineous accumulation of fluid between tissue planes.

Serrated: having a sawlike edge or border.

Shank: portion of a surgical instrument that connects the handle with the working end.

Shelf-life expiration: a method that uses a predetermined date that identifies how long an item should be considered sterile.

Shock: a condition of acute peripheral circulatory failure.

Short bowel syndrome: any of the malabsorption conditions resulting from massive resection of the small bowel.

Signalment: the part of the veterinary medical history dealing with the animal's age, sex, breed, and reproductive status.

Somatic pain: pain that originates from damage to bone, joints, muscle, or skin and is described by humans as localized, constant, sharp, aching, and throbbing.

Sphygmomanometer: an instrument for measuring blood pressure.

Splenectomy: excision of the spleen.

Sporicide: agent that kills spores.

Stenosis: narrowing or contraction of a body passage or opening.

Sterility: the absence of all living microorganisms, including spores.

Sterilization: the use of a process to rid an object of all living microbes.

Sterilize: To eliminate all microbes by death or inactivation.

Stranguria: slow and painful discharge of urine.

Strike-through contamination: contamination that occurs when liquids soak through a drape from a sterile area to an unsterile area, or vice versa.

Subluxation: partial or incomplete separation of a joint.

Supinate: to rotate the forearm to bring the palm face upward.

Surgery room: a separate room that should be used only for surgery.

Surgical conscience: the commitment of surgical personnel to adhere strictly to aseptic technique, because anything less could increase the potential risk of infection, resulting in harm to the patient.

Surgical hand rub: a scrubless, brushless, waterless antiseptic hand preparation product used during the process of scrubbing-in for surgery.

Surgical hand scrub: process of removing as many microorganisms as possible from nails, hands, and arms by mechanical washing and chemical antisepsis before participating in a surgical procedure.

Surgical nurse: sterile person who assists with surgical duties such as passing instruments, retracting tissue, and maintaining hemostasis.

Swage: to fuse, as suture material to the end of a suture needle.

Thermoregulatory: the physiologic process controlling the balance between heat production and heat loss in the body so as to maintain body temperature.

Traumatic: pertaining to, resulting from, or causing trauma.

Trichobezoar: hair ball.

Trocar: a sharp, pointed, needlelike instrument equipped with a cannula; used to puncture the wall of a body cavity and withdraw fluid or gas.

Urethrotomy: incision into the urethra.

Uroabdomen: presence of urine in the abdominal cavity; generally associated with a ruptured bladder.

Urolith: calculus or stone found in the urine or urinary system.

Urolithiasis: formation of calculi in the urinary tract.

Uveitis: intraocular inflammation.

Virucide: agent that kills viruses.

Visceral pain: pain that arises from stretching, distension, or inflammation of the viscera and described by humans as deep, cramping, aching, or gnawing without good localization.

Volvulus: rotation of an organ.

Wind-up: alterations in the nervous system that occur as a result of untreated or inadequately treated pain and lead to untreatable pain states; temporal summation of painful stimuli in the spinal cord. Mediated by C fibers and responsible for "second" pain.

Page numbers followed by f, t, and b indicate figures, tables, and boxes, respectively.